*Christopher H. Tebault,
Surgeon to the Confederacy*

Christopher H. Tebault, Surgeon to the Confederacy

ALAN I. WEST

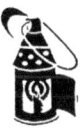

McFarland & Company, Inc., Publishers
Jefferson, North Carolina

ISBN (print) 978-1-4766-8082-8
ISBN (ebook) 978-1-4766-3884-3

Library of Congress and British Library
cataloguing data are available

Library of Congress Control Number 2020000397

© 2020 Alan I. West. All rights reserved

No part of this book may be reproduced or transmitted in any form or by any means, electronic or mechanical, including photocopying or recording, or by any information storage and retrieval system, without permission in writing from the publisher.

The front cover image of Dr. Tebault was first published in the 1914 *Confederate Veteran* as part of his obituary (August 1914, XXII (8): 372–373); *background* Confederate flag from the top of Dr. Tebault's medicine cabinet (photograph by author)

Printed in the United States of America

McFarland & Company, Inc., Publishers
Box 611, Jefferson, North Carolina 28640
www.mcfarlandpub.com

Table of Contents

Preface 1

1. Dr. Christopher Hamilton Tebault 5
2. The War 15
3. Medical Practice in New Orleans 46
4. Reconstruction 65
5. The Lost Cause 112
6. The United Confederate Veterans 136

Afterword 141

Dr. Tebault's Writings—A Selection 155

Chapter Notes 179

Bibliography 185

Index 193

Preface

My fascination with Christopher Hamilton Tebault began with an antique medicine box. In 1998 I purchased a walnut medicine chest from a Connecticut antiques dealer. It was manufactured by Savory & Moore, London, "Chemists to the Queen," with a label containing the notation "PRIZE MEDAL 1862 for Excellence of Manufacture." The chest included a number of original bottles with the labels of Thomas Roper, a 19th-century druggist who practiced in Ross-on-Wye, a small English town located in southeastern Herefordshire. But the most exciting part of the chest was its top, where a brass plate was engraved with a name.

C.H. Tebault, M.D.
—Surgeon—
10th S.C. Inf. Regt.
C.S.A.

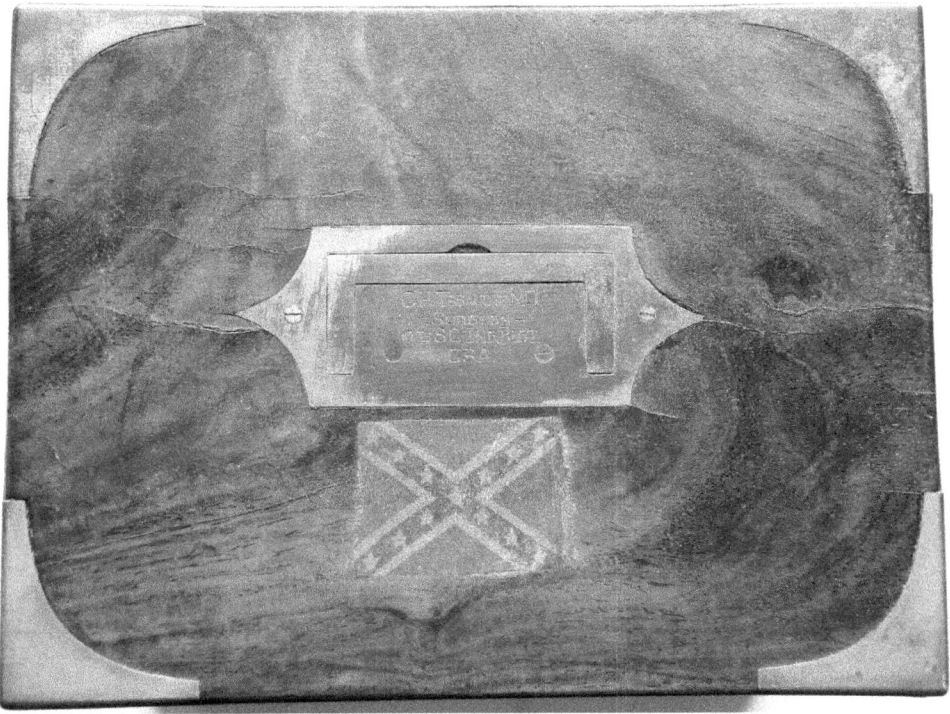

The brass plate reads "C.H. Tebault, M.D.—Surgeon—10th S.C. Inf. Regt. C.S.A." The purchase of the chest began a 20-plus-year journey to understand who its owner was. Photograph by author.

As the Savory & Moore label cited an 1862 prize, the chest had to have been purchased in 1862 or later, most likely from a Confederate blockade-runner. The wooden chest would have been expensive for its time. It is my belief that the case was presented to Dr. Tebault in honor of his promotion to surgeon of the 10th South Carolina Infantry Regiment in August 1862. The men of the regiment may have purchased it as a gift to an esteemed surgeon and colleague, but it is more likely that Dr. Tebault's father, Major Edward Tebault, procured it for his son. Blockade-runners auctioned their wares at southern port cities, such as Savannah, Charleston, Wilmington, Mobile and Pensacola. Interior states and cities rarely benefited from such goods. Major Tebault was financially well-off and connected politically, so he could easily have had access to those auctions.

How the chest wound up in the inventory of a Connecticut antiques dealer is still a mystery. The dealer had mentioned that the chest was purchased from a Connecticut estate. Somewhere during Dr. Tebault's travels, most likely during General Braxton Bragg's campaign in Tennessee, the chest may have been captured along with other supplies and eventually found by a Connecticut doctor. As it would have been too heavy for an enlisted man to carry or transport home, I believe it may have been used until the end of the war. Some of the bottles have handwritten labels that do not match Dr. Tebault's handwriting. But it is still one of those provenance mysteries that make collecting interesting.

Thus began a 22-year-long quest to understand the persona of Dr. Tebault. As I dug into his life, I discovered a complex individual. He was a creative and compassionate surgeon who utilized the meager resources available to Confederate surgeons to effectively treat the wounded and sick. After the war, he specialized in the diseases of children in New Orleans, perhaps as a respite to the devastation he faced during the war. His colleagues honored Dr. Tebault by choosing him as Surgeon General of the United Confederate Veterans in 1896. He worked to establish pensions and other benefits for aging Confederate veterans, he successfully fought the restrictive taxes placed upon Louisiana during Reconstruction, and he helped advance sanitation measures that successfully reduced outbreaks of disease in New Orleans. During reunions of the United Confederate Veterans, Dr. Tebault collected and compiled a significant amount of material regarding Confederate medicine that had been lost during the 1865 fires in Richmond. He published a number of often-quoted articles on Confederate resources, medicine, and the treatment of disease and injuries. Dr. Tebault was a friend of Confederate General P.G.T. Beauregard, and he moved in social circles with the elites of the South. He was one of the Confederate veterans chosen to escort Jefferson Davis's body to Richmond in 1893.

But Dr. Tebault was also a proponent of the "Lost Cause," an ideology that promulgated the belief that the cause of the Confederacy was just and heroic. While he was not a member of southern paramilitary groups such as the Ku Klux Klan and the White League, he did fight alongside the White League during the 1874 uprising of southern whites against the Republican government and a largely black metropolitan police force. His writings supported the notion that those living in the North failed to understand the "peculiar institution" of slavery as it was practiced "benignly" in the South.

I completed the first draft of his story a few years ago but could not finish it as I was conflicted. But, as I began to better understand the economic and political forces of Reconstruction and the social mores of the era, I developed a new respect for Dr. Tebault. The recent national controversies regarding Confederate monuments also made me want to revisit his life. I concluded that his story needed to be finished and told. A couplet that served as the tagline for the *Confederate Veteran* magazine summarized the southern ideal of respecting those veterans who had sacrificed so much:

> Though men deserve, they may not win, success;
> The brave will honor the brave, vanquished none the less.

The Lost Cause doctrine, however, went beyond simply honoring the brave and established the view that the South's cause was just, that the war was fought over states' rights and not the institution of slavery. How and why did such a doctrine arise? The vanquished of other wars came to terms with their participation; for example, Germany came to accept and reject their Nazi past and the atrocities of World War II. After researching this book and reading Dr. Tebault's many speeches and publications, I began to understand why southerners felt compelled to defend their actions rather than accept that their cause was flawed. Living in New Orleans during the years of Reconstruction must have been challenging for former Confederates. It was an era when black freedmen outnumbered the white citizens of the city, and many blacks were placed into political positions and made policemen, even though most were still illiterate. The city and state were under military rule by their former enemies, and New Orleans was controlled largely by a corrupt government of carpetbaggers and scalawags. It was certainly a tumultuous time.

It is my hope that this book is an adequate description of Dr. Tebault's life and his many contributions as a doctor and a man of compassion and strength, and that it provides the reader with a better understanding of the South following the war. Certainly, there is a difference between understanding a problem and excusing it. While we should never excuse the rise of groups such as the White League and the Ku Klux Klan, by understanding their evolution we can better appreciate how their rise affects even today's social environment. Sadly, racism is

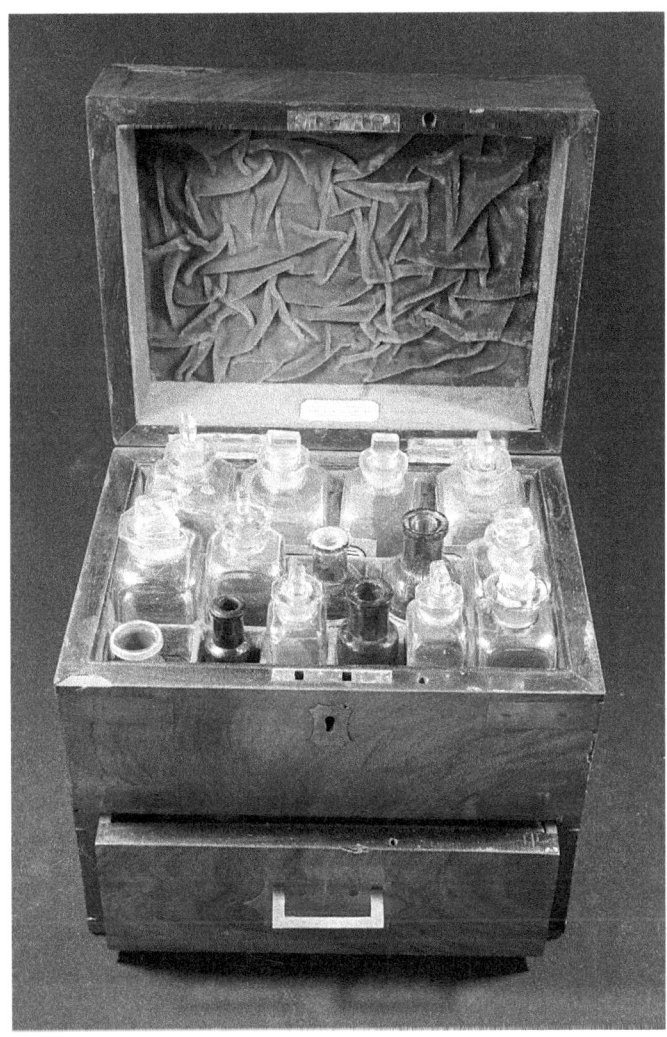

The chest was manufactured in 1862 by Savory & Moore, London, "Chemists to the Queen." Photograph by author.

still with us, but many of the forces that beget such prejudice began after the Civil War. Are the removals of Confederate monuments justified, or is doing so effectively erasing history? It is a question I personally have wrestled with, and I hope this book will help the reader better understand the issues behind the current debate.

Whenever possible, I have used original sources from the era. And, I have endeavored to let Dr. Tebault's own voice be heard and use extensive quotations. I have appended to this book four of his most important writings, which add to our knowledge of Confederate medicine and the tribulations of the men who served.

1

Dr. Christopher Hamilton Tebault

*"For the tenderest are the bravest,
The loving are the daring."*[1]

Standing five feet, 10 inches tall with penetrating hazel-colored eyes, Christopher Hamilton Tebault was a southern gentleman and patriot who became a prominent figure in the South both during and after the Civil War. During the war, he served as a surgeon on the staff of every southern commander in chief—Generals John B. Gordon, Stephen D. Lee, Clement A. Evans, George W. Gordon, and Bennett H. Young. Considered to be one of the top physicians serving the Confederacy, he distinguished himself as an assistant surgeon in the field and as the surgeon attached to a number of different Confederate hospitals. Later recognized for his medical contributions, he became Surgeon General of the United Confederate Veterans (UCV) following the war and used that position to collect and consolidate the history of Confederate medicine, advocate for Confederate veterans, and contribute to Confederate literature and the advancement of the "Lost Cause." He became actively involved in southern politics, participating in the Battle of Liberty Place in New Orleans on September 14, 1874; fighting the exorbitant taxes imposed on southern states during the Reconstruction period; and supporting efforts to establish pensions and relief for Confederate veterans. C.H. Tebault, as he usually signed his name, was personal friends with General P.G.T. Beauregard and served as a member of the honor guard that escorted President Jefferson Davis's body from New Orleans to his final resting place in Richmond. Dr. Tebault died in 1914, leaving behind a legacy of contributions to medicine, the City of New Orleans, Confederate veterans, and his family.

Born in Raymond, Mississippi, on November 12, 1838, Christopher moved with his family to Louisiana in 1844 at the age of six. His father, Major Edward John Tebault (1812–1886), was a banker and planter originally from Charleston, South Carolina. At the time of Christopher's birth, Edward was working as a planter on a sugar plantation in Mississippi and was also associated with banking in partnership with John A. Quitman. Quitman (1798–1858) was an influential politician who served under Zachary Taylor as a Brigadier General during the Mexican-American War. Quitman also served as Governor of Mississippi, first as a Whig from 1835 to 1836 and then as a Democrat from 1850 to 1851.[2]

Edward moved his family to Louisiana where he focused his efforts on banking, leveraging his relationship with Quitman and his network of associates. Edward initially was occupied in the liquidations of branch banks located in Napoleonville and Donaldsonville, Louisiana. A few years later, when Christopher had reached the age of 16, the family moved to New Orleans when Edward was offered the job of cashier of the prestigious Bank of Louisiana.[3]

One of Edward's relatives was Paul Charles François Adrien Henri Dieudonné Thiébault (1769–1846) who served under Napoleon as Lieutenant-General of the French army.[4] Thiébault married Elizabeth (Betsy) Walker, the daughter of Lady Mary Walker (1736–1821), a well-known Scottish author. Elizabeth's father was James Walker, a physician who led a troubled life, and her mother eventually became estranged from him. Elizabeth's mother then married George R. Hamilton, a cousin of Alexander Hamilton and whose last name she took and for whom Dr. Tebault was named. Some suggest that Lady Walker's first husband, James Walker, had not died as originally believed, leading to scandal as she had never divorced.[5] Lady Mary Hamilton was a strong advocate for educating women, and her stories may have influenced the English author, Jane Austen, who included in her writings several of Hamilton's character names.[6]

Christopher's mother, Caroline Hall (1819–1889), also came from an influential lineage. She was born in New York City and descended from some of the earliest settlers of the country. Included in her ancestry was Governor William Bradford, the first governor of the Plymouth Colony that would later unite with the Massachusetts Bay Colony. Caroline's father was Christopher Hall of Norfolk, Virginia, who served during the Revolution and was a warm personal friend to General Marquis de Lafayette, whom Hall entertained when Lafayette visited America.[7] Caroline's mother was Harriet Webber, who died after giving birth to five children. Her father, Christopher Hall, then married his cousin, Sarah Duyckinck (1796–1884).[8] The Duyckinck family was among the early settlers of New Amsterdam (New York City).[9] Evert Duyckinck became well known as a bookseller and publisher and helped establish New York City as a center for book printing and distribution throughout the young country.[10]

Christopher was named after his maternal grandfather, Christopher Hall, and Alexander Hamilton. Dr. Tebault was the oldest of seven siblings:

Elizabeth Tebault (1841–1870);
Richard Mansfield Tebault (1847–1913);
Edwin Tebault (1849–?);
B. Rutledge Tebault (1855–1880);
William Gartley Tebault (1859–1924); and
Virginia Caroline Tebault (1861–1908).

His brother, William Gartley Tebault (W.G. Tebault), would become a well-known furniture dealer in New Orleans. His store was located on Royal Street, and he became known as the "King of Royal Street" due to his poetic newspaper advertisements.[11]

As a result of his family's connections, young Christopher Tebault led a rather privileged childhood and attended private schools in New Orleans, graduating from the State High School. He then concentrated his educational efforts in the North at Georgetown College in the District of Columbia, studying literature and history.[12] He excelled in his studies and was honored by a presentation from President James Buchanan, who awarded him with a medal.[13]

Upon returning home to New Orleans, Christopher entered the Medical College of Louisiana, now known as Tulane University, to study medicine. The Medical College was founded in 1834 in response to concerns about the greatly feared diseases of smallpox, yellow fever and cholera that all too frequently tormented the city's populace in the warm and moist climate of New Orleans. Two years earlier, the *Amelia*, a ship sailing from New York to New Orleans, was wrecked off Folly Island just south of Charleston Harbor during a heavy storm. One hundred and twenty passengers made it to shore, but several were known to be infected with cholera. As soon as they recognized the danger of the situation, the city of Charleston quarantined the passengers on the island, fearing the spread of cholera to the city. Among the passengers was a young physician, Warren Stone. Dr. Stone (1808–1872) was born in Vermont and had earned his medical degree at the Berkshire Medical Institution in Pittsfield, Massachusetts. He had previously opened a medical practice in upstate New York where he treated cholera patients. Enticed by the idea of finding new ways to treat the disease, Dr. Stone decided to travel to New Orleans where cholera, yellow fever, and other diseases were common experiences.[14]

Hearing of the plight of the *Amelia* passengers, another young doctor, Thomas Hunt, joined Dr. Stone in treating the epidemic, and during that harrowing time they became fast friends. Thomas Hunt (1808–1867) was a native of Charleston and had studied medicine at the University of Pennsylvania. Together, the two men worked frantically to help the cholera victims and maintain the health of those still unaffected. Dr. Stone caught the disease while on the island, and when they both finally arrived in New Orleans, Dr. Stone was weakened and in poor health but gradually recovered. Both men settled in New Orleans.

Dr. Hunt fought additional outbreaks of cholera and became known in the city for his

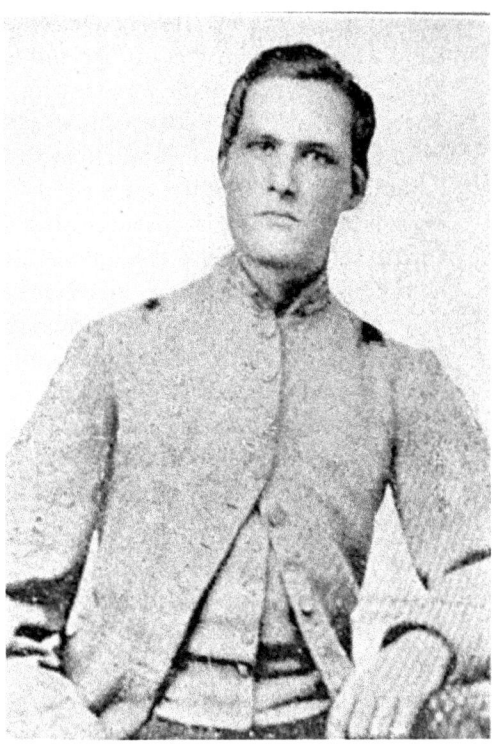

Dr. Tebault joined the 21st Louisiana as an assistant surgeon upon graduating from the Medical College of Louisiana in 1862. The 24-year-old was almost immediately pressed into service at Fort Pillow, arriving just as Union gunships began to bombard the fort.

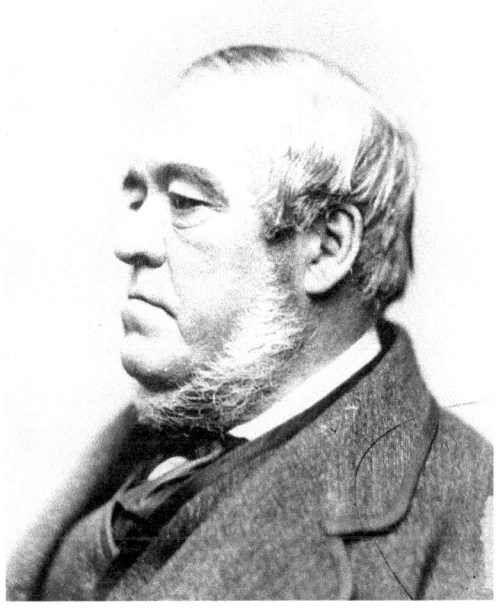

Dr. Stone was known as one of the most distinguished surgeons of the South. Image reproduced with permission from the Rudolph Matas Library of the Health Sciences, Tulane University.

war on the infectious disease. Dr. Stone became known as New Orleans's most prominent surgeon due to his unique surgical skills. Both men were elected to the staff at Charity Hospital, which was treating many patients with yellow fever and cholera. There they met Dr. John Hoffman Harrison (1808–1849), a kindred spirit originally from the District of Columbia, and the three men decided to create a new medical school to help relieve the frequent disease epidemics that plagued New Orleans. They astutely realized that to be successful, the school would need to be associated with the Charity Hospital where students could be exposed to its clinics and patients. Their honorable effort was not received well in the city by other physicians, who questioned how such young physicians could teach anything. All three were under 26 years of age at the time, and they were all new immigrants to the city. Ignoring the criticisms, the men proceeded to create the Medical College of Louisiana, built around the clinics of Charity Hospital. It became the second medical school in the South and the 15th in the United States.

That first-year session began on the first Monday in January 1835 and ended four months later. Eight medical school students were in attendance for Dr. Hunt's first lecture. Three years later, a School of Pharmacy was created. In 1843 the state legislature granted a ten-year lease for land to house the rapidly growing college provided (1) the faculty and students work at Charity Hospital without compensation, saving the state an estimated $24,000 annually, which it had been paying for medical services and (2) one indigent student from each parish in the state would be allowed to attend free. In 1845 the growing success of the college led the state to establish the University of Louisiana, with the Medical College being now a part of the larger public university. Within the Medical College were the separate departments of medical practice, chemistry, surgery, obstetrics, materia medica, physiology, anatomy, and demonstration of anatomy.

In the period prior to the outbreak of the Civil War, New Orleans was rapidly becoming renowned as one of the great medical centers in the United States. In addition to the University of Louisiana, the New Orleans School of Medicine had been founded in 1856 and was rapidly growing. During the 1859–1860 session, the University of Louisiana was 4th out of 42 medical colleges in terms of enrollment, and the two-year-old New Orleans School of Medicine was ranked 7th. The following is a list of the top schools and their student enrollment in the school year just before the war:

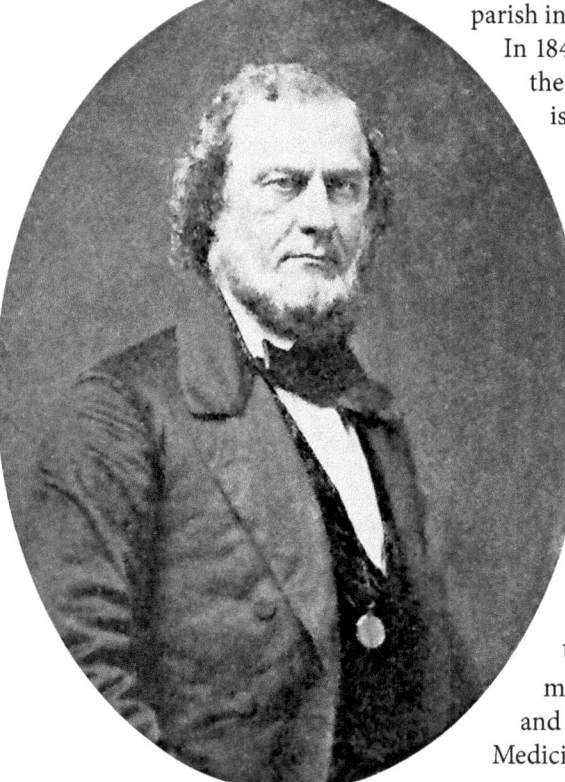

Thomas Hunt, co-founder of the Medical College of Louisiana (now Tulane University).

Table 1: Medical School Enrollment, 1859–1860

School	Total Students	Graduating Class
Jefferson Medical College	630	170
University of Pennsylvania	515	173
University of New York	411	138
University of Louisiana	401	113
New Orleans School of Medicine	216	63

Medical education augmented with clinical experience was almost unheard of during the mid–19th century. Typically, teaching was didactic only, with most medical schools lacking any affiliation with clinical facilities. The standard education course consisted of two terms of nine months followed by another term working with an experienced physician. The second term was often simply a repetition of the first. Laboratory and clinical instruction were rarely provided, and many states still banned dissection. Human dissection was not only controversial, but this was an era before cadavers were preserved in formaldehyde, so any dissections had to proceed rapidly as bodies quickly deteriorated. When dissections were offered as part of a physician's education, they were typically done during the winter months, when the cold served as natural refrigeration. The availability of cadavers was quite limited, however, and grave robbers were known to provide supplemental specimens.

In his diaries, medical student Charles Hentz described his dissection training at Louisville Medical Institute, which later became the University of Louisville:

> After supper, we returned to the college building, and dissected dead bodies in the suite of dissecting rooms that occupied the basement room of the large college building. The dissecting rooms were large; with brick floors; 6 or 8 of them, opening into each other, and into a hall that ran between them.... [Students] sat around the body on tall stools; some dissecting & some reading aloud from the Anatomy, to guide the matter of dissecting; the flesh & refuse matter left over after each night's work, was carried into the dead room, where there was an immensely deep dry well, into which it was dumped; & a close cover laid over the top; before returning home, we went through a vigorous process of ablution; there was a force pump of prodigious power, that knocked the filth and bad smell from the fingers; but it was very hard to get rid of; could sometimes, in spite of hard washing, smell the stench on our fingers even at the table.[15]

Such dissection was not without its hazards, as ungloved hands were prone to cuts and infections, and students could succumb to the same disease that had taken the life of the corpse they were dissecting.

Southern schools had essentially the same educational requirements as those in the North, although there were certainly educational differences between the two sections of the country. A North Carolina author wrote of the failings of the southern educational system. He noted that most educated men in the South owed their edification to northern colleges. "Not that there are no Southern colleges—for there are institutions, so-called, in a majority of the Slave States ... but as a general thing, Southern colleges are colleges in *name*, and will scarcely take rank with a third-rate Northern academy, while our academies, with a few exceptions, are immeasurably inferior to the public schools of New York, Philadelphia and Boston. The truth is, there is a vast inert mass of stupidity and ignorance, too dense for individual effort to enlighten or remove, in all communities cursed with the institution of slavery."[16] The medical college at the University of Pennsylvania was the first medical school in the colonies, founded in 1765. The nearby Jefferson Medical College was founded in 1827. Both Philadelphia schools were widely renowned. Many Philadelphia and northern-educated physicians residing in southern states wanted their sons to have the same training as they experienced, and thus northern schools enrolled many students from the South. Consequently, many considered the newer southern schools to be inferior to their more celebrated northern cousins.

Another problem facing southern schools was illiteracy. Many southern children worked on their parents' farms, and relatively few attended schools as compared to northerners. The following table illustrates the percent of illiteracy of the white population over twenty years of age in northern and southern states in 1860. Indiana and Illinois were the only two "Free States" that were bettered in terms of literacy by any "Slave State."

Table 2: Percent of Illiterate Whites, 1860

Northern States	Percent Illiterate	Southern States	Percent Illiterate
Connecticut	0.2%	Louisiana	2.6%
Vermont	0.2%	Maryland	3.7%
New Hampshire	0.3%	Mississippi	5.0%
Massachusetts	0.6%	Delaware	5.6%
Maine	0.9%	South Carolina	5.9%
Michigan	1.0%	Missouri	6.3%
Rhode Island	1.5%	Alabama	6.7%
New Jersey	1.7%	Kentucky	7.4%
New York	1.8%	Georgia	7.7%
Pennsylvania	2.0%	Virginia	8.0%
Ohio	2.3%	Arkansas	8.7%
Indiana	5.6%	Tennessee	9.1%
Illinois	5.9%	North Carolina	14.3%

The literacy in places such as New York, Rhode Island, and Pennsylvania was negatively influenced by the influx of a large number of illiterate immigrants; 69 percent of the 98,722 illiterate citizens of New York in 1860 were immigrants. In contrast, North Carolina, South Carolina, and Virginia had foreign illiterate populations of only 340, 104, and 1,137, respectively. Sixty percent of children between five and twenty years of age attended school in the North compared to only 8 percent in the South.[17] Ninety percent of southerners lived in rural areas, making it relatively difficult for children to travel to attend school. As newspapers were the primary source of news and opinion at the time, literacy was crucial to understanding the events of the day and their implications. Illiterate southerners had to rely on their more educated friends and associates for the assessments of events; thus, they were easily swayed by emotions and prejudiced opinions. Even so, it seems that the University of Louisiana Medical School was unique among Southern schools in the quality of the educational experiences they offered students. The only entrance requirement for college at the time was the ability to pay what was quite expensive tuition, so students were typically from well-to-do families who would have been able to afford better education for their children. Christopher Tebault was a good example of such a privileged and well-educated child.

George Bacon Wood (1797–1879) was a prominent physician in Philadelphia who authored numerous books, including the *Dispensatory of the United States* (1833), which was an important reference at the time that went through 17 editions. He also authored a two-volume medical text, *Treatise on Practice,* published in 1847, which ran through six editions, with the last published in 1867. He would meet his students nightly at his home, where he would examine them line-by-line and page-by-page through the two volumes of his own text. Medical students at other schools were typically less trained, as many schools only required a year of class instruction. Dr. Sample Ford served as a capable assistant surgeon of the 5th West Virginia Cavalry during the Civil War. He was born in Alexander, Pennsylvania, in 1827 and began his medical practice in Wheeling, Virginia (now West Virginia), in 1852, having attended only one term of lectures at Jefferson Medical College in Philadelphia and a few months of "medical reading" with Dr. R.H. Cummins in Wheeling. At the outset of the Civil War there was such a dire need for surgeons that many who entered the service had little training and clinical experience. Certainly, none were prepared for the traumatic wounds and sickness they would encounter. For many, including Dr. Ford, it was training under fire. Many poorly trained surgeons rose to the occasion, however, learning quickly how to treat gunshot wounds, amputate limbs, and tend to the sick.

The Medical College at the University of Louisiana started its first session in January 1835, with eleven students. A year later it issued its first degrees. Thomas Hunt served for 20 years on the staff (1834–1867) and died in 1867. Warren Stone served for 38 years (1835–1873). He died in 1873 and was the most famous surgeon of the institution at the time of his death.

Dr. Tebault's medical education was quite rigorous by 19th-century standards; not only did he attend a year of lectures, he also spent more than two years in residence at Charity Hospital, although at the time it was not a requirement for graduation. Originally named the Hospital of Saint John (L'Hôpital des Pauvres de la Charité), Charity Hospital was founded in 1736 as a hospital for treating the poor and indigent. Eventually, the hospital came under the management of the Sisters of Charity. In 1847 the Medical College was expanded into the University of Louisiana when a law school was added. The university was renamed Tulane University in 1884 when it evolved from a public to a private institution.[18]

The College's two famous founders, Thomas Hunt and Warren Stone, personally mentored the young Christopher Tebault.[19] Ominously, he earned his medical degree in April in the last session of the College just one month before the fall of New Orleans on May 1, 1862.

Confederate Medicine

In 1861, both sides were totally unprepared for the medical consequence of the impending war. In January 1861 there were a total of only 113 doctors—30 surgeons and 83 assistant surgeons—to support the 16,000 regular soldiers of the U.S. Army. When the war finally broke out in April, 3 surgeons and 21 assistant surgeons defected to the Confederacy, and an additional 3 were dismissed for disloyalty, leaving the Federal Army with only 86 doctors.[20] By April 1865 there were over 12,000 surgeons in the North and 3,200 in the South. Not only was the rapid education and qualification of such a large number of new physicians a remarkable achievement in itself, it is also notable that the quality of medical services improved as the war dragged on.

Aside from the small medical service, another reason for the poor medical preparations was the belief both sides shared that any conflict would be short-lived. Some volunteers worried that the conflict might end before they had the chance to join in on the action. Certainly, there were those who truly understood that a civil war would be both terrifying and costly in lives and gold.[21] But most in the media delighted in penning gallant prophecies on their pages. Horace Greeley in the *New York Tribune* boldly predicted that "the nations of Europe may rest assured that Jeff Davis and Company will be swinging from the battlements at Washington, at least, by the 4th of July. We spit upon a later and longer deferred justice."[22] Likewise, the *New York Times* proclaimed that "we have only to send a column of twenty-thousand men across the Potomac to Richmond, and burn out the rats there."[23] The *Philadelphia Press* presaged that "the rebels, a mere band of ragamuffins, will fly, like chaff before the wind, on our approach."[24] On April 15, 1861, President Abraham Lincoln called for 75,000 men to serve only three months of service, supporting the notion in the North that southerners would never stand and fight. His order for only a 90-day commitment further suggested a quick action.

Southerners were similarly convinced that the North would never truly oppose them, that northerners were undisciplined with no appetite for fighting. Edward Pollard, the prickly editor of the *Richmond Examiner*, published a southern history of the war in 1867 entitled *The Lost Cause*.[25] In the book he cites the delusions of both the North and South in believing that the war would be a short affair: "...[T]he war would be decided speedily, and its history be compassed in a few battlefields. It had been a theme of silly declamation that 'the Yankees' would not fight; and so-called statesmen of the South expounded the doctrine that a commercial community, devoted to the pursuit of gain, could never aspire to military prowess, and were unequal to great deeds of arms."[26] Southerners, rightly so, were convinced that they were better horsemen, and most had grown up in rural areas shooting rifles and so also considered themselves to be better marksmen; they were generally correct on both accounts, as many northern volunteers had never ridden a horse or fired a weapon. In fact, many northern volunteers viewed the cavalry as more desirable than other military branches because it appeared to be a more dashing and elite corps. To be effective, cavalry troopers had to train for months with their horses, as horse and rider needed to act as a single unit. In 1861, however, the northern men who volunteered for the cavalry were not selected as to their horsemanship or even their size and weight, and many had never ridden a horse.

The first Battle of Bull Run (Manassas), July 21, 1861, resulted in northern troops being severely routed, which confirmed the conviction of southerners that they were superior fighters. The *Richmond Daily Whig* bragged: "We are too close and too much influenced by the great events which are passing, to indulge much in philosophizing. But the rout and dispersion, at the great pitched battle near Manassas, bring into bold relief the great fact that the Yankees are humbugs, and that the *white people* of the slave-holding states are the true masters—the real rulers of the continent."[27] A popular southern book likewise boasted: "In almost every battle the Yankees have either, as at Manassas, marched away from the field, before the fight, to the sounds of our guns, or if they awaited the first shock, have been scattered like sheep by our gallant soldiery."[28]

The passions for war blinded logic and halted further debate on both sides.

The Medical Corps of the Confederate States Army was authorized by the first session of the Provisional Confederate Congress held in Montgomery, Alabama, on February 26, 1861, eight days after the inauguration of Jefferson Davis as President. The Act that was passed was entitled "An Act for the Establishment and Organization of a General Staff for the Army of the Confederate States of America." It called for a medical department consisting of a Surgeon General, four surgeons and six assistant surgeons. Later, on March 6, 1861, the Provisional Congress intended to require one surgeon and an assistant surgeon to serve in each regiment. The published Act was entitled: "An Act to provide for the Public Defence." The Act stipulated: "That the field and staff officers of a separate battalion of volunteers shall be one lieutenant-colonel or major, one adjutant with the rank of lieutenant, one sergeant major, one quartermaster sergeant, and a chief bugler or principal musician, according to corps; and that each company shall be entitled to an additional second lieutenant; and that the President may limit the privates in any volunteer company, according to his discretion, at from sixty-four to one hundred." Notably absent is any mention of medical officers. Due to a clerical error, the requirement for a surgeon, assistant surgeon and hospital steward was left off the official transcript, officially leaving the entire Confederate Army with only eleven doctors. The problem was quickly remedied, but the clerical oversight highlights the lack of careful medical planning and preparation.

Dr. D.C. DeLeon (1816–1872) was made the first Surgeon General of the Medical Corps, but he was quickly replaced by the more capable Dr. Samuel Preston Moore (1813–1889) when the Confederate capital was moved to Richmond in July 1861; Dr. Moore would serve in that capacity until the end of the war.[29] Moore faced the unenviable task of creating from scratch the new medical corps and its organization. Southern physicians were generally from rural areas and had little experience in surgery and hospital administration. Many were poorly trained and had received only a year of lectures and/or short apprenticeships. Moore was known as a strict disciplinarian, however, and quickly created the Army Medical Board to administer examinations to screen out incompetent or unqualified surgeons.[30]

The Army Medical Boards utilized both written and oral examinations. In the first months following the outbreak of the war, admission standards for surgeons were quite low due to the dire need to recruit medical officers. Adding to the problem was the fact that there was a dearth of new medical school graduates, as every southern medical school closed its doors during the war with the two exceptions of the Medical College of Virginia and the University of Nashville, although Federal soldiers occupied Nashville on June 6, 1862. The Medical Board examinations varied in their intensity from state to state, but they were all generally criticized as focusing on subjects that were easily tested rather than more practical knowledge that would truly measure a surgeon's ability in treating the myriad of diseases and trauma they would face in the field. One Confederate surgeon recalled a painful examination before the board: "The examinations were oral, and were harrowing experiences for eager, although nervous, doctors. On one occasion the victim of Yandell's intense grilling about gunshot wounds brightened when asked what he would do for a 'shot right through there,' the Medical Director pointing to his own knee." (David Wendel Yandell was president of Kentucky's Medical Board.) "Well, Sir, if it was you that was shot through there, I would not do a damned thing," announced the applicant.[31] It is not known whether that particular applicant was given a passing score.

The ineffectiveness of the Medical Boards was not a complaint only of the Confederate medical service; the North had similar problems with unqualified surgeons and also instituted examination boards who were at times inconsistent and overly harsh. *The American Medical Times* published an article on June 22, 1861, entitled: "The Right Man for the Right Place." In the article, the author wrote:

> The State Boards of Medical Examiners have proved, in many instances, either negligent, or culpably ignorant of their duties. We may estimate by hundreds the numbers of unqualified persons who have received the endorsement of these bodies, as capable Surgeons and Assistant-Surgeons to regiments.

Indeed, these examinations have in some cases been so conducted as to prove the merest farce. Irregular practitioners, "retired physicians," disabled "political doctors," physicians unable to obtain a livelihood in civil practice from sheer incapacity, have emerged from the "Green Room" full-fledged Army Surgeons. The result of this official ignorance is now apparent; the Secretary of War has recently called the attention of the Surgeon-General of the United States to the reported incapacity of regimental surgeons of the volunteer forces at Washington, and directed a re-examination, with a view to the dismissal of those found incompetent.[32]

By the end of 1861 the Medical Boards were rejecting almost 80 percent of Confederate applicants.[33] In spite of all the difficulties and challenges in quickly organizing a medical corps, Surgeon General Moore was able to grow the medical departments of the Confederate Army and Navy to over 3,300 men by the end of the war.[34]

On September 26, 1862, the Committee on Military Affairs presented to the Confederate Congress the names of 108 surgeons and 234 assistant surgeons who had passed review by the Medical Boards. The Congress approved the resolution giving the men their commissions. Christopher Tebault's name was among the assistant surgeons thus approved.[35] This was fortunate, as Dr. Tebault was already engaged with the 10th South Carolina in Kentucky at the time.

2

THE WAR

"seventy-five times seventy-five thousand men cannot conquer us."[1]

War Frenzy and Passions in New Orleans

Southerners' nationalistic spirit had been slowly building over several years with talks of states' rights and secession. Debates regarding the legality of secession had been going on for years prior to the attack on Fort Sumter in April 1861. Most believed that they had the legal right to do so. Southerners also were angered that northerners had distorted views of the "peculiar institution" of slavery as it was practiced in the South. Harriet Beecher Stowe's popular book, *Uncle Tom's Cabin*, was viewed as northern propaganda.

> It is a caricature of slavery. It selects for description the most odious features of slavery—the escape and pursuit of fugitive slaves, the sale and separation of domestic slaves, the separation of husbands and wives, parents and children, brothers and sisters. It portrays the slaves of the story as more moral, intelligent, courageous, elegant and beautiful than their masters and mistresses; and where it concedes any of these qualities to the whites, it is to such only as are, even though slaveholders, opposed to slavery. Those in favor of slavery are slave-traders, slave-catchers, and the most weak, depraved, cruel and malignant of beings and demons.[2]

The book's popularity in the North was further viewed as hypocritical; while southern slaveholders were demonized, radical abolitionists in the North, including "brutes" like William Lloyd Garrison, were applauded. (William Lloyd Garrison [1805–1879] was a staunch abolitionist who helped form the New England Anti-Slavery Society in 1852 and published an anti-slavery newspaper, *The Liberator*.)

Northerners had made a hero of John Brown, even though he had been fomenting a slave rebellion that would result in the murder of innocent women and children in the South had it succeeded. While denouncing slavery in the South, northern industrialists abused poor factory workers who were subjected to what many southerners considered to be much worse conditions than those experienced by southern slaves. Northerners completely ignored the "benevolence" of plantation owners to their slaves. And, they had disregarded Federal law by refusing to return runaway slaves, in spite of the Supreme Court's Dred Scott decision and the Fugitive Slave Act of 1850. Consequently, many in the South believed that if northerners could ignore the U.S. Constitution and its laws, then the South was well within its rights to secede and create its own Constitution and laws.

While New Orleans prepared for the 1860 holiday season with its celebrated parties and Christmas gaiety, there was a nervous undertone from Abraham Lincoln's recent election. Even before the holiday season commenced, South Carolina announced its secession.

Following in South Carolina's footsteps, Mississippi, then Alabama, then Georgia quickly joined the new Confederacy. Not wanting to wait for the Louisiana Convention to determine their State's position, the Washington Artillery was sent to Baton Rouge on January 9, 1861, to take over the Federal arsenal located there. Other seceding states had also been actively seizing Federal forts and arsenals and collecting any arms they might find.[3] When General P.G.T. Beauregard attempted to similarly take over Fort Sumter located in the middle of Charleston Harbor, Major Robert Anderson, its Federal commander, refused. On April 12, 1861, the Fort was fired upon. Anderson's surrender of the Fort the following day ignited passions on both sides. Once President Lincoln called for 75,000 volunteers to crush the southern rebellion, secession fever grew enormously in response to what was viewed as northern aggression and threats, and those originally opposed to secession now either advocated for it or remained silent. While many southerners had not been in favor of secession, Lincoln's call for troops was viewed as an affront and inflamed calls for other southern states to secede and organize an army to oppose any "invasion" from the North. Local newspapers helped ignite the passions of those citizens, now all too eager to join the fray.

In Richmond, Virginia, there were grand celebrations over the news of Fort Sumter's surrender: "Many of the houses were brilliantly illuminated from attic to cellar; flags of the Southern Confederacy were abundantly displayed from roofs and windows; the streets blazed with bonfires; the sky lighted with showers of pyrotechnics; and, until midnight, crowd after crowd found speakers to address them from balconies and street corners."[4] In Louisiana, the press believed that the majority of northerners would not follow the lead of the "Black Republicans," congressional abolitionists whom many in the South regarded as acting so fanatical as to represent only a very small minority of those in the North.

> The patriotic fires which have been lying dormant in the hearts of the people of the Border Slave States, have burst forth in all their splendor, and soon we shall see the whole South united to repel the fanatical myrmidons of the Black Republican Confederacy.... Every man is resolved to fight in defense of his home and fireside, and will die in his tracks rather than surrender or retreat from the Black Republican army.... We do not believe that there has been any such uprising of the people of the North, as the briefings of the press have telegraphed abroad, for the purpose of intimidating the Southerners and causing them to ground their arms and "disperse." We know that there are many at the North who are opposed to the insane measures of the Black Republican administration, which are destined to bankrupt the country, and then to end in a humiliating and disgraceful defeat.... That the North may do us great injury in a long and bloody war, we do not deny; but they never can subjugate us—NEVER. In the language of our eloquent Vice President [Alex. H. Stephens], "seventy-five times seventy-five thousand men cannot conquer us."[5]

As in the South, the northern press had been arousing nationalistic pride with their own belligerent exclamations. A month before the first shots echoed in Charleston Harbor, a Pennsylvania newspaper exclaimed: "We have borne with treason as long as it is possible to do so. Talk of tearing down our fair fabric of government! Never! Never! Jeff Davis is on the road to the gallows, and his followers had better be careful."[6] Following the news of the bombardment and surrender of Fort Sumter, the northern press breathlessly reported the excitement observed in northern cities. The *New York Herald* exclaimed: "The war spirit is fully aroused in this city. Stars and Stripes are flying in all directions, and all parties are in favor of sustaining the government."[7] Another New York paper noted: "Party lines disappeared—party cries are hushed or emptied of meaning—men forget that they were Democrats or Republicans in the newly aroused and intense consciousness that they are Americans."[8] A few days later, the *Herald* summarized the feelings of many in the North:

> The people of the Northern States are a unit. They are actuated by one thought, one sentiment, one soul—the solemn resolve that whatever the cost may be, *the integrity and unity of this great republic*, for all future time, shall evolve out of the present political chaos. The thunders of a dozen batteries, maned by seven thousand men, against a handful of half-starved soldiers in Fort Sumter, awaken the North to the conviction that they had been cruelly deceived, and that self-respect as well as sound policy demanded an instant resort to arms. The fires of Vesuvius never burst with greater suddenness from its crater, than did the war spirit, from the previously inert and passive surface, in this city and elsewhere in the free States....[9]

The war frenzy in the North surprised most southerners. Some southerners tried to rationalize all the northern flag waving rhetoric: "This peculiarly Yankee exhibition in flags pervaded nearly every square mile of the country, and was carried even into the sanctuary ... and even in distant parts of the country flags floated from gate-posts and tops of trees, as evidence of 'loyal' sentiments and marks for protection against 'vigilance committees.'"[10] While some in the North no doubt felt pressure to conform to the patriotic spirit displayed by their fellow citizens, southerners failed to appreciate the genuine reaction of many in the North.

After the war, Dr. Tebault remarked that the bombardment of Fort Sumter was from a southern viewpoint an unavoidable response to the Federal Government's unlawful seizure of the property of South Carolina. "The Fort was within the jurisdiction of South Carolina. It was built especially for her protection, and belonged to her."[11] So why were Yankees viewing a bloodless attack to take back property owned by a southern state as a traitorous attack on the Union? This was a question that many in the South failed to understand, even long after the end of the conflict. In their minds it was the Federals who tossed aside negotiation and compromise and forced the hand of the South to take action, an act that they also believed the U.S. Constitution supported. Southerners who were more politically savvy noted with sadness the loss of support from some of their Democratic friends in Congress, a party "which had so long professed regard for the rights of the Southern States, and even sympathy with the first movements of secession. The party now rivalled the Abolitionists in their expressions of fury and revenge."[12] Neither party understood the passions of the other. And, neither believed the other side to be so principled that they would actually fight.

The 21st Louisiana

Dr. Tebault's class of 1862 would be the last class to graduate from the Medical School until after the war. Many of his classmates and professors had already gone to join the Confederate forces. After receiving his medical degree from the University of Louisiana, Dr. Tebault was recruited by John B.G. Kennedy to join the 21st Louisiana Regiment in February 1862. Brigadier General John B. Villepigue commanded the regiment. Before Dr. Tebault joined the regiment, approximately 7,000 men of the 21st had marched to Island Number 10 on February 23, 1862, to begin the arduous work of erecting batteries for heavy artillery pieces under the command of Major General John P. McCown. The balance of the regiment later joined them mid–March, and Villepigue moved some of the men down the Mississippi to garrison Fort Pillow, splitting his command.

Following the fall of Forts Henry and Donelson, Confederate forces found it increasingly difficult to defend the upper Mississippi River Valley. Brigadier General Ulysses S. Grant succeeded in capturing Fort Henry on February 6, 1862. The fort had been built to prevent the Union from using the Tennessee River and was located on its eastern bank.

Following the fort's defeat, the Union was now able to freely move along the Tennessee River. Six days later, Grant attacked Fort Donelson, which was built on the Cumberland River, about five miles east of Fort Henry. After four days, Fort Donelson also surrendered on February 16. That surrender now opened the Cumberland River to enable Federal forces to take the important southern city of Nashville on February 25.

Island Number 10 was located on a tight double bend on the Mississippi River near New Madrid, Missouri. It was named as being the tenth island in the Mississippi River downstream of where the Ohio joined the Mississippi. Now that Grant had opened the Tennessee and Cumberland Rivers, his next step was to free up the Mississippi, with Island Number 10 representing the northernmost resistance. On March 15, 1862, Union gunboats and floating mortars laid siege to the island's defenses, shortly after the 21st had helped complete them. After three long weeks, the appearance of Federal ironclads tipped the balance of power, and an unusually well-coordinated attack with Flag Officer Andrew H. Foote of the Navy and General John Pope of the Army succeeded in outflanking the Confederate defenses. Seeing his only means of retreat cut off, Brigadier General Mackall surrendered the island garrison of about 4,500 defenders on April 8, 1862. The fall of Island Number 10 effectively opened the Mississippi River from Cairo, Kentucky, in the north to Vicksburg, Mississippi, in the south. The only remaining resistance that now stood in their way was the city of Memphis, with Fort Pillow guarding the city from the north. The remnants of the 21st had retreated to the fort and now waited for the inevitable assault by Federal forces.

Brigadier General Gideon Johnson Pillow had built the fort named after him in early 1862 to guard the river traffic and protect Memphis, 60 miles to the south. The fort stood on a high bluff overlooking the Mississippi and commanding the river for two or three miles above and below the fort. The bluff descended to the river's edge precipitously, its side being covered with trees, bushes and fallen timber. Ravines extended back from the river on both sides of the bluff. These natural fortifications were augmented by a semicircle of entrenchments in front of the fort's four-foot thick parapet. The protective thickness of the parapet, however, would prove to be a detriment to the fort's defenders as they could not fire upon advancing troops without climbing onto its top, thus exposing themselves to enemy fire. Additionally, its thickness meant that the fort's six artillery pieces found it difficult to depress their barrels sufficiently to fire upon attackers once they moved close to the fort's walls.

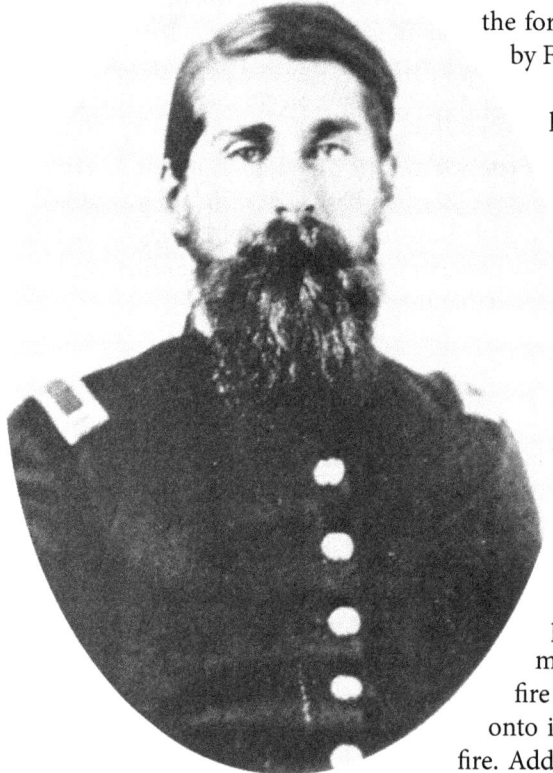

Brigadier General Villepigue commanded the 21st Louisiana. The photograph is copied from Miller's *Photographic History of the Civil War* identifying Villepigue as "The Defender of Fort Pillow."

Twenty-four-year-old Dr. Tebault arrived at the fort just as a Union fleet of gunboats and ironclads threw the first shells against it on April 10. He was immediately required to exercise all the surgical skills he had learned, as the constant bombardment of exploding shells took its toll on the Confederate defenders. The bombardment would continue until June 4.

Dr. Tebault's training and creativity were challenged by an incident that occurred one month after he arrived at the fort. Under the direction of Union Commodore Charles H. Davis, 200 Confederate prisoners were delivered to the fort on May 20 as part of an exchange of prisoners. These men had been imprisoned at Alton, Illinois, and some were sickened with smallpox. Believing that these men would communicate the dreaded disease to the rest of the garrison at the fort, General Villepigue sent an urgent dispatch describing the situation to General Beauregard, who was encamped in nearby Corinth. Beauregard immediately wrote back with instructions to return the sick prisoners to the Federals. General Villepigue quickly sent a dispatch to Davis.

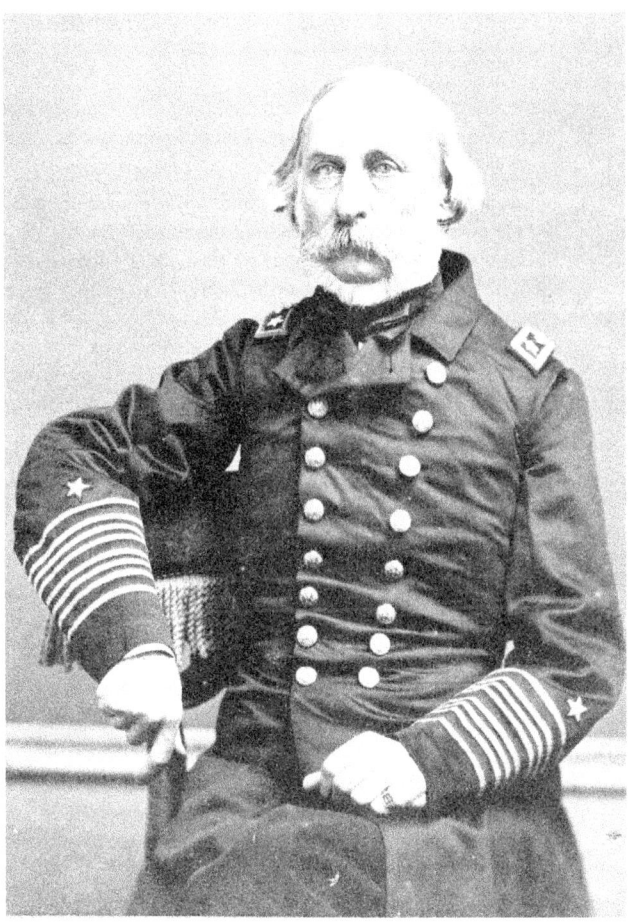

Commander of the Western Flotilla on the Mississippi River, Captain Davis delivered 200 exchanged Confederate prisoners to Fort Pillow, some of the men being ill with smallpox. Library of Congress, Prints & Photographs Division, Civil War Photographs, CPH3c04940.

Captain C.H. Davis, Commanding Western Flotilla, Mississippi River

CAPTAIN: On yesterday evening while temporarily absent from my headquarters the second in command, Colonel A. Jackson, Jr., through inadvertence or carelessness, received at this post 202 Confederate prisoners of war just from an infected prison at Alton, Ill., with two or three cases of small-pox among them, in exchange for the same number of U.S. prisoners turned over to your authorities some time ago free from infection.

While I do not presume that you are in any way responsible for so barbarous an act as sending released prisoners to communicate to my command the loathsome and infectious disease of small-pox, I demand that your Government disown the act by receiving these prisoners back into its lines and caring for them until every symptom of the infection had disappeared from their midst.

I am, captain, with high respect, your obedient servant, John B. Villepigue, Brigadier-General, Commanding.[13]

Captain Davis refused to take back the prisoners. He replied in a dispatch to General Villepigue:

Letter from C.H. Davis, Captain, Commanding Western Flotilla, Mississippi River, to Brig. Gen. John B. Villepigue, Commanding Fort Pillow, Tenn., May 21, 1862:

Your letter of 20th instant has been received. I have not a sufficient knowledge of the circumstances of the case—as for example, the condition of the building at Alton, Ill., in which the prisoners referred to have been confined, the health of the prisoners at the period of their release or the possible change of health they may have undergone on their way to this place—to render it worthwhile for me to enter into the details of the subject. In order, however, to remove any grounds of complaint and to make a suitable provision for an unexpected emergency, I propose that a temporary neutral hospital be established for the benefit of the prisoners suffering from smallpox. The place for this hospital may be determined by Captain Dove, the bearer of this letter, acting for me and such officer as you may designate on your part. I have the honor to be, general, very respectfully, your most obedient servant, C.H. Davis.[14]

When the prisoners heard of their proposed return to Union forces, they expressed outrage that their comrades in arms would even think of returning them back to the enemy and voiced fear that they would die in a Union prison were they to be returned. General Villepigue subsequently sent another dispatch to General Beauregard informing him of the state of affairs, which Beauregard forwarded by telegram to General Henry Halleck:

Corinth, Miss., May 20, 1862

Maj. Gen. H.W. Halleck, Commanding U.S. Forces

GENERAL: I have this day been informed by Brigadier-General Villepigue, commanding the Confederate forces at Fort Pillow, that 200 exchanged prisoners were sent to him yesterday and that these prisoners had the small-pox amongst them. I have directed General Villepigue to return them forthwith. I presume that all this has been done without your knowledge, as your communication on the subject of exchange of prisoners I regarded as an agreement on fair and equal terms. To send us prisoners afflicted with contagious diseases of a dangerous and deadly character is in my judgment violative of all ideas of fairness and justice as well as humanity. For all prisoners therefore surrendered by Confederate officers I shall insist, general, that they are entitled by every claim of fairness and justice to demand in exchange an equal number of prisoners in like condition of those sent back to you.

Very respectfully, your obedient servant,
P.G.T. BEAUREGARD, General, Commanding.[15]

General Halleck wrote back to General Beauregard that he thought the story was a "fabrication" but that he would investigate the matter further if provided with more details. General Villepigue again replied to Beauregard:

Fort Pillow, May 22, 1862

General Beauregard:

The transaction is no myth, but from what the prisoners say looks very much like an attempt to communicate the small-pox to my command. They were taken at Pea Ridge and are just from an infected prison at Alton, Ill. They were received by the second in command while I was reconnoitering. I endeavored to get Flag Officer Davis to take them back but he refused. Will send by first boat all the papers and correspondence.

JOHN B. VILLEPIGUE, Brigadier-General, Commanding.[16]

The contention that the prison in Alton was infected with smallpox was correct. An earlier dispatch from the commander of the prison at Alton describing the health of the Confederate prisoners confirmed such:

Alton, Ill. May 18, 1862

ASSISTANT ADJUTANT-GENERAL

Department Headquarters, Saint Louis, Mo.

SIR: I have the honor to transmit a list of prisoners received. released, &c., from the 1st to the 10th of May 1862.... I respectfully recommend that no more prisoners be sent to this prison until the small-pox has abated. There are now about twenty cases, and though not severe it is probable some will terminate fatally. I will send you a list of the Pea Ridge prisoners in a day or two, as soon as it can be prepared. No list of these prisoners was ever sent here and all the information we have we obtained from the prisoners themselves. The exchanged prisoners left yesterday morning. There were 199. The three officers from Columbus did not arrive to go with them.

Very respectfully, your
obedient servant, S. BURBANK
Lieutenant-Colonel Thirteenth
Infantry, Commanding.[17]

It seems likely that there was no deliberate conspiracy on the part of the Federals to infect the Confederate command at Fort Pillow by transferring infected soldiers. Neither was there an effort, however, to avoid doing so as they knew that some of the men were infected.

Under the care and direction of Dr. Tebault, the smallpox victims were quickly quarantined on Hatchie Island located on the

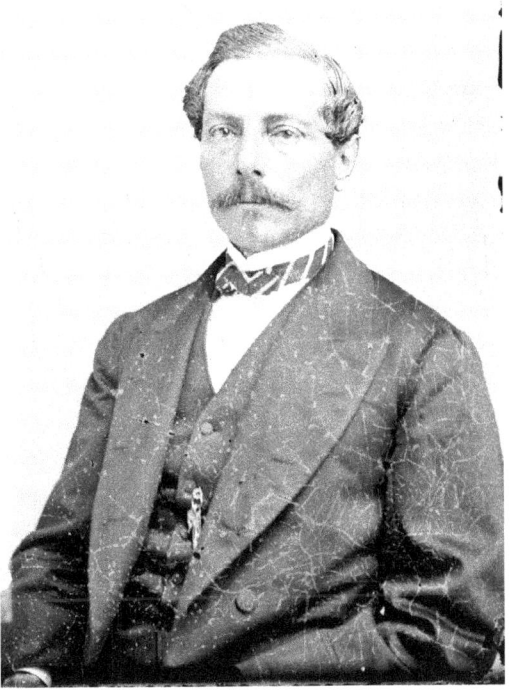

General Pierre Gustave Toutant-Beauregard was the Commanding General of the Confederate Army and a friend of Dr. Tebault's from New Orleans. He accused Union General Halleck of a deliberate attempt by the Union forces to infect his men at Fort Pillow with smallpox. Library of Congress, Prints & Photographs Division, Civil War Photographs, cwpb-05517.

Mississippi a few miles south of Fort Pillow. Lacking any vaccination matter, he recalled from his own observations while at Charity Hospital in New Orleans that it was seemingly impossible to successfully vaccinate a young child exclusively fed with milk. As there happened to be a cow on Hatchie Island, he conceived the dangerous idea of diluting smallpox lymph taken from one of the sick men with milk and using this "modified" vaccine to inoculate. In addition to the garrison at Fort Pillow, he used the weakened virus on himself. This risky experiment proved quite successful, with the men thus vaccinated exhibiting the typical vaccination response and none catching the dreaded disease. He would later successfully repeat this experiment with milk-weakened smallpox virus while at Ocmulgee Hospital in Macon, Georgia. There had been other such experiments with smallpox inoculation. In the early part of the 19th century a Prussian physician used smallpox lymph to inoculate a cow, and then used the lymph from the cow's lesions to successfully inoculate children. He later described a means of doing the same without the direct involvement of the cow by preserving the smallpox virus for 10 days then adding milk to the weakened virus and using it for inoculations. It is not clear, however, whether Dr. Tebault knew of this earlier work or if he first tried to weaken the smallpox matter before dilution. Regardless, the efforts show the doctor's creativity and resolve to help his patients and the men of the regiment, given the difficult conditions within which he worked.

Dr. Tebault's friend Dr. Joseph Jones later described the modified inoculations as being effective but also expressed concerns regarding the procedure's maintaining the inoculated individual's contagious nature:

> Dr. C.H. Tebault practiced Modified Inoculation or the engrafting of equal parts of cow's milk and variolous matter taken from the pock in the vesicular stage in October 1864 upon some thirty Confederate soldiers in the Ocmulgee Hospital at Macon, Georgia. Dr. Tebault states that he engrafted one soldier after another with the modified lymph until thirty-odd had swelled the list of my experiments. Of thirty-five persons thus successfully inoculated there only exhibited a few additional pocks in no case more than six in addition to the seat of puncture. Additional pocks are not characteristic of the vaccine disease, but they are characteristic of inoculated small pox.... Inoculation whether performed with pure small pox matter or with a mixture of variolous matter with cream or milk induces a comparatively mild and harmless disease to the individual; but it keeps alive the contagium of small pox, and involves the health and lives of all unprotected persons in contact.[18]

(After the war, Joseph Jones [1833–1896] became one of the renowned experts on infectious diseases in the country. He taught at the University of Louisiana and was appointed the first Surgeon General of the United Confederate Veterans [UCV] until his death in 1896.)

Surgeon General Samuel P. Moore had assigned Dr. Jones to conduct medical studies of the major southern hospitals and military prisons. He previously served as a visiting physician at Charity Hospital during the time that Dr. Tebault was studying there. Dr. Jones would later be elected Surgeon General of the UCV in 1889, and Dr. Tebault would replace him in that position following Jones's death in 1896.[19]

While Dr. Jones's concerns regarding modified inoculations were valid, Dr. Tebault had no other option at the time he first utilized the procedure on Hatchie Island, there being no vaccination matter available. It is also noteworthy that he volunteered to personally care for the former prisoners and first tried the modified inoculation on himself, placing himself in danger of infection. His quick actions in the face of adversity most likely saved many of the soldiers from becoming infected and earned Dr. Tebault their respect and loyalty.

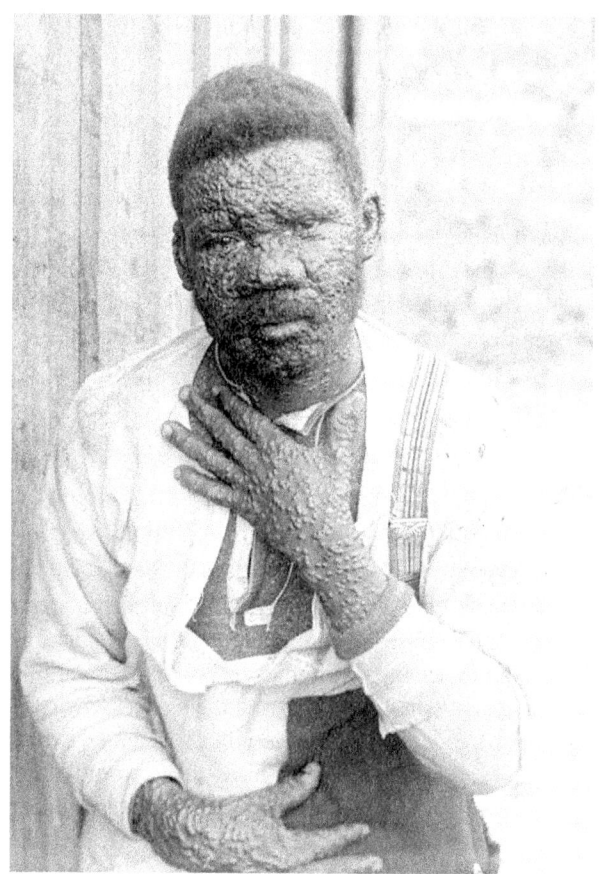

Smallpox, while greatly feared, was largely kept under control during the war with vaccinations and inoculations. Initial symptoms include a skin rash that leads to fluid-filled blisters resulting in deep, pitted scars and disfiguration. Florida, State Board of Health collection Series 46, Administrative Files, 1889–1926; Box 44, folder 6.

Corinth, Mississippi

Meanwhile, General Beauregard had assembled a force of 70,000 in nearby Corinth, Mississippi. The Union army had been slowly advancing on his position, moving only five miles in three weeks. Instead of attacking, they were cautiously entrenching and preparing to lay siege to Corinth. Positioned on the high ground within a thousand yards of the Confederate defenses, Union artillery began shelling the earthworks, supply bases and railroad facilities in the city.

In 1862 Corinth was more a hamlet than a city. Incorporated in 1856, it had a population of only about 1,000. Once the fighting started, the city became an important rallying point for troops and supplies. Albert Sidney Johnston and his army arrived there after the fall of Forts Henry and Donelson in February 1862, bringing with him more than 40,000 soldiers. A significant number of the men were ill or became ill while in Corinth. When General Beauregard arrived following the battle of Shiloh, he added to the city's plight with additional troops, many of whom were suffering from wounds inflicted at Shiloh or from illness. Corinth had essentially become a vast hospital, with most houses sheltering the injured and sick.

On May 28, General Beauregard wrote General Villepigue to inform him that he was withdrawing his army from Corinth away from the river with hopes that the Federals would follow and stretch out their supply lines, giving the Confederates an advantage. "Wishing to take the enemy farther into the interior, where I hope to be able to strike him a severe blow, which cannot be done here, where he is so close to his supplies, I have concluded to withdraw on the 30th [of May] from this place for the present before he can compel me to do so by his superior numbers."[20] General Beauregard had previously considered Corinth to be critical for the defense of the South. "If defeated here, we lose the whole Mississippi Valley and probably our Cause."[21] However, his position at Corinth had become untenable, with the added difficulty of illness caused by a poor water supply that had been fouled by the army's waste. He knew that the longer he stayed at Corinth, the more likely that typhoid fever and dysentery would further devastate his force. And, he now faced prospects of being surrounded and stalled there by a siege. General Beauregard therefore changed his mind about holding the city at all costs and retreated south to a new base of operations at Tupelo, Mississippi. His withdrawal left Fort Pillow vulnerable to being overrun from a flanking land attack, which would then guarantee the fall of Memphis, a situation that Beauregard fully understood: "Whenever you shall be about to abandon the fort you will telegraph the commanding officer at Memphis to burn all the cotton, sugar, &c., in the vicinity of that city.... You will necessarily destroy all Government property—arms, guns, &c.—that you will not be able to carry off with you."[22]

General Villepigue had wanted to abandon Fort Pillow almost a month before finally receiving Beauregard's message, so he wasted little time. On May 28 he ordered the infantry to vacate the fort, which they did in the midst of heavy rains and mud. Edwin Sessel, one of the fort's last defenders, described the evacuation after the infantry had moved out in a letter he wrote to his cousin Kate Cumming. (Kate Cumming [1829–1909] was a Confederate nurse whose diary and writings have become valuable sources of information concerning Confederate nursing and medical care.)

> Abbeville, Miss., August 14, 1862
>
> My Dear Cousin: As you wish to hear the particulars of the evacuation of Fort Pillow, I will give them as near as I can remember. On the 28th of May last the order was issued for the infantry to

move, which they did under trying circumstances, the rain pouring in torrents, and the mud awful. However, the infantry did move, leaving one artillery regiment to cover their retreat. The next afternoon the Yankee fleet made its appearance around the point, and was received by our double-shotted guns in a becoming manner, and it was driven back. That night the artillery regiment left, and we commenced the work of destroying our guns and property. First we set fire to the quartermaster's stores; next, the commissary, and then every "shanty" on the "hill." We blew up all the guns, except two which would not burst. It was a terrific sight—the rain pouring down, the thunder rolling midst the lightning flashes, while the Yankees were pouring a stream of fire, making the sight sublime, though terrible.

After the work of destruction the general, a portion of the staff and officers on horseback, the adjutant-general, myself, and a few others got on board the *Golden Age* at Fulton, and made double-quick time down-stream, the Yankees keeping uncomfortably close behind us. They were stopped at Memphis by our fleet, and we kept on to Vicksburg, where we had to undergo another stream of fire from the Yankees.[23]

Later, on June 11, General Beauregard issued General Order No. 67 praising Villepigue and his men:

The commander of the forces calls the attention of the army to the prolonged defense of Fort Pillow by Brig. Gen. John B. Villepigue and the gallant soldiers under his command. The defense was conducted with skill, vigor, and intrepidity. Week after week he and his resolute comrades in arms in open batteries kept back the enemy's superior land and naval forces, and when the purposes and designs of the campaign had been accomplished, under circumstances of difficulty which also attest the ability of the general, he brought off his command in the face of superior numbers with a success equaled only by the brilliancy of his defense. Such devotion of duty is worthy of appreciation and the approval of the country.[24]

Once Fort Pillow had been abandoned, the Union fleet was able to quickly approach Memphis. Following a desperate naval battle watched from the muddy shoreline by the city's anxious inhabitants, the city surrendered on June 6. The fall of Memphis represented a terrible blow to the South.

A portion of the 21st Louisiana regiment met up with General Beauregard's army at Corinth as it was still withdrawing from that city and followed them to Tupelo. The withdrawal from Corinth was skillfully carried out based largely on a hoax perpetrated by General Beauregard. Some of his men were given three days' rations and ordered to prepare for an attack. As expected, deserters and spies, perhaps some of them fake, sent word to the Federals of an imminent attack. Meanwhile, Confederate forces began evacuating the city by railroad on the night of May 29. When an empty train arrived, it would be greeted by cheering Confederate troops as if reinforcements were coming in. Campfires were kept burning and buglers and drummers played, giving the impression of a significant force and allowing the rest of the men to slip away. When Union patrols cautiously approached the city the next day, they found it empty of Confederate soldiers.[25]

During their brief stay in Corinth, illness had swept through the 21st Louisiana regiment and further reduced its strength. On July 28, General Braxton Bragg ordered the regiment disbanded and the men assigned to other Louisiana units in the army. Dr. Tebault was promoted to surgeon and assigned to the 10th South Carolina Volunteer Infantry.

The 10th South Carolina Volunteer Infantry

Only two days after Dr. Tebault was assigned as surgeon of the 10th South Carolina, the regiment left Tupelo in preparation for campaigning in Kentucky. Federal forces occupied Kentucky, and the Confederates believed that liberating it would swell the ranks of

Confederate volunteers and restore the Confederate government in the state. However, as in western Virginia during 1861, their fanciful hopes of finding sympathetic new recruits in borderline states would go unrealized.

General Braxton Bragg's invasion of Kentucky, however, had other purposes. While the Union was busy dealing with a Confederate threat to Washington and the demoralization following the Second Battle of Bull Run, General Bragg planned to move his forces around those of Major General Don Carlos Buell's by splitting them into two armies, both driving north about 100 miles apart from each other. Their plan was to take back Kentucky and extend the Confederate border to the Ohio River.

On August 25 the regiment crossed the Tennessee River at Harrison's Landing, entering Kentucky at Tompkinsville. They advanced to Glasgow and went to cut the Louisville and Nashville Railroad (L&N) at Proctor's Station. The Confederates wanted to prevent Buell's use of the railroad line without totally destroying it, as they themselves would need it once they liberated Kentucky. After they cut the railroad line they moved towards the Federal garrison at Munfordville, about 30 miles north of Glasgow.[26] On September 18, the 10th moved ahead of the Brigade and met scattered resistance from Federal pickets as they advanced. General Bragg was able to surround the town, and that night the city surrendered without a shot being fired. Just south of Munfordville an important bridge for the L&N traversed the Green River. The bridge had been completed in 1859 just before the outbreak of the war and was an impressive 1,200 feet long and 125 feet tall; it was considered an engineering marvel at the time and was built by local men. Importantly, the bridge allowed the L&N to complete the link between Louisville and Nashville. After Munfordville was taken the destruction of the bridge was ordered, but only the southern end of the bridge was destroyed as many of the men were local to the region and resisted its total destruction. The bridge ultimately survived the war and is still in use today.

Two days later, the 10th South Carolina moved northeast to meet up with the forces of Major General Kirby Smith. Thus began a strenuous march of 50 miles over 55 hours.[27] In spite of the forced march, the two Confederate armies would not unite in time. General Bragg, realizing this and fearing a confrontation with General Buell's larger Union force, turned his army to the east and encamped in Bardstown.

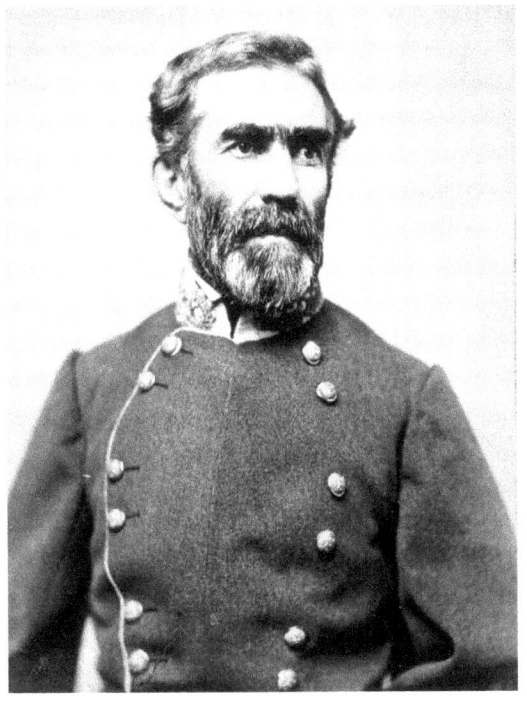

General Bragg's invasion of Kentucky in 1863 was overshadowed by the more newsworthy battles at Gettysburg and Vicksburg. Bragg's failure to retake the state and the critically important Chattanooga railroad began the ultimate deathly spiral for the Confederacy. Library of Congress, Prints & Photographs Division, Civil War Photographs, CPH 3g07984.

"With only three days of provisions, we marched to this place (59 miles) and reached here after some privation and suffering. It is a source of deep regret that this move was necessary as it has enabled Buell to reach Louisville, where a very large force is now concentrated.... We are sadly disappointed at the want of action by our friends in Kentucky. We have so far received no accession to this army.... We have 15,000 stand of arms and no one to use them."[28] General Bragg as well as President Davis had been assured that between 25,000 and 50,000 new recruits would join the Confederate army as it moved into Kentucky. General Bragg was so convinced of that assurance that he carried with him 15,000 rifles for the new recruits.

Finally, at urgings from Washington, General Buell reluctantly moved his forces out of Louisville on October 1 with 80,000 men divided into three corps spread out on separate roads. Due to a summer drought that year, clean water was a scarce commodity, and both sides searched for a clean supply. Portions of both armies would inadvertently run into each other while searching for water at the town of Perryville on October 8. General Bragg led about 16,000 of his soldiers in an attack on approximately 25,000 Federal soldiers, driving them back until the advance was checked by General Phil Sheridan's artillery. While he had defeated a portion of the Union army at Perryville, he realized that tackling the entire Union army the next day might result in a different outcome. General Bragg and the 10th began to retreat south, a march memorable due to its hardship of traveling 168 miles in twelve days. "Often did the hungry Confederate gather into his haversack the dirt where some horse had been fed by the roadside, to sift out, when reaching camp, for the few grains of corn which it contained. Parched corn was for days the staple diet of all, from private to Major-General. We reached Knoxville footsore, scantily clad, hungry, and we luxuriated there on full rations, rest and a plenteous supply of clothing, sent us by the ladies of Carolina."[29]

General Bragg's invasion of Kentucky had not achieved its dream of returning the state to the Confederacy and recruiting soldiers sympathetic to the South, but it had kept Federal forces from reinforcing George McClellan as Robert E. Lee's men threatened Washington. Forty thousand Southern troops had kept many more Union troops busy for almost two months.[30] General Bragg's refusal to fight and his retreat from Kentucky was matched by Buell's unwillingness to challenge the Confederates as they retreated. The capabilities of both men were being questioned at home. Following a visit to President Davis in Richmond, Bragg returned to Tennessee feeling vindicated, with Davis's support. He now prepared to occupy middle Tennessee and await the Federals and chose Murfreesboro as his base.

Major General Ulysses S. Grant now prepared to move deep into the Confederacy and take Vicksburg, opening the Mississippi River to the north and splitting the Confederacy in two. He reorganized his army as the newly formed Department of Tennessee and convinced General-in-Chief Henry Halleck to replace Don Carlos Buell with William Rosecrans to head up the newly formed Army of the Cumberland. In early November, General Grant moved his forces south, east of the Mississippi, to prepare for his assault on the fortress at Vicksburg.

After recuperating in Knoxville, the 10th moved first south by the Nashville and Chattanooga Railroad rail, which twisted tortuously through the Cumberland Mountains and left them off at Stevenson, Alabama, about 50 miles southwest of Chattanooga. From there they marched about 60 miles north on foot to Tullahoma, a vital link along the Nashville and Chattanooga Railroad. Following a brief stay there, the regiment finally moved 40 miles towards Murfreesboro. There the regiment was ordered to go into winter quarters, General Bragg being generally unconcerned about a winter offensive from the Federals.

While in Knoxville, Dr. Tebault came down with a debilitating case of dysentery and requested a 30-day sick leave.

Camp near Knoxville, Tenn.
October 28, 1862

Lt. Col. Prestley, Comdr 10th SC
Dear Sir,

I beg leave to ask at your hands a leave of absence of thirty days in order to recruit my health, considerably reduced by means of an obstinate & violent attack of Dysentery. I have given the disease a fair opportunity to get well without having to solicit a leave of absence, but finding work out of the question, I have with great reluctance been constrained to resort to the above.

Very respectfully, CH Tebault, Act Surg 10th SCV.[31]

Camp Near Knoxville, Tenn.
Headqrts, Med Depart Brigade
Oct. 29th, 1862

Acting Surgeon CH Tebault of the 10th S. Car. Vols, having applied to me for a certificate in which to submit an application for leave of absence, I do hereby certify that I have carefully examined the officer and find that he is suffering from acute dysentery which is intractable & not amenable to treatments in camp & that in consequence thereof he is in my opinion unfit for duty. I further declare my belief that he will not be able to resume his duties in a less period [of] time (30) thirty days. I will therefore recommend that said leave of absence be granted.

W. H. Hawkins, Sr. Surg 4th Brigade.

(Surgeon William H. Hawkins was originally surgeon of the 19th South Carolina Volunteers, which later consolidated with the 10th South Carolina.)

Dr. Tebault was granted the leave and was sent to the Division Hospital in Cleveland, about 80 miles southeast of Knoxville. Dysentery and diarrhea were common ailments during the war for both sides. The lack of camp sanitation, especially during the early part of the Civil War, encouraged the spread of diseases. Diarrhea was commonplace, with about 2.5 million cases in both armies.[32] Loose stools were a constant complaint among soldiers, and the affliction was attributed to the eating of unripe fruit and uncooked vegetables. The poor quality of the diet that frequently included spoiled meat must have contributed significantly to the problem. *Gunn's New Domestic Physician* was published in 1858 and definitively stated that diarrhea was caused by "the action of the summer heat upon the system. This disease prevails most in the season when fruit and vegetables of all kinds are most abundant. Green Corn, Beans or Cucumbers, and other garden vegetables are a prolific cause of it."[33] Emetics such as Ipecacuanha were given to induce vomiting and removal of the offending contents. "Cold water may be drank, but not in too great a quantity, or it will increase the disease."[34] Such treatments were almost certain to cause further dehydration that would lead to additional complications. Opiates were frequently given as well, which would have been marginally effective in calming the actions of the bowels.

Civil War surgeons often used the terms "diarrhea" and "dysentery" to mean the same thing, although the term "dysentery" was usually used when bloody stools were present. Remarkably, the disease was not often fatal although it could reduce the number of men well enough in a regiment to enter a battle. Victims of the disease had to quickly answer the urgent call of nature wherever they were, and there was an unwritten rule honored by both Confederate and Federal troops not to shoot a man when he was unlucky enough to be in such a compromised position.[35]

The Confederate forces found Murfreesboro to be a charming and welcoming place to winter. A combination of unusually warm and clear weather along with General Rosecrans's unwillingness to assault Murfreesboro in early December allowed the soldiers to enjoy themselves.[36] "Christmas in camp—our first since leaving home—was a merry day. All ranks were leveled, and every one joined in its sports. The country was ransacked for our Christmas dinners—dinners served with the best sauce, a good appetite. The condition of the Regiment was splendid. We had received new clothes and full rations, and the health of the command was fine. On 10th December the sick list was only 15."[37]

In Washington, Lincoln sought a victory with which to end 1862 and dissuade the English and French from recognizing the Confederacy. General Ambrose Burnside's bloody defeat at Fredericksburg and the frustration of Grant and Sherman to take Vicksburg left Washington looking towards Tennessee. Rosecrans, however, was slow to move.

WAR DEPARTMENT
Washington, December 4, 1862

Major-General Rosecrans, Nashville, Tenn.:

The President is very impatient at your long stay in Nashville, the favorable season for your campaign will soon be over. You give Bragg time to supply himself by plundering the very country your army should have occupied. From all information received here, it is believed that he is carrying large quantities of stores into Alabama, and preparing to fall back partly on Chattanooga and partly on Columbus, Miss. Twice I have been asked to designate someone else to command your army. If you remain one more week at Nashville, I cannot prevent your removal. As I wrote you when you took the command, the Government demands action, and if you cannot respond to that demand someone else will be tried.

H.W. HALLECK, General-in-Chief[38]

The threats from Washington finally had an effect, and General Rosecrans reluctantly agreed to move. As Christmas drew to a close, his Federal units were approaching Murfreesboro from the direction of Nashville in the north.

The second battle of Murfreesboro, also known as the Battle of Stones River, opened just before daybreak on December 31, with each army planning on attacking their opponent's right flank. General Bragg struck first, successfully overrunning the Union right. General Sheridan had his men located in the right of center of the line and was able to repulse the attack, preventing a collapse of the Federal line, which backed up to the Nashville Turnpike. Repeated Confederate attacks were repulsed from this concentrated line. The fighting resumed on January 2 with General Bragg assaulting the now well-fortified Union line located to the east of Stones River. Repulsed once again with heavy losses due to Union artillery, the 10th South Carolina advanced towards two of the batteries, which they took at great cost, losing 118 killed and wounded. Bragg finally decided to withdraw his army to Tullahoma on January 3, having learned of Federal reinforcements arriving. The battle took a heavy toll, with almost 13,000 Federal casualties and 12,000 Confederates. As a total of only 76,000 men were engaged, the battle had the highest percentage of killed and wounded of any Civil War battle. While inconclusive, Rosecrans claimed victory as the Confederates had withdrawn from the field. The battle thus boosted morale in the North. President Lincoln telegrammed Rosecrans for his hard-won victory: "God bless you and all with you! Please tender to all, and accept for yourself, the nation's gratitude for your and their skill, endurance, and dauntless courage."[39]

Exhausted from the fighting and exposure to the weather that had turned cold and damp, the regiment retreated to winter quarters in Tullahoma near Shelbyville.[40] For the next six months while General Bragg was in Tullahoma, General Rosecrans was encamped in Murfreesboro, resupplying his army. There would be several cavalry skirmishes as both sides tested the other, but General Rosecrans made no effort to move his men against Bragg. Washington made numerous entreatments to Rosecrans to leave Murfreesboro. Henry Halleck first politely tried to push Rosecrans:

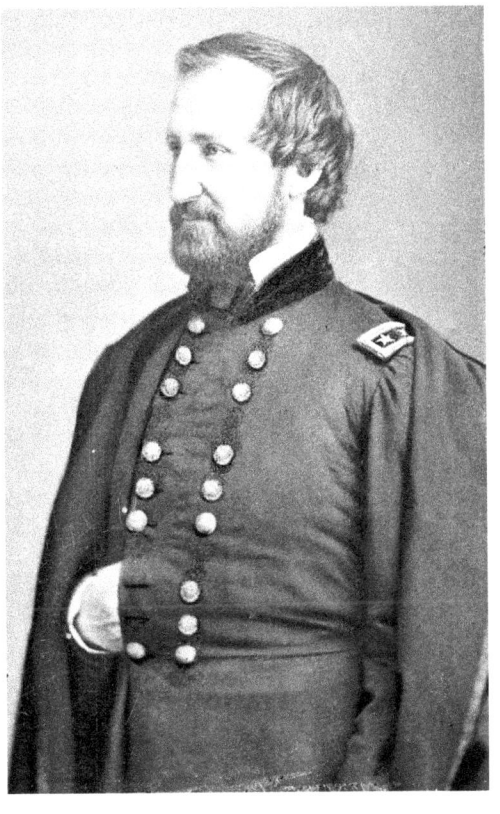

WAR DEPARTMENT
Washington, June 12, 1863

Major-General Rosecrans, Murfreesboro, Tenn.
GENERAL:

... If you say that you are not prepared to fight Bragg, I shall not order you to do so, for the responsibility of fighting or refusing to fight at a particular time or place must rest upon the general in immediate command.... If you do not deem it prudent to risk a general battle with Bragg, why can you not harass him, or make such demonstrations as to prevent his sending more reinforcements to Johnston. I do not write this in a spirit of fault-finding, but to assure you that the prolonged inactivity of so large an army in the field is causing much complaint and dissatisfaction, not only in Washington but throughout the country.

H.W. Halleck, General-in-Chief.[41]

General Rosecrans's gruff and argumentative style earned him General Grant's and Secretary of War Stanton's animosity and distrust. The importance of his success in Kentucky against General Bragg was not fully recognized at the time due to the concurrent Battle of Gettysburg and the fall of Vicksburg. Library of Congress, Prints & Photographs Division, Civil War Photographs, LC-BH82-4455.

Washington was concerned that Bragg was reinforcing Johnston against Grant who was besieging Vicksburg. Halleck earlier had suggested that if Rosecrans was not going to attack, some of his men should be moved south to reinforce Grant. Later, a still-frustrated Halleck would again implore Rosecrans to act:

WAR DEPARTMENT
Washington, June 11, 1863—3 PM

Major-General ROSECRANS

I deem it my duty to repeat to you the great dissatisfaction that is felt here at your inactivity. There seems no doubt that a part of Bragg's force has gone to Johnston.

H.W. Halleck, General-in-Chief.[42]

A few days later, Halleck again telegrammed General Rosecrans:

WAR DEPARTMENT
Washington, June 16, 1863—2 PM

Is it your intention to make an immediate movement forward? A definite answer, yes or no, is required.

H.W. HALLECK, General-in-Chief.[43]

Rosecrans finally responded four and a half hours later with a terse reply:

> MURFREESBORO, TENN
> June 16, 1863—6:30 PM
>
> Maj. General H.W. HALLECK, General-in-Chief:
>
> In reply to your inquiry, if immediate means tonight or tomorrow, no. If it means as soon as all things are ready, say five days, yes.
>
> W.S. ROSECRANS, Major-General.[44]

Finally, eight days later, Rosecrans moved. His plan was to divert Bragg's attention to his front by attacking the strongly fortified town of Shelbyville while Rosecrans would attack Bragg's right flank and rear with his main force. General Bragg continued to wait at his Tullahoma headquarters. However, his staff had little faith in General Bragg's ability, and General Leonidas Polk recommended a retreat, to which Bragg concurred, leading his men during the night of June 30. Bragg appeared to be broken by a combination of Rosecrans's advance and his uncooperative generals, and he additionally suffered from painful boils that made riding his horse almost impossible. The Confederates retreated to Chattanooga, finally coming to a rest at Lookout Mountain on July 7.

The Tullahoma Campaign of 1863 did not get much attention due to the Battle of Gettysburg and the simultaneous fall of Vicksburg, which were considered to be more newsworthy events. The results of Rosecrans's strategy, while painfully slow in unrolling, were at least as important as the Battle of Gettysburg and siege of Vicksburg. The loss of men, agricultural provisions, and the critically important Chattanooga rail center commenced the ultimate deathly spiral for the Confederacy.

On August 24, 1863, while resting in the vicinity of Lookout Mountain, Dr. Tebault received orders to report to Dr. Hill at Quintard Hospital in Griffin, Georgia, to serve there as assistant surgeon:

> Office Surgeon in chg. Hospitals
>
> Cleveland, Tenn, July 16th, 1863
>
> Sir
>
> You are hereby ordered to report for duty to asst. Surgeon S.V.D. Hill in charge of Quintard Hospital
>
> Very Respectfully, Your Obt. Svt.,
> Wm. Cha. Nichols, Surg in charge
> of Hospitals, Cleveland, Tenn.[45]

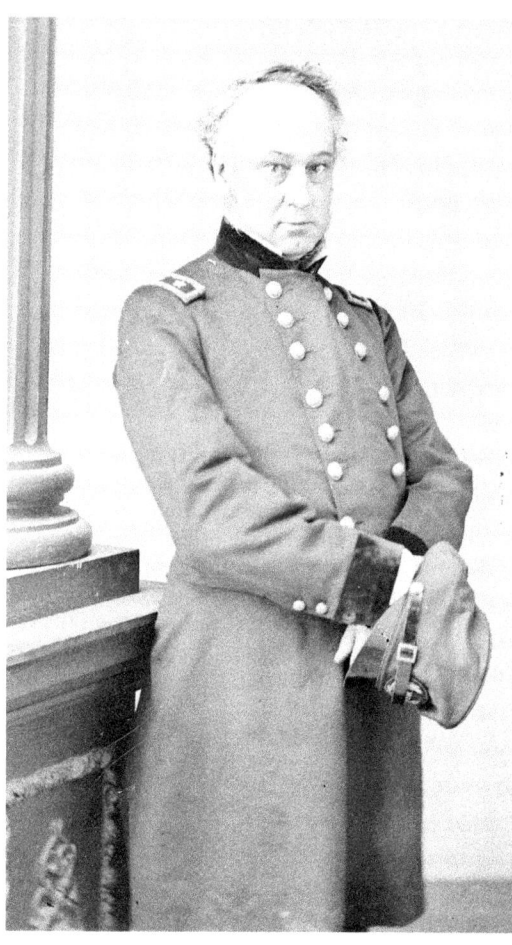

In 1862 Halleck was appointed General-in-Chief of all the Union forces. He was known as an expert in logistics and military strategy, although President Lincoln became frustrated by his cautious manner and inability to get his Generals, like Rosencrans, to move more aggressively against Confederate forces. Library of Congress, Prints & Photographs Division, Civil War Photographs, LC-B813-6377A.

(William Charles Nichols was Surgeon in Charge of the Hospital at Cleveland, Tennessee. Later he became Assistant Medical-Director of the Army, Department of Tennessee.)

Leaving the regiment was not Dr. Tebault's idea, and his appointment to the hospital service most likely was due to Dr. Samuel Van Dyke Hill, the surgeon in charge of Quintard. Dr. Hill had been in charge of the Division Hospital in Cleveland and may have become familiar with Dr. Tebault during his month-long recuperation from dysentery. The hospital was named after Charles Todd Quintard, the Second Bishop of Tennessee who served as both Chaplain and Surgeon of the Army of Tennessee. Quintard had marched into Kentucky with Bragg's men, helped treat the wounded at Murfreesboro, and was with Bragg's army when they retreated to Lookout Mountain.[46] Dr. Quintard also may have met Dr. Tebault during those campaigns. So, it is probable that Drs. Hill and/or Quintard were responsible for Dr. Tebault's assignment to the general hospital service. Dr. Quintard described in his memoirs a wedding he performed in Griffin in February 1864 in which he remarked that he was "in attendance at the hospitals in Griffin at the time."[47] Thus, had Quintard not known Dr. Tebault before he was assigned to the hospital at Griffin, Quintard certainly would have known him once he was there.

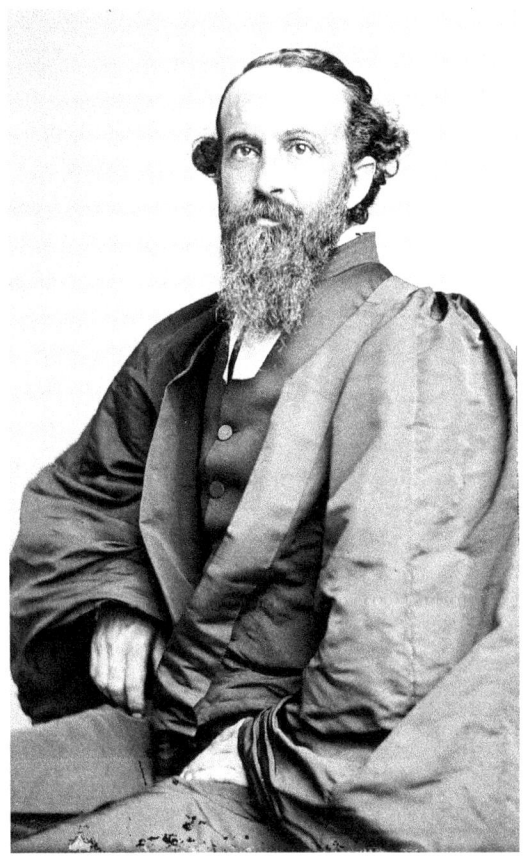

Charles Quintard served as both Chaplain and Surgeon of the Army of Tennessee. The hospital in Griffin, Georgia, was named in his honor. Library of Congress, Prints & Photographs Division, Civil War Photographs, LC-BH82- 5376 A.

Quintard Hospital, Griffin, Georgia

The town of Griffin is located about 50 miles south of Atlanta along the Macon and Western Railroad. Camps Stephens and Milner were strategically located there and were mobilization points for Confederate infantry and cavalry, respectively. Because of the railroad line, trainloads of sick and wounded poured into hospitals, public buildings, the courthouse, stores, colleges and even private homes in Griffin. Susan G. Pope had been a student at Synodical College in Griffin where Quintard Hospital was established. She recollected:

> After the long years of anxiety, it was terrible to see each train that came into Griffin bring dozens of wounded and sick soldiers. Soon the hospitals overflowed, and the Courthouse, public buildings, stores, colleges, and even private homes, were filled with the cots and the patients made as comfortable as possible with the limited means we possessed. Already we had used our linen underwear, sheets and

table linen for bandages, and revealed them into lint for wound dressings. Griffin was not in the track of Sherman's march to the sea, and so escaped the destruction suffered by so many towns, and it was probably for that reason that she had the heavy burden of caring for such large numbers of wounded soldiers. Most of these were brought from a distance, as the nearest fighting that took place occurred in the battles of Jonesboro and Atlanta. I am not sure, but my impression is that many of the wounded were brought from the battlefields of Virginia.[48]

While Quintard Hospital was the largest hospital in the town, a home owned by David Jackson Bailey was also used as a hospital. Bailey was 1st Colonel of the 30th Georgia Infantry. He had been a member of the Georgia Secession Convention in 1861 that passed the Ordinance of Secession. Colonel Bailey also had served throughout the Indian War with the Seminoles and Creeks. He previously had served as the Speaker of the House of Representatives and President of the Senate in the U.S. Congress. Interestingly, Colonel Bailey and Dr. Tebault's grandfather, the Honorable Seaton Grantland, were both in Congress at the same time, one a Whig and the other a Democrat.[49] In 1859 he had commenced work on building his home in Griffin. The large house was not completed until the middle of the war due to supply shortages. Bailey's wife and his two daughters, Sallie Bradford Bailey and Annie Tinsley Bailey, helped with nursing the wounded. The house still stands and is now known as the Bailey-Tebault House.

Samuel Van Dyke Hill had been in charge of the General Hospital at Cleveland, Tennessee, during the time of Tebault's convalescence from dysentery in 1862. Dr. Samuel H. Stout later placed Hill in charge of Quintard Hospital in Griffin, Georgia. The hospital was largely comprised of a collection of tents and sheds adjacent to one large building, which had previously been used as a college for women. One of the college's students later recalled

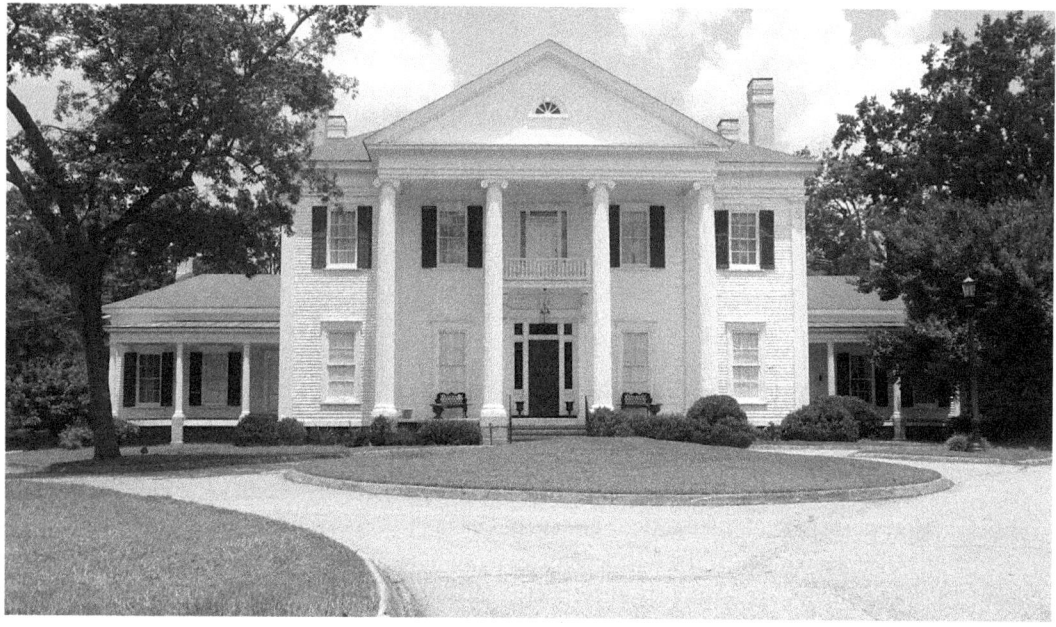

Bailey-Tebault House. David Bailey began construction on his home in 1859. During the war the house, along with every available building in Griffin, was used as a hospital to treat the many wounded who were arriving by rail. In 1866 Dr. Tebault married David Bailey's daughter, Sallie, who later inherited the house. The historic mansion is now the home of the Griffin-Spalding Historical Society (author's collection).

the sadness of being forced out of the school's building to make way for the hospital: "The girls in the Synodical College left the building in order to make room for the wounded. It was a sad procession when the line of weeping girls, laden with book and other school supplies, wended their way from the old Synodical College, where I was a student, to the Presbyterian Church, where, we were told, we would have to end our school year."[50]

Kate Cumming, a nurse visiting the hospital, described the layout of the building: "There [was] one nice, large ward in the upper room. There are many rooms downstairs, one a fine linen room."[51] There were also several smaller buildings used for kitchen, dining bakery, etc. Quintard Hospital had originally been located in Rome, Georgia, north of Atlanta, but was relocated to Griffin as the war around Atlanta moved dangerously closer to Rome.[52]

In the early months of the war, the ablest of surgeons, such as Dr. Tebault, were assigned field service with regiments, leaving the hospitals managed chiefly by inexperienced contract physicians.[53] Experience taught both sides to become better equipped and organized to attend to the extraordinarily large numbers of wounded men following battles. When General Braxton Bragg took command of Johnston's Army of Tennessee, he wisely chose Stout as superintendent of all the general hospitals of the Army. In 1863, Stout became Medical Director, reporting directly to the Surgeon General in Richmond, and was responsible for all the hospitals in the District of Tennessee. Early in 1864, Stout was working from headquarters at Atlanta and continued there more or less until July when he moved to Macon. In October 1864 he moved on to Columbus, Georgia, and apparently stayed there through the end of the war. Stout, however, was on the move a good deal in connection with inspections of hospitals. His contributions to the efficiency and organization of the medical care of the Confederacy are comparable to Jonathan Letterman's contributions in the Union Army. Dr. Stout instituted required examinations for new physicians, weeding out individuals who were incapable of running the hospitals and/or caring for the wounded and sick.

While at Quintard Hospital, the enterprising Dr. Tebault established a separate hospital devoted to the treatment of erysipelas and hospital gangrene, two common diseases that appeared at the time to be related by similar symptoms. The hospital consisted of an encampment of tents, providing isolation of the sick along with plenty of fresh air. Infected cases were sent to Quintard from other hospitals or directly from the field. Erysipelas is a bacterial infection affecting the skin and cutaneous lymphatic system. A rash on the face and legs is most common along with the symptoms of high fever, fatigue, headaches, vomiting, pain and general malaise. During the Civil War, erysipelas was considered to be a contagious, eruptive disease:

> Of the causes which operate in producing erysipelas, this much is known: Erysipelas is often the product of dissecting wounds—of wounds received in skinning diseased cattle, or in skinning the putrefying carcasses of those killed by accident. It is often seen to result, in the form of puerperal peritonitis, from the infection upon the hands of the midwife, as in the historical German cases. It is often associated with injuries and diseases of the bones, especially with caries, a disease remarkable for the persistent fetor of the discharges.... Erysipelas, too, seems to be engendered in over-crowded and ill-ventilated apartments, reeking with foul emanations of the human body; in rooms receiving exhalations from drains and cesspools, especially from the former. It is producible by miasma emanating from the bodies of those having the disease. The bodies of those having erysipelas, in some of the worst epidemics of the disease, have been known to emit a putrid odor.[54]

We now know that erysipelas is caused by a streptococcus bacterium often originating from even minor wounds to the skin where the bacteria, possibly from strep bacteria in one's nasal passages, can cause the infection. Surgical incisions may also have played a

Diagrams showing the Monthly Rates of Prevalence of Small Pox and Erysipelas among the White and the Colored Troops per thousand of strength.

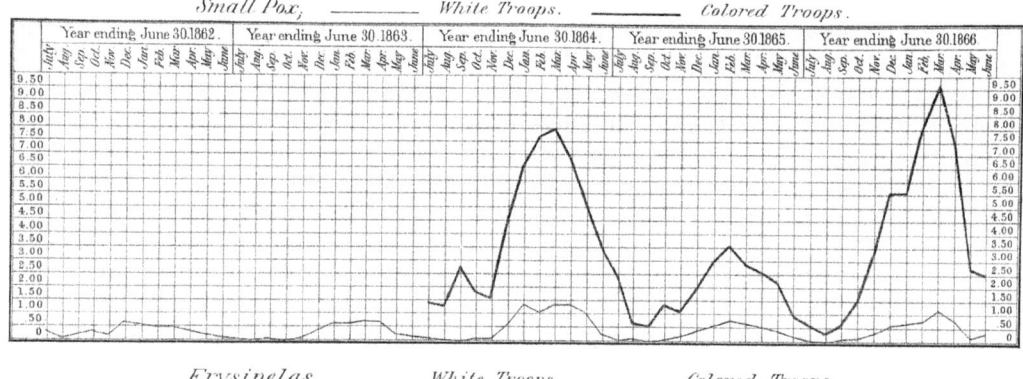

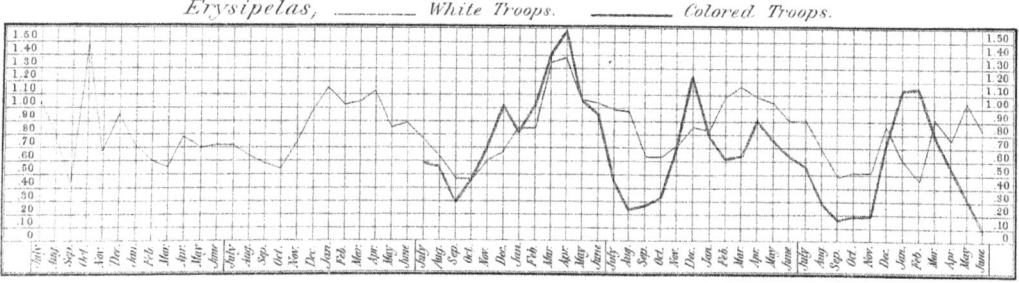

Table 3: Smallpox and erysipelas. Black troops were often not vaccinated, leading to a higher incidence of smallpox than with white troops. Erysipelas, however, affected both equally throughout the war. (Chart taken from Barnes et al., *The Medical and Surgical History of the War of the Rebellion*, part 3, vol. 1, 624.)

role in causing erysipelas as the disease was noted to be a "scourge of the hospital wards rather than the regimental camps."[55] It was thought to be extremely contagious, undoubtedly spread by the dirty hands of the caretakers. It also was common to see erysipelas in a patient already weakened by typhoid fever, measles, or pneumonia, adding to the difficulty in establishing the exact cause of death. While the death rate from erysipelas is unknown, it has been estimated to be as high as 8 percent.[56] The incidence of erysipelas was typically overestimated, as the diagnosis also included cellulitis that extended locally around the infected wounds. Table 3, which is taken from *The Medical and Surgical History of the War of the Rebellion*, shows erysipelas to be a relatively constant problem during the war years, with the summer months showing the lowest incidence, perhaps due to lighter clothing and more frequent bathing. There is little difference in the incidence of erysipelas between white and black soldiers. Smallpox, on the other hand, plagued black soldiers significantly more than whites, most likely due to a lack of or poorer vaccinations amongst the black soldiers.

Dr. Tebault described his treatment of erysipelas: "When erysipelas had proceeded to the formation of pus, free incisions were made for its ready escape and these openings were syringed with properly diluted chlorinated water solutions, properly weakened tincture of iodine solutions, or solutions of tannic acid, once, twice, or thrice daily, according to the severity of the case."[57] Camphorated oil would also be applied topically to provide cooling relief from the pain. Dr. Tebault also used quinine, which was given to relieve the fever. A diet of "eggs, milk, concentrated broths, and stimulants … together with an abundance of pure outdoor, fresh air."[58] For severe pain, he administered gum opium, a name describing the raw opium resin. Unlike morphine, gum opium was not thought to disturb the patient's appetite or stomach.

As with erysipelas, hospital gangrene also appeared to attack and spread along the skin. It was also thought to be contagious as it was noted to spread quickly in overcrowded wards that were poorly ventilated. "Of the causes which produce hospital gangrene, this much is known: hospital gangrene arises spontaneously in wards where the wounded are crowded together—where the wards, are filled with the stench of traumatic profluvia, and receive the air of sewers and cellars. That the spread of gangrene is propagated by the ever produced new gangrenous matter is obvious to the most superficial examination."[59] Today we understand gangrene to be a necrosis of tissue due to a lack of blood flow and an associated immune response. Symptoms include swelling, a color change to the skin from red to brown to black, pus formation and a foul smell, and high fever. If the bacteria get into the bloodstream, septic shock and death typically follow. Hospital gangrene was much feared by recuperating soldiers and had a 45 percent mortality.[60]

Dr. Tebault describes a similar medical treatment for hospital gangrene as he offered for erysipelas:

> The best treatment for hospital gangrene was found to be the same internal medication, nourishment and stimulants mentioned for erysipelas, with fresh outdoor air in abundance.... The local treatment was as follows: In the gangrenous stump, for example, cotton saturated in turpentine short of dripping was pressed into the gangrenous mass, completely plugging it. Over this was bandaged a poultice thus made—pulverized charcoal, ... carrots reduced to a pulp with hot water and flax seed meal when procurable, but generally cornmeal in suitable proportions. These dressings were changed three or four times during the day and night. It was magical to see how soon the rotten mass would melt away, leaving behind a healthy wound.[61]

The active ingredient in Dr. Tebault's poultice was turpentine, a medicine commonly used during the 19th century as a stimulant, diuretic or laxative when taken internally. It was also externally applied to the skin as a rubefacient, producing dilation of capillaries and increased blood flow.

Dr. Tebault would later be asked by Dr. Stanford E. Chaillé to write his thoughts regarding hospital gangrene while he was at Ocmulgee Hospital. Dr. Chaillé was the medical officer in charge of the hospital and had previously met Dr. Tebault when he was at the University of Louisiana in New Orleans.[62] Dr. Chaillé was born on July 9, 1830, in Natchez, Mississippi. Educated in the North, he graduated from Phillips Academy in Andover, Massachusetts, in 1847. Chaillé then received a bachelor's degree in 1851 from Harvard College and later earned his medical degree from the Medical Department of the University of Louisiana in 1853.[63] Before the Civil War, Dr. Chaillé worked as a resident student in the New Orleans Charity Hospital and then served as a resident physician at the United States Marine Hospital and at the Circus Street Infirmary. He taught anatomy at the University of Louisiana from 1858 to 1860, during which time he met the young Dr. Tebault. During the war, he served in the Confederate Army in multiple capacities. He initially enlisted as a Private in the New Orleans Light Horse (1861–1862); then became the acting surgeon general of the state of Louisiana (February–May 1862); surgeon and medical inspector of the Army of Tennessee (May 1862–July 1863); surgeon in charge of Fair Ground No. 2 Hospital in Atlanta, Georgia (1863); and surgeon in charge of Ocmulgee Hospital in Macon, Georgia (January 1864–May 1865), when he was captured and paroled.[64] Dr. Chaillé served as Dean of the Tulane Medical School (1885–1908) and chair of the school's Department of Physiology (1868–1902). He has been referred to as the "father of hygiene and health education," having gained such fame when he led the 1879 U.S. Yellow Fever Commission to Havana, Cuba. His microscopic studies of the blood of yellow fever victims helped identify the *Aedes aegypti* mosquito as the vector causing the dreadful disease.[65] A nationally recognized physician, Dr. Chaillé spent much of his life pushing for numerous sanitary improvements to be made in cities: better sewage and drainage systems, paved streets, clean water supplies, and the control of mosquitoes.

Dr. Chaillé kept meticulous notes on disease statistics and therapies and asked Dr. Tebault to record his experience with hospital gangrene in one of his many notebooks.[66]

> The first case of Gangrene coming under my work prior to the opening of the Special Ward occurred in Griffin, Ga, where I was stationed sometime in September 1863. As far as I am able to judge I would say if anything Hosp Gangrene has rather increased of late. Regarding its severity, I have not discovered any disposition to increase in this respect or the reverse.... Anorexia is minimally complained of by the patient as long as the wound remains unhealthy. Returning appetite is a very favorable omen—it is more it is an infallible evidence that the wound is once more resuming healthy action.... In regard to Hospital Gangrene as a local disease, I have this to say—I have accidentally inoculated myself some thirty times, and in no instance did I experience any constitutional disturbance. I never suffered the disease to take any permanent hold upon me but at once set to work to avoid its farther progress. Many of my nurses took the disease in the same way with like results.... We have in turpentine an agency quite equal to the disease and far less painful in its application. I recommend as the best mode of applying it to mixing our with it a sufficient quantity of charpie to cover the entire diseased tissue, oiling the healthy tissue around the wound. [Charpie is a lint bandage.] The application should be kept up until every vestige of disease has been removed.... To stimulate the border of the wound to healthy action with the topical application of Tinct. Iodine three times a day I found to be an excellent treatment.

His recommendation to apply tincture of iodine to the wound would have undoubtedly helped in controlling the infection, even though germ theory and the actions of antiseptics were unknown concepts at the time. Finally, Dr. Tebault discussed in his notation the "constitutional" or systemic treatment of the disease: "While I do not believe the disease is amenable to constitutional treatment alone, I do think that partially local treatment might be made to bring about the desired results. The most expedient and proper in my mind is to treat the wound both constitutionally and topically. The best constitutional treatment I believe to be easily digested & nutritious aliments such as beef tea, broths, soups etc. and stimulants to excite and keep alive the appetite."

Dr. John C. Gunn described a somewhat similar treatment method in his popular text, *Gunn's Family Physician*:

> The first and principal thing to be done is to arrest the spread of the disease; while at the same time the patient's strength must be upheld, and nature assisted in separating the mortified parts from the living, so as to prevent absorption of the poisonous matter into the system. If the mortification is external, as of a wound, the most powerful antiseptic washes and poultices must be applied. The part should be thoroughly bathed with tincture of Myrrh and Pyroligneous Acid, equal parts, mixed, and a poultice applied composed of Elm bark, Hop yeast, and powdered Charcoal. [Myrrh is the resin of the tree species of the genus *Commiphora* and is a natural antiseptic, currently used in many mouthwashes and liniments. In the 19th century it was thought to be a "deobstruent," having the power to clear or open natural ducts of the fluids and secretions of the body. Pyroligneous acid is also commonly referred to as wood vinegar and is made from wood distillation. Elm bark has been used as a tea for a range of health issues such as coughs, gastritis, and typhoid fever.]
>
> This is an excellent poultice for all cases of gangrene and mortification. It should be removed often, bathing the injured part well each time with the above liquids. A decoction of the Wild Indigo is also a powerful antiseptic, and is good to wash the part with, and also to make a poultice with Elm bark, or

with corn meal. Balsam of Peru may be added to the tincture of Myrrh and Pyroligneous Acid. [Wild indigo is a perennial plant native to North America and was a favorite medicine of indigenous people as a topical treatment for burns and wounds. Balsam of Peru is a tree found growing in South and Central America. Extracts of the wood have been used for treatment of wounds and ulcers as it acts as a natural antiseptic.] It is also recommended to sprinkle Sulphate of Zinc freely on the part previous to applying the poultice. As fast as the mortified flesh becomes loose, it should be removed, and the remedies applied again.[67]

It is interesting to note that Gunn frequently uses the term "antiseptic." While some of the ingredients in his poultices were natural antiseptics as we know them today, Gunn defined the term as meaning: "that which resists or removes putrefaction or mortification."[68]

It is difficult to believe that Dr. Tebault's remedy of turpentine would do much to a gangrenous stump that had become a "rotten mass" as he described, but turpentine does have antiseptic properties. At the 1902 UCV Reunion held in Dallas, Texas, Dr. Tebault further described the treatment of wounds using a tincture of iodine: "The healthy wounds were washed very generally with an infusion of red oak bark, a most valuable treatment. They were often stimulated with a brushing over with the tincture of iodine and were always well nigh hermetically sealed by water dressings on which fresh water constantly dripped except when being dressed."[69]

The doctor's recollection was penned by him in 1902, and the memory of such successes may have become somewhat distorted by time. Some of these 19th-century poultices, however, contained natural antiseptic agents and may have had remarkably good results, especially if the patient was provided with a good diet as part of the therapy. While one can argue the effectiveness of some of these procedures he described on erysipelas and gangrene, one cannot deny that Dr. Tebault exhibited forethought and creativity in establishing a separate hospital focusing on these two diseases, for which there was much unknown. This effort is reminiscent of his work in isolating smallpox patients at Fort Pillow and devising a novel method of inoculation using weakened smallpox virus rather than vaccination with cowpox matter, which was unavailable to him at the time.

Dr. Tebault also noted the value of fresh air, water and sunshine, which undoubtedly had a positive effect on an ailing soldier. He also wrote about the adverse role that he believed oxygen played: "There is a constituent from which the open wound must be carefully guarded from for any length of time as a rule. Oxygen is the element to which I here allude. It is the active principle of the atmosphere and is destructive in all its effects."[70] As an explanation, he went on to discuss the negative effects of oxygen on fruit such as peaches and noted that fruit keeps longer if kept sealed in a container from which the oxygen has been removed.

> An animal dies. The oxygen is on the alert, and the instant the victim expires, and sometimes a little sooner, this agent so anxious to commence, begins by removing that which would soon be an offense to all sensitive nostrils. We accidentally cut our finger and soon the unwelcome oxygen begins at the quivering nerve beneath. The keen throb with which the unexpected hollow in a tooth is revealed to us, announces the entrance of this foe at an unguarded breach. It was the practice of Confederate surgeons and assistant surgeons to hermetically seal up all wounds as soon as practicable, and it was the almost universal adoption of this surgical procedure in all wounded cases that yielded us our splendid results in wound surgery.[71]

To seal a wound from the effects of oxygen, water dressings were frequently used. There was some debate over whether warm or cold water was better, but generally all agreed that a wet dressing promoted healing. The use of cold water had the additional effect of soothing an infected and "hot" injury, with evaporation of the water keeping the dressing cool. "Cold water is the only proper and universal antiphlogistic [anti-inflammatory] that can be applied to wounds."[72] By keeping the wound cool, the water dressing would counteract the heat of inflammation. On the other hand, warm water dressings were observed to encourage suppurations and laudable pus formation. Unfortunately, the use of non-sterile water, frequently obtained from contaminated sources, added to the certainty of wound infections. Some physicians complained that wet dressing led to tissue sloughing. Following the Battle of Gettysburg, the only available treatment for many of the Confederate wounded was exposure of their wounds to the air with a noted positive effect that was somewhat surprising at the time.[73]

A variation of water dressing was the hermetic sealing of wounds espoused by Surgeon John Julian Chisolm during the latter part of the war. Dr. Chisolm was known for publishing the definitive manual for Confederate surgeons in 1861, which he revised in 1862 and 1864.[74] In September 1864 he published an article in the *Confederate States Medical and Surgical Journal* espousing the benefits of hermetically sealing gunshot wounds entitled "Conversion of Gun-Shot Wounds into Incised Wounds as a Means of Speedy Cure."[75] After the war Dr. Chisolm wrote about his advice in 1867 for hermetically sealing gunshot wounds:

> I observed that when a ball struck the outer and upper portion of the thigh, so as to make a log course, and finally become embedded and lost, if the orifice of entrance be so located that the tension of surrounding tissues could close the opening immediately after the passage of the ball, excluding air from the track, the entire passage ... would heal by quick union.... From these observations I inferred that any gun-shot wound placed in a similar condition of exclusion from atmospheric air would heal in the same way.... I adopted a plan for healing all gun-shot wounds by the first intention, viz: by hermetically closing their orifices. At my suggestion, an order was issued to Field Surgeons of the Confederate Army to adopt [the method].... The suggestions were tried and failed. Although they were hermetically sealed, matter would soon accumulate and reopen the cicatrized wound. In other cases the pent up pus produced ... painful abscesses.[76]

Dr. Chisolm's approach was not described until September 1864, late in the war. Thus, Dr. Tebault's recollection about the almost universal adoption of Chisolm's approach would not have made a great impact, even if the technique had been proven sound. Dr. Tebault's theory regarding the negative effects of oxygen on a wound, however, is an interesting one, and again demonstrates his thoughtful, if inaccurate, approach. We now know that the opposite is true; a lack of oxygen can delay healing and increase the likelihood of infection.

During Dr. Tebault's stay in Griffin he met Sallie Bradford Bailey, the strikingly beautiful 20-year-old daughter of David Bailey, most likely because her family home had been turned into a hospital where she helped nurse the wounded and sick. Sallie was an accomplished artist and had studied for two years at the Philadelphia Academy of Fine Arts, where she excelled in painting and sculpture. "Only her marriage prevented her from becoming one of the greatest sculptors of America."[77] After the war, Sallie's artwork was admiringly described: "Some of Mrs. Tebault's work with the brush was exhibited at the World's Fair and at the Atlanta Exposition.... Two notable paintings in her exhibit are panels of a satiny, gold-colored surface, the natural tint of some beautiful ash timber that grew upon her father's place in Georgia. The borders are elaborately carved, and upon the sheen of the center surface of each, birds of different plumage hang as if just placed there by the hunter, so faithfully are the colors of their feathers reproduced."[78] Dr. Tebault and Sallie would marry three years later in 1866.

While they never lived in the Bailey-Tebault house in Griffin, they did frequent the town following the war. In a letter dated September 5, 1867, the Reverend John Jones writes to his sister: "Yesterday I saw Dr. Tebault of New Orleans, who is passing some weeks here with his wife, formerly Miss. Bailey. His last letters from New Orleans are favorable."[79]

As a member of the Daughters of the American Revolution, Sallie would later describe her ancestry sometime in the 1890s as part of the record of the Louisiana State Regent:

> My ancestors on both sides are among the first settlers of Virginia. One of my ancestors was William Bradford, first Governor and for twenty years Governor of Massachusetts. My maternal Grandfather Honorable Seaton Grantland, and my father, David Jackson Bailey, were both members of Congress, and were leading men of Georgia. My mother was Mary Susan Grantland of Georgia, which is my native state. My maternal ancestor Thomas Tinsley was a Colonel in the Revolutionary War, his bachelor brother Samuel Tinsley was a Captain in the cavalry. Thomas Tinsley my great, great grandfather was also a member of the House of Burgesses. My paternal ancestor Robert Bailey joined the Revolutionary Army at the age of eighteen years. I was educated in Baltimore and Philadelphia and graduated with the highest honors of the school, also took a gold medal for painting and sculpturing. My father was a Colonel in the Confederate Army, and my husband Dr. C.H. Tebault was a surgeon in the Confederate Army and is now on the Staff of General Stephen D. Lee, as Surgeon General U.C.V. Dr. Tebault's family Duyckinck was among the first settlers of New York. [Evert Duyckinck settled in New Amsterdam (now New York) in 1638.] I am installed to be a Colonial Dame. [The Colonial Dames of America is an organization of women who are descended from an ancestor who lived in colonial America during the period prior to the revolution and who had been of service to the colonies by holding public office or as a member of the military or militia.] I am a Daughter of 1812, also a Daughter of the Confederacy, and a Daughter of the American Revolution. I have recently been elected for the sixth time as the Louisiana State Regent D.A.R. I have three children, Dr. C. Hamilton Tebault, Jr. who had charge of the Officers Hospital in Santiago, Major Grantland L. Tebault now on our Governor's Staff is a lawyer, and Miss Corrine S. Tebault who two years ago was Chief Sponsor for the South U.C.V.[80]

Ocmulgee Hospital, Macon, Georgia

After the battle of Atlanta in July 1864, Dr. Stout moved south, setting up hospitals away from danger to service the wounded. An important consideration to their location was the availability of rail service to move the injured rapidly and with as little pain as possible. The ambulances and roads at the time caused much suffering from the jolting rides while rail travel was considerably smoother and certainly faster.

Shortly after the fall of Atlanta, Dr. Tebault was ordered to leave Quintard Hospital for duty at the hospital in Albany, Georgia. Albany was located at the southern terminus of the Southwestern Railroad that ran from Americus to Albany and enabled the rapid movement of cotton and supplies.[81] An additional advantage that Albany had was that the Flint River ran through the city providing other means of transportation as well as plenty of fresh water. Dr. Tebault did not stay long in Albany, and only a few months after his arrival he was again ordered to move to Macon, Georgia, about 100 miles to the north towards Atlanta.

"C.H. Tebault is relieved from duty in Albany Ga. On Oct 6 1864 will report without delay to Surgeon S.E. Chaillé for duty in Ocmulgee Hosp."[82]

Ocmulgee Hospital was located on Walnut Street near the banks of the Ocmulgee River. It was one of the largest hospitals in Macon, Georgia, and was established in December 1863 as an appendage of Floyd House Hospital. In January 1864 the name was changed to Ocmulgee.[83] The hospital was housed in four buildings, which in the summer of 1864 cared for 500 patients.

The Confederate medical service was stressed at the outset for medical supplies, which had to either be manufactured in the South largely using less effective substitute plants and materials or purchased from blockade-runners. Blockade-runners were private enterprises not working for the government, so drugs and supplies brought by them were typically auctioned in cities such as New Orleans, Galveston, Mobile, Charleston, Savannah, Pensacola and Wilmington. The gulf cities received much of their supplies from Cuba while Texas was able to take advantage of smugglers carrying goods across the Rio Grande. Interior towns, such as Albany, rarely received any benefit from these supply routes and had to rely on medicines manufactured by local druggists from roots, herbs, barks, and medicinal plants.[84] One medicine not in short supply was whiskey due to the enterprising moonshiners' stills.

Francis Porcher, the surgeon in charge of hospitals in Charleston and an expert on materia medica, published a book on substitute plants found in the South: *Resources of the Southern Fields and Forests, Medical, Economical and Agricultural, being also a Medical Botany of the Southern States, with Practical Information on the Useful Properties of the Trees, Plants and Shrubs*.[85] The book was prepared by the direction of Samuel Stout, the Surgeon General of the Confederate States, and recommends such substitutes as motherwort and American hemlock for opium; wild jalap and Carolina hipps for Ipecac; and dandelion, pleurisy root or butterfly weed for calomel (mercuric chloride). One of the most commonly prescribed and welcome remedies was a tonic and anti-malarial concoction consisting of barks and "medicated whiskey."[86] No doubt the whiskey helped soldiers swallow the tonic. Even beeswax was substituted with berries from low-bush myrtle providing a wax that could be made into candles.[87] The effects of the blockade and the use of indigenous plant remedies may have spared many Confederate soldiers from the effects of the more toxic "standard" medicines, which included poisonous mercury, antimony and lead compounds.

Dr. Tebault reminisced after the war that one of the benefits of the blockade, not recognized at the time, was the absence of surgical sponges.[88] Absorbent sponges were used to absorb blood and fluids, and often a sponge would sit in a bloody basin all day during which it would be used on multiple patients. As real sponges were in short supply, Confederate surgeons were forced to substitute rags, typically made of cotton. Once saturated, such rags would quickly lose their ability to absorb blood unless they were washed. Because blood would quickly clot in them, the most efficient washing method was to throw them into boiling water, thus inadvertently sterilizing the rags.

At the beginning of 1865, Dr. Tebault wrote Sallie's mother, Susan Bailey, a letter while he was in Macon describing the holiday festivities in Macon and the more somber conditions he experienced in Griffin:

Macon Jan. 5th 1865

Mrs. Susan Bailey

Dear Madam

I am in receipt of your very friendly letter and cannot but acknowledge myself as decidedly undeserving of the many kindly sentiments expressed in my favor.

I at once attended to the little business entrusted to me. I was informed at both offices that a paper would be mailed to you by the same mail which bears this.

I have little of interest in the way of news—Macon has been exceedingly gay of late & thus invited to most of the numerous parties have as yet been present at none. I am in receipt of a very interesting letter from Miss Sallie to which I hope to respond at length in a few days. Paid a flying visit to Griffin on New Year's—was away to find Miss Mary quite sick—she is, however, improving at present—Miss Limbuton another lady friend of mine was also confined to the same room. The place to me appears sadly altered—Made a pilgrimage to my old stand—to the feasted mansions of my friends but soon turned my back upon them for the gloom was too terrible for long contemplation.

Here we have presented a vivid picture of the great uncertainty of human institutions. The most magnificent structures of today may in the morrow be buried and lost to sight in the bowls of an Earthquake.

A few days back, I was surrounded by many a cheerful face & friend—Schemes for the winter's enjoyment were numerous and many; in an hour's time all these plans were subverted and grounded into dust, an order, a peremptory command transferred them far away in absence—leaving only me. Kindest regards to all the members of your family & trusting that the papers may reach you in one course & regularly.[89]

Francis Trevelyan Miller in his ten-volume *Photographic History of the Civil War* devoted a volume to *Prisons and Hospitals*. C.H. Tebault is described in that tome as one of four distinguished Confederate surgeons Miller recognized. "The Confederate medical service had to contend with lack of medicines, supplies, and ambulances, but the resourcefulness, energy, and tact of its members rose superior to all obstacles. Dr. Tebault served as a field surgeon with the 21st Louisiana and 10th South Carolina regiments, and afterwards as a hospital surgeon."[90]

During the war, the Confederate Surgeon General's office was located in Richmond and was destroyed by fire in April 1865 as the Confederates abandoned the city. In his first address in 1896, Dr. Tebault reflected on the loss of medical records but remarked that with respect to the Army of Tennessee, Confederate surgeons A.J. Foard and S.H. Stout maintained their own personal records that were duplicates of some of the ones lost in Richmond. Foard, the Medical Director of the Army of Tennessee, kept four books containing the names of the medical staff reporting to and assigned by him during the war, amounting to some 1,248 surgeons.[91] Stout became the Medical Director of the Hospitals of the Department of Tennessee initially acting under Dr. Foard but later in the war reporting to Confederate Surgeon General Moore. During the time Stout was thus engaged, he kept meticulous records of his reports and circulars.

Confederate Hospitals

At the 1902 United Confederate Veterans Reunion, Dr. Tebault described the organization and operation of Confederate hospitals during the meeting of the Association of Medical Officers of the Army and Navy of the Confederacy, which ran concurrently with the Reunion of the United Confederate Veterans. His paper entitled "The Hospitals of the Confederacy" has become one of the seminal works of its time for historians as it describes in some detail the organization and functioning of the Confederate medical service. In it, Dr. Tebault focuses on a number of different issues related to the medical care provided to the sick and wounded, of which the following excerpts have been extracted.[92]

At the opening of the war, much confusion existed regarding the medical service on both sides due to their lack of preparations: "Confusion very largely prevailed at first. The ablest surgeons and assistant surgeons, the most experienced, were in the field, while the hospital service was chiefly under the management and direction of the little experienced contract physicians, not immediately connected with the service. The required examinations that shortly followed as the service became better organized, weeded many of these out, and placed in charge of established medical posts, and in immediate charge of the Confederate hospitals, our very ablest surgeons and assistant surgeons."

Whenever there was advanced notification of an impending battle, the medical corps sprang into action:

On the moment of an expected battle a telegram would be sent by the Medical Director of Hospitals to the hospital post surgeons within easy and rapid communication with the expected battlefield, to forward to the more distant hospital posts all the sick and wounded who could bear transportation, and immediately to telegraph for available supplies for the impending emergency. The able Medical Director in the field was always in instant official communication with the Medical Director of Hospitals. Thus there obtained no loss of time or confusion in knowing where to send the sick and wounded on such instant and momentous occasions, and hospital posts were thus always in readiness to receive and care for our wounded and desperately sick comrades whenever a battle was joined between the contending armies; and our unequalled women, God bless them all, likewise duly notified, were also prepared with the needed delicacies possible to provide with their own dainty and loving hands that our straightened circumstances permitted. When the wounded and sick were received, all who could stand a bath were given one, and those who could not were carefully sponged off, and all were dressed in clean cotton material for the bed and placed upon neat and comfortable bunks.[93]

Dr. Tebault went on to describe the responsibilities of different individuals:

Every hospital had its officer of the day, who was in authority on that day. Each hospital surgeon and assistant surgeon discharged in turn this important office, and concluded his day's inspection with a written report which was strictly examined by the surgeon in charge of the hospital, and then transmitted by him to the surgeon of the hospital post. The surgeon in charge of the hospital had highly responsible duties; he received and disbursed all money under proper vouchers, looked after and cared for all hospital belongings, drugs, instruments, etc., bought all provisions and made regular monthly reports to the surgeon of the post. The surgeon of the post supervised the entire hospitals at the post, received and gave all post orders and transmitted the hospital reports to our vigilant Medical Director of Hospitals. The assistant surgeons were the real active workers among the hospital sick and wounded.... Chickens, eggs, butter, vegetables, etc., were foraged for by convalescent soldiers detailed for this purpose who frequently were out for a week at a time.[94]

The belief in the importance of fresh air to aid in the healing of the sick and wounded contributed to the recovery of many soldiers. Fresh air was a response to the belief at the time that sickening miasmas were the cause of most disease.

In the Confederate Hospitals it was the daily custom when the weather permitted to remove all bedding from the building and expose it to the sun and air. Those too ill to leave their beds were carried out in their bunks and placed in the shade of the hospital, or in the sun if desired, or under the shade of trees. Thus the hospitals were frequently cleaned and scrubbed and thoroughly ventilated and kept neat and sweet. Hospitals frequently conducted vegetable farms by renting land in near reach which was worked by the convalescents; and fresh vegetables thus secured for the sick and wounded. Every day committees of Southern ladies would visit the hospitals, bringing the delicacies wrought by their ever busy hands, and as they passed from bunk to bunk speaking kind, cheering and comforting words to the occupants, and so ministering as loving and Christian and especially only Southern womanhood could.[95]

Smallpox was a much feared disease that never gained a significant foothold in either the North or South due to strict calls for vaccinations and a practice of isolating infected victims. "Smallpox cases were treated in tents properly floored, with due regard to drainage, and for heating when necessary, strictly and inflexibly isolated under wise and well guarded precautions. The surgeons and assistant surgeons assigned to such encampments were restricted to these patients."[96] Physicians at the time knew that proper vaccinations could prevent the disease. Although they were still unsure as to its cause, they understood the highly contagious nature of smallpox and used the isolation of patients and previously vaccinated caregivers as effective measures to control its spread.

Proper nutrition was also understood as critical for convalescing patients, although shortages in the South created difficulties. "The diet was eggs, milk, concentrated broths, and stimulants to meet the requirements of each case. This treatment gave most satisfactory results; together with an abundance of pure outdoor, fresh air. Occasionally for a short time where pain was a factor to be prescribed for, an opiate would be exhibited, say, preferably, gum opium in grain doses every one, two, three, or four hours, or at longer intervals to control this symptom, and given no longer than absolutely required."[97]

Due to the northern blockade, many Confederate surgeons had to make do with whatever they either had or could take from northern supply wagons.

> All medical supplies and instruments, and everything else required by us, were made contraband of war in spite of the immense number of prisoners of war held by us, and whose exchange was persistently refused on the part of the United States government. These hospitals were furnished with from forty-eight to sixty-four bunks with well calculated distances between them. They contained but two doors, a large front and a large rear door, and at the rear end two or more small rooms for the necessary hospital use. The bedding and all other material for equipping these bunks and all other washing and bed material were kept by the hospital stewards in separate rooms disconnected from these wards, and the most rigid rules of cleanliness enforced. The laundry work was performed some distance from the hospitals, and the cooking also was done at a proper interval from the sick and the wounded, and these and all else of importance were daily closely inspected and reported upon as stated, by the medical officer of the day.[98]

The system Dr. Tebault describes was no doubt well intentioned and organized, but his recollections in 1902 may have been enhanced by time and a desire to leave an outstanding legacy of service. The Confederate medical service faced severe shortages and strains, and surgeons, hospital stewards, and nurses undoubtedly made numerous sacrifices to assist the sick and wounded. "The hospitals constructed under the direction of the Confederate Surgeons, and their management of them, stand even at this date unequalled in the matter of ventilation and in the method of caring for the wounded."[99]

In his report at the 1896 meeting of the United Confederate Veterans, Dr. Tebault discussed the effectiveness of the Confederate medical system:

> Every battalion, every company of artillery had its assistant surgeon; every regiment its surgeon and assistant surgeon; and this applies alike to both the infantry and to the cavalry arm. On the staff of every major general, of every lieutenant general and of every general, there was a medical director. At every hospital post was a surgeon of the post, and every hospital had its surgeon and assistant surgeons. The navy was likewise provided with her corps of surgeons and assistant surgeons.
> On the more than two thousand battlefields the Confederate surgeon's duty called him where the battle waxed the hottest, and where the dead and wounded lay the thickest. His mission required him to be calm, self-possessed, and unawed where death's messengers filled the very air he breathed, with no weapon in his hand save his surgical instruments.
> The Confederates had 53,773 killed outright, and 194,026 wounded on the field of battle. More than one-third of the 600,000 Confederates were, therefore, confided to the Confederate surgeons for battle wounds. For the nineteen months—January, 1862, to July, 1863, inclusive—over 1,000,000 cases of wounds and sickness were entered upon the Confederate field reports, and over 400,000 cases of wounded upon the hospital reports. It is estimated that all of the 600,000 Confederates were, on an average, disabled for greater or lesser periods by wounds and sickness about six times during the war. The heroic, untiring, important part thus borne by the skillful Confederate surgeons in maintaining in the field an effective army of unexampled Confederate soldiers must challenge particular attention.[100]

Dr. Tebault was quoting from the memoirs of Joseph Jones, in which he states that between January 1862 and July 1863 the total number of Confederate sick and wounded was 1,057,349 with a mean monthly strength of officers and able bodied men of 160,231.[101]

Most surgeons on both sides of the conflict made numerous sacrifices. In many cases, they worked to heal both their own soldiers as well as their enemies. Surgeons achieved remarkable success, given the lack of sepsis and the trying conditions under which they worked. Of the 174,000 wounds to the extremities reported in the *Medical and Surgical History of the Rebellion*, 17 percent required amputations with 76 percent of those patients surviving.[102]

End of the War

Union Brigadier General James H. Wilson was in charge of an effort to destroy southern manufacturing. In a similar effort to General Sherman's march to the sea, his cavalry unit, known as "Wilson's Raiders," moved through the South destroying railroad and manufacturing facilities. On April 20, 1865, they were just 13 miles from Macon when a flag of truce came from the city to announce the armistice signed by General Joseph E. Johnston and William Tecumseh Sherman in North Carolina. The April 18 armistice called for an end of hostilities with the details of the capitulation to be worked out—the actual surrender occurred six days later on April 26. There being no further resistance, Wilson took possession of Macon. Just before his death in 1911 Dr. Chaillé recalled his capture by Wilson's Raiders and said that he "was treated by General Wilson's medical director with marked consideration and to many favors … and he urged me to continue in charge, on Federal pay, retaining my Confederate inmates, and admitting to separate wards Federal sick and wounded. My feelings were then too bitter to accept his generous offer."[103]

Dr. Tebault, who had been serving with Dr. Chaillé in Macon, must also have felt bitter regarding the surrender and decided to leave Macon shortly afterwards. He was considered to be a paroled prisoner of war and received a Pass on May 2 to enable him to return to New Orleans, which he reached on May 22.[104] Dr. Tebault walked from Macon to Mobile, Alabama, a distance of 350 miles and a journey that must have been extremely arduous. From Mobile he met up with his old friend, General P.G.T. Beauregard. The General had surrendered with General Joseph E. Johnston on April 26, and Beauregard left Greensboro, North Carolina, in a small army wagon train containing provisions such as tobacco, nails, thread and yarn that they were able to trade along the way to Mobile for food.[105] He and Dr. Tebault booked passage from Mobile on a U.S. naval transport bound for New Orleans, arriving in their home city on May 22.[106]

One can only imagine the emotions and bitterness that Dr. Tebault and his comrades were feeling as they slowly journeyed home through a devastated country. His army had surrendered, and all the years of personal sacrifice and blood had been for naught. He was returning home to an economy in ruin with paper money that was now worthless. According to the U.S. Census Bureau, in 1860 47 percent of the total population in Louisiana was made up of black slaves, while Mississippi and South Carolina had more slaves than whites at 55 percent and 57 percent, respectively. These former slaves were not only now free according to the 13th Amendment to the Constitution, they were also full U.S. citizens by the 14th Amendment. Cities like New Orleans were inundated with black refugees seeking food, shelter and jobs. Dr. Tebault was also returning to a state and city ruled by his former enemies. In 1867, Phil Sheridan was appointed in charge of the states of Louisiana and Texas, which made up the 5th Military District during Reconstruction. Even before that time, northern soldiers dressed in blue were seen patrolling the city streets. Such an affront must have been terrible to bear as former Confederates journeyed home to re-start their lives. Twenty-seven-year-old Christopher Tebault would not simply assimilate into the streets of New Orleans, however—he would dedicate the remaining years of his life to teaching, the medical profession, politics, and preserving the medical history of the Confederacy. The end of the war was only the beginning of his illustrious and at times contentious career.

Efforts to identify, rebury and count the dead began almost immediately after the war ended. However, such a task was thwarted by incomplete records from both sides. Men were missing. Hospital and prison records were imperfect. The dead were frequently buried in unmarked graves. With no official notification from the government, widows and families were forced to conjecture about the death of a loved one who never returned home. Lieutenant Thomas Livermore was a New Hampshire native who served in the 5th New Hampshire Infantry among others during the war. He is best remembered as the author of the often-quoted reference, *Numbers and Losses in the Civil War in America 1861–65*.[107] For years Thomas Livermore's estimates have been widely accepted as fact: a total of 618,000 men died during the war, 360,222 from the North and 258,000 from the South. Livermore's data came largely from unit muster rolls and other official sources. Recently, however, David Hacker challenged those longstanding numbers by recalculating them based on an extensive survey of 19th-century census data. Hacker's new estimates are 20 percent higher, with a new assessment of 752,000 total deaths.[108]

3

MEDICAL PRACTICE IN NEW ORLEANS

"It is of vital importance to the inhabitants of Southern cities to weigh well all the facts relating to the origin, causes, and means of prevention of yellow fever."[1]

Following the war, Dr. Tebault served as Professor of Anatomy at the University of Louisiana's Medical College. He also joined the staff at Charity Hospital, becoming Adjunct to the Chair of Obstetrics and Lecturer on the diseases of children.

The Charity Hospital could treat annually 10,000 in-patients—"indoors"—and another 20,000 out-patients—"outdoors." In 1868 students at the Medical College were, for the first time, required to add clinical instruction in Charity Hospital as part of their education. In the early years there were no requirements for enrollment into the college except for the ability to pay for the classes. In 1893 a minimum educational qualification was for the first time required for admission to the University of Louisiana; the minimum qualification was a "second grade teacher's certificate." In the 19th century and the beginning of the 20th century, teachers were certified as third, second or first grade. A First Grade Teaching Certificate was more rigorous than a Third Grade Certificate. In Louisiana, to obtain a Third Grade Certificate, one "must be found competent to teach spelling, reading, penmanship, drawing, arithmetic, English Grammar, geography, the history of the United States, the Constitution of the United States, the Constitution of the State of Louisiana, physiology, and hygiene, with special reference to the effects of stimulants and narcotics upon the human system, and the theory and art of teaching." To obtain a Second Grade Certificate, "the applicant must be found competent to teach all the foregoing branches, and also grammatical analysis, physical geography and elementary algebra." Finally, an applicant for a First Grade Certificate "must be found competent to teach all branches required for a third grade and second grade certificate, and also higher algebra, natural philosophy and geometry...."[2] So a medical student applying to the Medical School had to at least have the educational fundamentals of the Second Grade.

In 1898 Charity Hospital treated 7,734 admissions (4,716 white, 3,018 black), of whom 6,599 patients were discharged and 1,117 patients died. In its out-patient (outdoors) clinic, the hospital treated 20,635 patients and gave 70,879 consultations.[3] The Lying-In Department recorded that year a record number of births (276) with a death rate of 13.4 percent, a rate that would be considered staggering by today's standards. Table 4 shows hospital admissions and deaths recorded from 1832 through 1898. The years 1850–1852 saw peak admissions of over 18,000 annually to the hospital. Much of this rise in admissions can be related to epidemics of typhus, which became endemic from 1847 through 1853.[4] Large number of immigrants infested with Rickettsia-infected body lice were entering the city during the period. In addition to typhus fever, there were constant cases of cholera, small-

3. Medical Practice in New Orleans

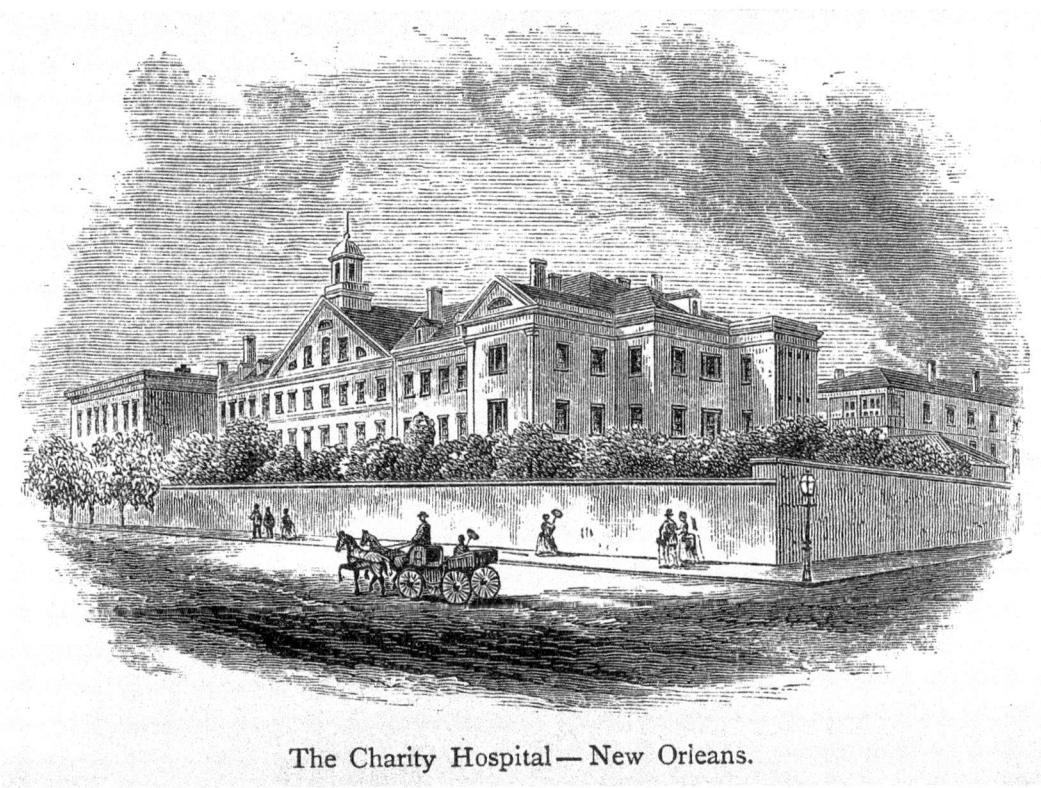

The Charity Hospital — New Orleans.

Charity Hospital was founded in 1736 for the treatment of the indigent. The hospital later was administered by the Sisters of Charity, during which time it became affiliated with the Medical College of the University of Louisiana. Charity Hospital, New Orleans, Louisiana. Wood engraving. The Wellcome Collection.

pox, and the much-feared yellow fever. It is estimated that 40,000 residents of New Orleans were stricken with yellow fever in 1853, or about 27 percent of the population, and more than 8,000 died. "New Orleans streets were deserted; stores were closed; people remaining in the city, huddled in their houses, making pitiful attempts to fight off the disease. It was a city of the dead."[5]

Yellow fever was a constant problem in New Orleans, with most years recording at least a few deaths from the disease. Table 5 shows years when there were major yellow fever epidemics. For each of the seven years shown in the table the epidemic claimed more than a thousand lives. As many of its victims succumbed at home, the death toll from yellow fever was much larger than that seen in the hospital's records, which only includes the city. As previously mentioned, the 1853 epidemic infected an estimated 40,000 residents of New Orleans. The 1878 outbreak spread up river from the city and infected over 100,000 people with 20,000 deaths.

Some of the yellow fever outbreaks in New Orleans were so virulent that student enrollments at the Medical College were reduced. "Although no medical student has ever died of yellow fever during a collegiate session, nonetheless this disease has most unfavorably influenced the number of students attending. The great epidemic of 1867 was followed by a decrease of 28 percent, due chiefly, if not wholly, to this cause."[6]

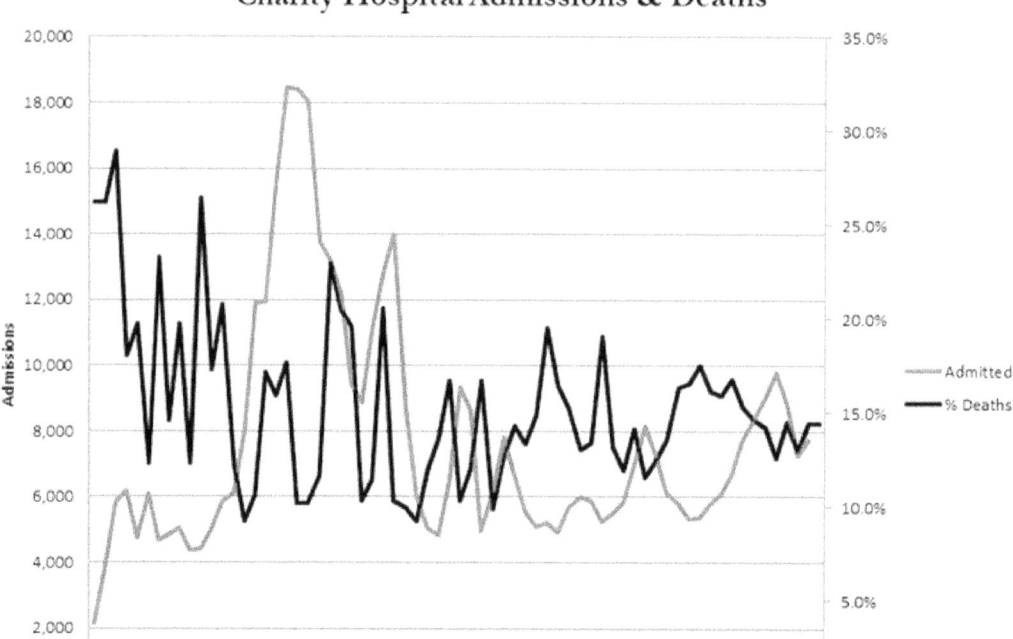

Table 4: Hospital admissions largely corresponded to the outbreak of diseases endemic to New Orleans, including yellow fever, cholera and typhus. Major yellow fever epidemics hit the city in 1853 and 1858, as can be seen in the admissions for that year. The death rate of admitted patients dropped from a high of 29 percent in 1833 to about 15 percent. Data extracted from Augustine, *History of Yellow Fever*.

The Civil War and its consequences also greatly influenced the attendance of students. From 1834 to 1859 the number of students enrolled at the Medical College increased from 11 to 276 by normal growth. In 1861, the number increased rather dramatically to 404; this was largely due to an influx of students who had been attending medical schools in the North. Many southern students left northern schools and returned to the South as their home states voted to secede. April 1862 saw the last classes as many students and teachers enlisted in the Confederate Army and Navy.

Medical equipment was frequently lacking from medical schools in the early years; Harvard University's medical school purchased its first stethoscope in 1868, 30 years after its invention. Even so, physicians during the Civil War became quite adept at auscultation and percussion to listen to abnormalities of the chest. In his book on civil war medicine, Dr. Alfred Bollet suggests that the detailed physical examinations of hearts and lungs noted in the *Medical and Surgical History* could have only been made with the use of a stethoscope.[7] While medical schools also did not own any microscopes, the microscopic analysis of diseased tissues had developed significantly before 1861. Oliver Wendell Holmes used his own microscope to teach students at Harvard starting in the 1840s. Harvard purchased its first teaching microscope in 1869.[8]

Table 5: Major Epidemics of Yellow Fever in New Orleans

Year	Total Yellow Fever Deaths	Charity Hospital Deaths
1847	2,306	2,037
1853	7,849	3,164
1854	2,425	2,702
1855	2,670	2,391
1858	4,845	2,290
1867	3,107	1,438
1878	4,046	1,120
Total	27,248	15,142

The medical thermometer was another new innovation not generally used during the war. Glass thermometers were delicate to carry into the field, and temperatures were measured from the patient's armpit, which would have required a significant amount of time. Thermometers were, however, sometimes used in hospitals. Confederate surgeon Joseph Jones described his experiences with traumatic tetanus while at the Confederate General Hospital in Augusta, Georgia, during the early part of the war. The first case he describes is that of a Confederate soldier named Gilstrap who received a bullet wound to his arm on June 16, 1862. "The wound suppurated freely, and appeared to be doing well, until July 6th, when the suppuration was sensibly diminished, and the patient complained of spasmodic twitching's and painful sensations in the muscles of the wounded arm.... July 8th, 12 o'clock M—Says that he feels a little better; just now the spasms do not appear to be so violent; pulse 82, soft and full; respiration quiet and regular between paroxysms; disturbed and almost entirely arrested during the spasms. Temperature of hand, 37.6° C. (99.2° F); temperature of axilla, 37.9° C. (100.2° F)."[9] From Dr. Jones's descriptions, it is apparent that not only was he using a thermometer, but he also was using auscultation, most likely with a stethoscope.

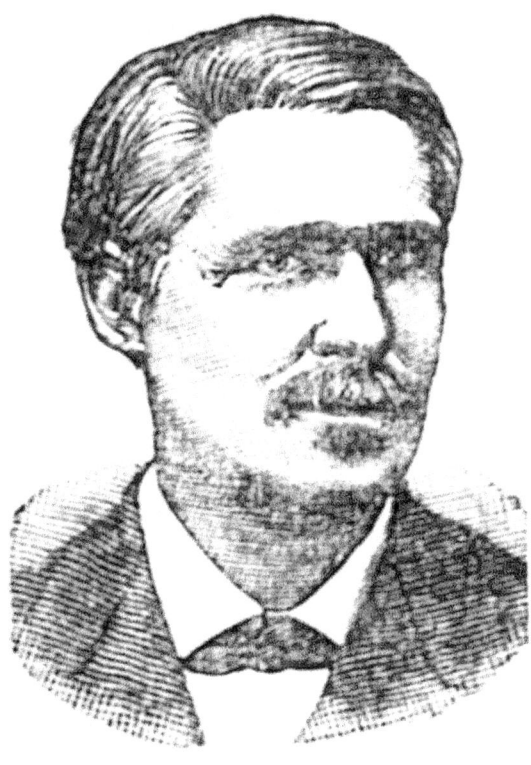

Dr. C.H. Tebault, 1887. In 1887 the *Times-Picayune* published a biography of Dr. Tebault and his family. The article was entitled: "Physician, Soldier and Public-Spirited Citizen." December 25, 1887, 16.

Upon reopening the university following the war, the university fell on hard times due to the economic depression in the South during the Reconstruction period. Paul Tulane (1801–1887), a prosperous businessman who made his fortune in dry goods, clothing and real estate, was a local philanthropist who donated large tracts of land in support of education, leading to the creation of the Tulane Education Fund (TEF). The Fund's board decided to support the University of Louisiana rather than try to create a new school. As a result of the TEF's efforts, the state legislature transferred control of the university to the TEF in 1884, creating Tulane University as a private school—one of the few state schools to have become privatized. There perhaps was a sinister reason for the legislature's actions, however. The 1868 Louisiana Constitutional Convention had desegregated public schools, upsetting many southern whites who were indignant over the idea of their children attending an integrated school. Therefore, the privatization of the university was a solution to that dilemma.

Many of the university's board members, professors, and administrators were former Confederates, including Drs. Tebault, Stanford E. Chaillé, and Joseph Jones. William P. Johnston, Tulane's first president (1884-1899), was formerly a Colonel in the Confederate Army and a member of Jefferson Davis's staff during the war. His successor, William O. Rogers, had also been a Confederate officer. The legacy of segregation at the university was thus difficult to change, and Tulane would remain a segregated school until 1961.[10]

The Scourge of Yellow Jack

Yellow fever was a truly devastating and frightful disease, and today it is difficult to imagine the sheer terror that outbreaks of "yellow jack" had on the population of the cities and states where it frequented. The disease began with a high fever and accompanying headaches, nausea and chills. The infection attacked one's internal organs, causing the victim's skin and eyes to turn yellow as their liver failed. Bleeding would then commence from the eyes, nose and mouth, and one of the last symptoms before death was uncontrolled vomiting—black vomit, resulting from partially digested blood in the stomach. Watching a victim die of yellow fever must have been horrendous. The date of the first cases of yellow fever in the United States is difficult to ascertain due to the paucity of records in the 18th and early 19th centuries and the difficulties in making accurate clinical diagnoses. The first outbreak that was officially recognized occurred in Philadelphia in 1793, most likely brought to the city from the West Indies or Africa.[11] That epidemic occurred between the warm months of August and November and took more than 5,000 lives.[12]

Yellow fever was greatly feared as its cause and spread was not understood in the 19th century. During the 19th century, there were two opposing theories on the spread of yellow fever. Proponents of the first theory believed that yellow fever was highly contagious and could spread easily from person to person. Cities therefore quarantined those suffering from the disease in order to prevent its spread. Advocates of the contagion theory likened the disease to smallpox, cholera, and the plague—diseases thought at the time to be highly contagious.[13] Ships arriving in many southern cities during the "dangerous months" of late summer and early autumn were automatically quarantined, as it was believed that sailors as well as cargo might be carrying the disease even if no one onboard was symptomatic.

A second theory supported the idea that yellow fever was not, in fact, contagious but caused by unsanitary conditions, stagnant waters, and the resulting miasmas. Dr. Benjamin Rush (1746-1813) was an advocate of this theory. Dr. Rush was one of the most prominent surgeons in the United States in the early 19th century. He believed that quarantine laws did nothing but cause tremendous grief and economic loss. "Thousands of lives have been sacrificed, by the faith in their efficacy, which has led to the neglect of domestic cleanliness."[14] Dr. Rush, one of the signers of the Declaration of Independence, was also a champion of the so-called *heroic medicine* that was widely followed before the Civil War—i.e., bleeding, purging and vomiting. Insects were not known at the time as possible vectors for disease, but Rush had observed that yellow fever disappeared upon the first frost or after a heavy rain. He also noted that "unwholesome exhalations" accompanied yellow fever outbreaks, and while in New York during an outbreak of the disease in 1780, he keenly observed that "muschetoes were uncommonly numerous during the autumn."[15] Dr. Rush further observed that clearing an area of trees created an unhealthy situation; such clearings usually had numerous pools of stagnant water where tree stumps had been excavated. On the other hand, cultivating the land ridded it of filth and pooled water and was noted to stop or slow the disease.[16] We now can relate all of Dr. Rush's observations to conditions ideal for mosquito infestations, but no one at the time thought that the pesky insects could cause disease.

Dr. Tebault was on the side of Dr. Rush. He noted that naval vessels, in particular, appeared to carry the disease but that holding the sailors and others on board in quarantine failed to stop the disease from spreading to the nearby city. "Yellow fever, the most dreaded scourge of New Orleans, was unequivocally generated in a large number of filthy and unventilated gunboats and other naval vessels lying idly at anchor within a mile from the densest portions of the city, [and] by fomites or some other material agency the infection of yellow fever was communicated to the guard and to certain other persons who were exposed in a narrow district at the Naval Hospital landing in Erato Street and near New Levee and Tchoupitoulas streets." (A fomite is a non-living object capable of carrying infectious organisms. Examples of fomites include clothing, bowls, buckets, shovels, etc.) "[The] infected vessels ... discharged no cargoes [and] were under an armed surveillance and discipline and were seemingly incapable from the circumstances of diffusing their own infection except by the clothing and dunnage of the sick when taken ashore."[17]

Dr. Benjamin Rush. A signer of the Declaration of Independence, Benjamin Rush (1746–1813) was an important 18th-century physician and proponent of "heroic medicine" (bleeding, blistering, purging, vomiting). He espoused the theory that yellow fever was caused by miasmas (Library of Congress, Prints & Photographs Division, Civil War Photographs, CPH 3b46235).

Dr. Tebault published a detailed report in 1889 on the drainage system and resulting health problems peculiar to New Orleans.[18] In his report he details what he considered to be the causes of yellow fever:

> The removal of the entire surface drainage of a city by pumping is very exceptional, there being no other instance in this country in which it is necessary. Hence, but few observations on this subject have been made or recorded. The importance of a careful study in this case is therefore apparent.... Rainfalls of six inches are of sufficient frequency to make it necessary to provide for the removal within twenty four hours of such part as is not retained by cisterns, absorbed by the soil, or consumed by vegetation. Assuming the mean or average lift from the interior canals to the level of the lake as three feet, there would be required for the removal of this volume of storm drainage an aggregate of six hundred and seventy four horsepower....
>
> It is of vital importance to the inhabitants of Southern cities to weigh well all the facts relating to the origin, causes, and means of prevention of yellow fever. Only through the accumulation of a large number of well observed and undoubted facts can we reach a correct knowledge of the laws which govern yellow fever and all other diseases.... Let me add that shortly after the occupation of New Orleans by the United States forces the most stringent sanitary requirements were promulgated and an efficient sanitary police established. Following is from Dr. Elisha Harris's report [Elisha Harris (1824–1884) was president of the American Public Health Association and became sanitary superintendent of New York City and served on the U.S. Sanitary Commission. Harris was active in fighting epidemics of yellow fever and an advocate of the contagious nature of the disease.]:
>
> "Throughout the entire period, upwards of two years, the Provost Marshal, the Military Governor, the Mayor and appointee of the provisional government, together with the Medical Director of the post and certain subordinate health officers, have vigilantly administered the regulations relating to municipal hygiene and cleanliness in New Orleans and its vicinity.... The conditions under which the Crescent City has obtained this remarkable immunity from a doom which her own bitter experience seemed to fasten upon her are now as well understood as were the apparently inexorable causes of her former insalubrity."

There had been a general assumption that people who had become accustomed to the wet climate and humid temperatures of New Orleans had somehow become immune or acclimated to many of its scourges of disease. It was thought (and hoped by southerners) that northern soldiers would not have resistance and would succumb to the disease, as Dr. Tebault noted:

> During all that period [of Federal military control] the accustomed scourgings of yellow fever have been suspended in that city while the dire forebodings and prophecies of the inevitable pestilence that would quickly destroy the Northern soldiery on reaching the Gulf coast remain unrealized.... First, the relentless rigor and precision of a military government precluded the ordinary violations of quarantine regulations while it gave peculiar certainty to the execution of sanitary regulations in the city. Second, the official usages and the armed discipline of the naval fleet in the harbor of New Orleans and upon the river enabled the medical officers to trace to its source every case of yellow fever that occurred in the gunboats. Third, that the climate of the city and of the river districts during the past three years was not perceptibly different from the climate of previous years and the periods of yellow fever epidemics the same evils from imperfect culture and drainage, imperfect levees and extensive crevasses flooding and subsequent evaporation from vast areas of overflowed land continued to recur in the latter as in the former years. In short all the physical conditions that are supposed to promote the prevalence of yellow fever, excepting only such as are immediately controllable by a sanitary police, prevailed continually and abundantly in the delta of the Mississippi during this period of immunity from that dread[ed] disease.[19]

Dr. Tebault continued in his report the notion that yellow fever could be held in check by strict sanitation:

> Such immunity from her accustomed scourgings of yellow fever had not been enjoyed by New Orleans the last half century. Even her wisest hygienists had been generally discredited, and often derided, when they publicly taught, as Fenner, Barton, Simonds, and Bennett Dowler had most faithfully, that

3. Medical Practice in New Orleans

the active and localizing causes of yellow fever and the high death rate in that city were preventable. [Erasmus Darwin Fenner was a visiting physician to Charity Hospital and had published a book in 1854, *History of the Epidemic Yellow Fever at New Orleans*; Edward Hall Barton was Chairman of the Department of Materia Medica and Therapeutics at the Medical College; J.C. Simonds was a noted sanitation expert in New Orleans who tracked the statistics of yellow fever; Bennett Dowler was Editor-in-Chief of the *New Orleans Medical and Surgical Journal* and had published a history of epidemics in New Orleans.]

There was a truthfulness worthy of the medical profession in the words of Dr. Barton, who as President of the New Orleans Sanitary Commission, sitting in grave and scientific consultation upon the terrible visitations of yellow fever, unhesitatingly declared the causes of that pestilence and the city's excessive insalubrity entirely susceptible of cure. But how few persons appreciated the truth of Dr. Barton's words of prophecy when he said that upon the broad foundation of sanitary measures we can erect a monument of public health, and that if a beacon light be erected on its top and kept alive by proper attention, this city will be second to none in this first of earthly blessings.

...It will be shown that for two successive years the threatening pestilence was localized in a fleet of gunboats moored so close to the city's levees that they menaced the streets with death. It will likewise appear that by the exercise of absolute and relentless military authority, an impregnable system of quarantine was maintained, restraining all the exotic causes of yellow fever, and controlling such causes at a distance of nearly seventy miles from the city, and yet that this dreaded scourge originated spontaneously in more than twenty of the gunboats that were moored in the river opposite the city, also that those naval vessels were uniformly filthy, ill ventilated, and overcrowded, that of the more active cleanly and less crowded steamboats, 120 in number, employed in quartermaster's service, no yellow fever occurred, that in all the city not more than three or four cases of yellow fever occurred each year, and that the cause of such immunity from the pestilence of former years was as certainly the direct result of civic cleanliness and the hygienic care of the poor, as its accustomed visitations were the result of neglect of these public duties.

...The Summers of 1862 1863 1864 and 1865 have now passed without any sign of epidemic disease except from paludal malaria being manifested at New Orleans, save only the outbreak of smallpox last Winter. That epidemic was at once controlled by a house to house visitation by a corps of medical inspectors armed with vaccine virus.

Malarial fever and the ordinary diseases of the climate, not dependent upon a medical police, continued to prevail but the diarrheal and infantile maladies were less fatal than in former years.[20]

In his article, Dr. Tebault reasserts his views concerning the transportability and the infectious nature of yellow fever:

With the peculiar and abundant experience of yellow fever in the ports of the North fresh in mind, the history of this malady at New Orleans and in our naval fleet on the Mississippi was investigated, with all the predilections which such experience could justly impart in favor of the theory of the exotic and imported origin of the disease. Well marked and fatal cases of yellow fever occurred in New Orleans in the Autumn of 1863, and in the Autumn of 1864. In the former year, the Charity Hospital received two cases, both of which proved fatal. Both were boat hands from the steamer *J.H. Hancock*, a river tug. In 1864 there were five undoubted and fatal cases of yellow fever terminating in black vomit. The writer conversed with the physicians who attended the patients viz.: Professor Crawcour, Dr. Bennett Dowler, and Dr. Smythe; and Dr. Huard has furnished notes of a case that occurred in the parish prison. [I.L. Crawcour was Professor of the Principles and Practice of Medicine at the Medical College; John Smythe was on the staff of the Presbyterian Hospital of New Orleans as well as the Charity Hospital.] These five cases occurred in persons who resided or daily visited in the vicinity of Erato, Tchoupitoulas, and New Levee streets. They were exposed to known causes of the fever. Other cases may have occurred; if so they have eluded all search.

...Filthiness, crowding, excessive heat and moisture, lack of ventilation, and the stagnation incident to anchorage in a tideless stream constitute the leading facts relating to the infected vessels. To test the merit of this view of the spontaneous origin of the fever, the writer has obtained the written history of every case of which any note was made at the Naval Hospital and elsewhere. He also obtained from the quartermaster in charge of water transportation a record of the 120 steamers and sailing vessels that were under his control. Of these active vessels only one had yellow fever onboard. That these ordinary mercantile and transport vessels, under control of the quartermaster, were open ventilated and moving briskly about from place to place, yet infinitely more exposed to all sources of exotic infection, is the only comment this point in our record requires. Our records show that not less than 191 cases of yellow fever occurred onboard the twenty five vessels we have mentioned in the fleet at New Orleans in the year 1864, and that of these, fifty seven proved fatal. Also, that in addition to these there were twelve cases and three deaths among employees and guard at the Naval Hospital and landing on Erato Street. Five other cases of black vomit occurred in citizens exposed to the same cause in the vicinity of the landing.

... It should be stated that this sanitary work, under the military occupation of this city was not performed by the large forces on duty here—it was done by non-military employees of the city government, and paid for out of the city treasury. It is proper, however, to say that the city government was conducted through military appointments, control, or direction. The most rigid sanitary regulations during the four years of military control began and ended in the simple and strict enforcement of the privy and drainage systems of our city. Nothing new was practiced or even suggested—not an addition was deemed necessary to be added thereto. Our two peculiar systems just above mentioned were found capable of meeting the most exacting requirements and the very highest duty in the interest of, possibly, the most scrupulous and inflexible sanitary discipline that was ever invoked on the top of the earth, and the constant spur of apprehended danger never relaxed, thus evidencing results never before attained, much less equaled, in any known large community. Indeed it is well averred, "so clean a city had never before been seen upon the continent."

... The occupation of this city was a matter of crucial importance, and the very fact that no fault was ever found with its sanitary system, its drainage, etc. pleads eloquently from this source in the splendid and continuous good health of this large army of invasion for the maintenance of our unsurpassed system if rightly administered, and its careful and intelligent perfection to keep pace with our enlarging and growing requirements.

Our open ditches and open canals flushed with our exceedingly pure (from an analytical standpoint) Mississippi River water, and exposed, as they are, to the constant influence of one or the other of Nature's three greatest and perfect disinfectants, to wit: the general atmosphere, the sunshine, and our heavy rainfalls, it is impossible for noxious and poisonous gases from this source to attack our people, as is too often the case in sewered cities. The ensuing from a high authority is pertinent: The exhalations from the lungs and skin of a single human body vitiate or spoil for breathing ten cubic feet of air per minute, or about 90,000 gallons per day. This foul air, together with that formed from innumerable other sources of contamination, is perfectly removed by diffusion (an unfailing chemical law) and the atmosphere is thus preserved respirable and pure.

The drainage canals were in a bad condition when the city was occupied by the military, hence the larger expenditure in 1862. In a future contribution, if this meets with a favorable reception, we may have more to say on this subject. We might, with pardonable pride, close with the inquiry, where may we look to find a system equal to our own."[21]

There were numerous epidemics of yellow fever prior to the Civil War—twelve occurred between 1829 and 1852 with 22,884 total deaths, or 888 deaths per year on average. In contrast, the years 1862–1865 during the Federal occupation of the city passed without any epidemic outbreak of the disease.[22] (See Table 4 showing the number of deaths in Charity Hospital during those years.)

There was a concerted effort to discover the yellow fever "germ." As many physicians began to throw out the concept of miasmas and turn to mosquitoes as the method by which the disease spread, there was widespread condemnation of such ideas. A Cuban doctor, Carlos Finlay, was the first to suggest that mosquitoes were the cause of disease transmission.[23] Tebault strongly disagreed.

I am indebted to a prominent gentleman of this city for the loan of a letter just received by him from Dr. George M. Sternberg, dated Baltimore, April 13, 1888, from which I am permitted to make the following extract [George M. Sternberg (1838–1915) was an assistant surgeon in the U.S. Army during the war and is considered to be the first U.S. bacteriologist, publishing the *Manual of Bacteriology* in 1892.]: "We have no exact knowledge of the yellow fever germ, and my recent researches have, unfortunately, only shown that the claims of the physicians in Brazil and in Mexico, who claim to have discovered it are without foundation." Professor Stanford E. Chaillé and Dr. George M. Sternberg authoritatively visited Havana, Cuba, to investigate the germ question and to make every effort where yellow fever exists the enduring year to discover the yellow fever germ. The search was diligently, zealously, and faithfully made.[24]

The trip to Cuba that Dr. Tebault mentions was the U.S. National Board of Health Commission that was sent to Cuba in 1879. It was led by Dr. Tebault's associate and friend, Stanford Chaillé. His partner, Dr. George Sternberg, was a U.S. Army bacteriologist. The Commission was created largely in response to the devastating epidemic that occurred in Louisiana the prior year (1878). Most epidemics of yellow fever were thought to occur in August and the early fall when cold weather and frosts would eventually end the outbreak. The 1878 epidemic, however, ravaged the population of Louisiana and the South throughout the summer. It was believed to have started from a steamship, the *Emily B. Souder*, that arrived at New Orleans from Havana.[25] Cuba was considered by many at the time to be the source of most yellow fever epidemics. The 1878 outbreak spread from New Orleans upriver and along the railways infecting over 100,000 people and taking more than 20,000 lives in 100 different cities and towns. Those who could flee the cities moved to rural areas or northern cities seeking safety, while others huddled in their homes in self-imposed quarantines. Commerce in the region ground to a halt.[26] The purpose of the Commission was to investigate the sanitary conditions in Cuba that appeared to sustain the disease so that sanitary measures might be taken to prevent ships from Cuba from becoming infected and spreading the disease to southern ports.

The Committee found sanitary conditions in Cuba almost non-existent. In his testimony to the National Board of Health following the trip, Dr. Burgess, a sanitary engineer, stated:

> Havana is admirably located on elevated ground which readily admits of excellent drainage and sewage; yet, while perhaps one-tenth only of the streets have sewers, these are so defective that they are for sanitary purposes worse than useless; large pools of dirty water, pregnant with filth, suspiciously embossed with green, all kinds of slop and urine, are found in many of the streets. Heaps of excrement, garbage, and dead animals, putrefying in the tropical sun, are common in and around the city. The universal household receptacle for human excrement and household slops is merely an excavation in the rear of the house. The effluvia therefrom pervades the houses, and the fluid content saturates the soil and the soft porous coral rocks on which the city is built. Hence, all well-water is ruined, and every ditch dug in the streets exhales an offensive odor. Thus Havana may be said to be built over a privy.[27]

The Committee recommended that strict quarantine be utilized for any ships from Cuba during the yellow fever months.

In 1897, the *Lafayette Gazette* published an interview of Dr. Tebault, who suggested a remedy for preventing yellow fever.

> In 1866–67 I was health officer of this city and had just returned from the confederate army. I was unacclimated, like all these who returned. The epidemic of 1867 was the most general epidemic this city has ever had and it was the mildest, because of the reacclimation of its returning citizens. Being in the midst of it as health officer, and in connection with my own practice, I concluded to test the possibility of avoiding taking it and put myself under treatment while actively engaged in my work. I escaped, not only that year, but several years afterwards under that treatment, and only finally had the disease after I had stopped the treatment for the purpose of reacclimating myself by braving it. Since then, during the various epidemics we have had of this fever, I have repeatedly given it with success to patients who are unacclimated.[28]

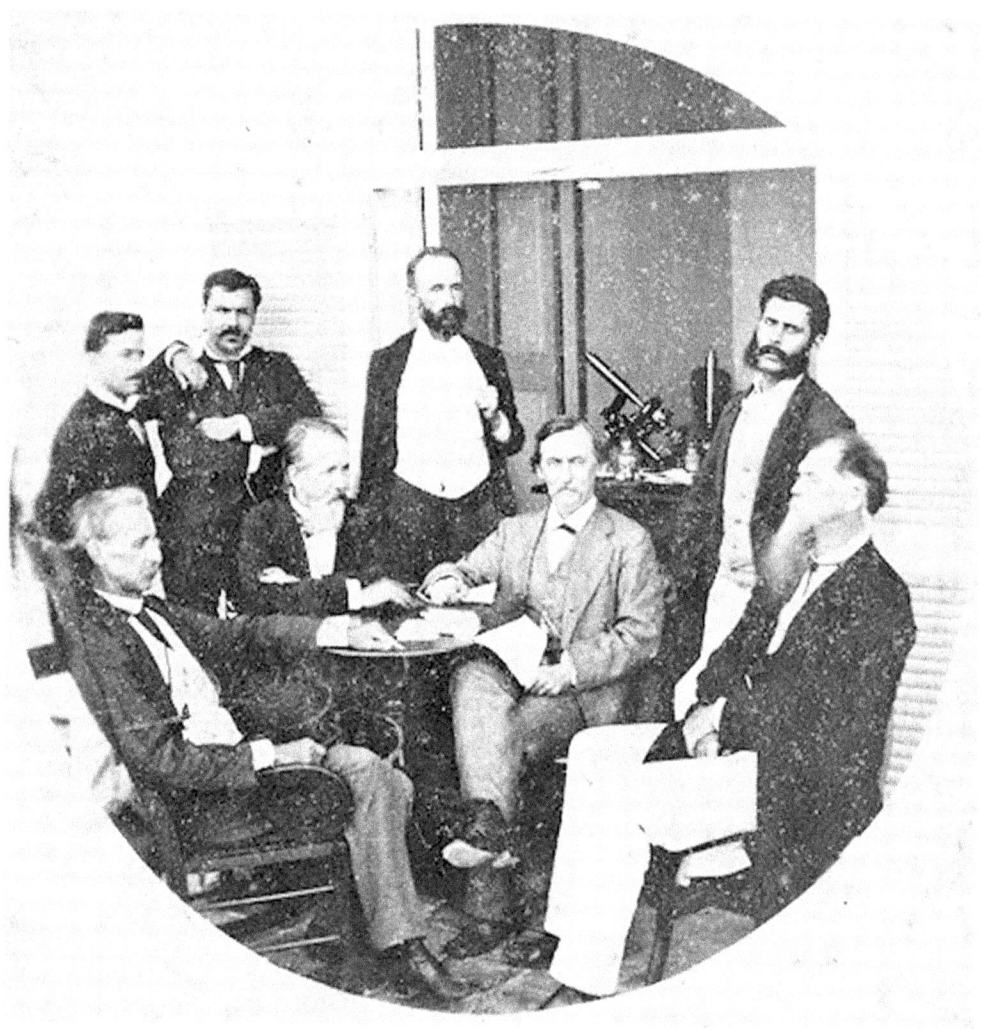

Yellow Fever Commission of 1879. Seated, from left to right: Mr. Hardee, an engineer; H.C. Hall, U.S. Consul to Havana; Dr. Stanford E. Chaillé, chairman of the Commission; Dr. D.M. Burgess, sanitary inspector. Standing, left to right: Mr. Henry Mancel, photographer; Mr. Rudolph Matas, clerk; Dr. George Sternberg, secretary; and Dr. J. Guiteras. The Commission traveled to Cuba to study the sanitary conditions at the ports that caused yellow fever to thrive, and to identify measures to prevent the spread of the disease to U.S. ports. The cause of the fever was still unknown in 1879, and most believed it to be contagious. Public domain—copied from Finlay, *Carlos Finlay and Yellow Fever*, 55.

The following is Dr. Tebault's prescription that was published and for which he encouraged pharmacists and physicians to prepare the formulations and make the treatment available to the public:

Quinine Sulph., gr. C.
Cinchonydiae Sulph., gr. C.
Pulv. Lactopeptine, gr. L.
Mixed.
Ft. Capsules No. C. (made into capsules)
S. One three times a day, one hour before or one hour after meals.

The above is for adults or children able to swallow a capsule. For children of five years and under, the following formula was suggested:

> Tincturae Xanthoxyli, 1–2 drachm.
> Glycerine, 1–2 drachm.
> Batley's Liquor Cinchoniae. 7 drachms.
> Mixed.

> This seems very simple, but the simple things sometimes do a great deal for us, and as nothing is suggested by anyone better than this, I give it as the result of my own experience for the benefit of those who chose to try it. I would recommend all infected places, or supposed to be infected, or under surveillance, to adopt this treatment at once and give it a thorough test. This treatment is distinctly recommended not to the sick but to those who are perfectly well, and before any symptoms are presented. As yellow fever commences with a distinct chill, this treatment would prevent that chill if taken on time, and, of course the following fever.[29]

Dr. Tebault's entreatments for pharmacists to compound his yellow fever remedy were apparently heard, and the advertisement in Figure 20 was printed in the *New Orleans Times-Democrat* on September 18, 1897, a few days following Dr. Tebault's interview.

DON'T WAIT
UNTIL YOU HAVE
YELLOW FEVER.
Prevent It
BY USING
DR. TEBAULT'S
YELLOW FEVER REMEDIES
— FOR SALE BY —
EUGENE MAY, Canal and Chartres Streets

In 1897 a newspaper advertisement was printed for Dr. Tebault's remedies for preventing and treating yellow fever. Eugene May, the pharmacist running the ad, was compounding medicines based on Dr. Tebault's prescriptions. Public domain—copied from the *New Orleans Times-Democrat*, September 18, 1897.

In the same interview Dr. Tebault described the symptoms of the disease in rather graphic detail based on his experience and observations:

> Yellow fever is an [infectious], acute and eruptive fever. The eruption is so faint in some cases that it is overlooked before the physician sees the case, but if seen early and a close inspection is made an eruption will be found on the skin and on the mucous membrane of the mouth and fauces. The eruption indicates that there is something of an irritant character in the blood, and doubtless the cause of the changes found in the internal viscera, especially the stomach and kidneys, producing in the stomach that softened condition found in its mucous coat, which thus produces black vomit which is a mixture of the mucous of the stomach associated with blood and the gastric juice. This irritant substance circulating in the blood damages the kidney and is the cause of the albumen found in the urine associated with this disease. Yellow fever has three stages, the first febrile, is ushered in suddenly with a chilly sensation, and often a distinct rigor. Fever rises rapidly; there more or less headache and other pains, and more or less irritability of the stomach, with nausea. The first stage lasts from twenty-four hours to three days. This is followed by a remission, or second stage, where the fever subsides, pains disappear, and the patient either rapidly convalesces or merges into the third stage, known as the stage of collapse. In this stage the fever becomes very much higher; the gastric irritability increases into great nausea and repeated vomiting. Albumen is found in the urine, and frequently blood oozes from all the mucous surfaces and is passed by the bowels. Black vomit is associated with this stage, the patient dying from exhaustion or gradually recovers by slow stages.
>
> In the first stage, the peculiar odor of yellow fever is found about the second day, and the eyes and capillary circulation are congested. All of these are intensified in the third stage.[30]

Dr. Tebault also mentions in the newspaper article the observation that "one attack affords an almost certain immunity," an observation noted earlier that presaged the yellow fever vaccinations available today.

Several years later, in 1905, there was still debate of the cause of yellow fever, with a medical journal extolling a paper by Dr. Tebault that further discounted mosquitoes: "Another refreshing paper is by Dr. C.H. Tebault. Dr. Tebault lives in New Orleans where they do not believe that mosquitoes convey yellow fever because they have mosquitoes all the time and yellow fever only part of the time. Dr. Tebault does not believe in the specificity of tubercle bacillus or any other parasite. He agrees with Dr. B. Ward Richardson, Braxton Hicks, Sir Thomas Watson, and other good souls who would be shocked out of their shrouds if they knew it." (Benjamin Ward Richardson [1828–1896] was a Fellow of the Royal College of Physicians who studied yellow fever and other diseases and wrote numerous articles discounting the contagious nature of tuberculosis; John Braxton Hicks [1823–1897] was also a Fellow of the Royal College of Physicians who became renowned for his work in childbirth, the first painless contractions known by his name; Thomas Watson [1792–1883] was famous for his lectures on the practice and principles of medicine, which were published in Philadelphia and widely read. He felt that tuberculosis was not contagious.)

The title of Dr. Tebault's paper is "The Parasitic Origin of Phthisis Pulmonalis (pulmonary tuberculosis)."[31] Dr. Tebault argues that the disease is not contagious and is therefore not carried by a "parasite" (i.e., bacteria); rather the more likely causative factors are miasmas and a lack of fresh air, similar to what he believed to be the causes of yellow fever. The editors of the magazine obviously favored Dr. Tebault's theories.

Due to the high number of yellow fever deaths during the Spanish-American War, Dr. Walter Reed, along with George Sternberg, led a number of army doctors in research into the disease and was the first to prove Dr. Finlay's mosquito theory, publishing on the theory in 1901 upon his return from Cuba.[32] Dr. Tebault and many of his compatriot physicians in the South still fought Reed's findings well after their discovery was announced.

In 1855, Louisiana had established the first Board of Health in the United States, largely because of the devastating yellow fever epidemic of 1853 that occurred along with an epidemic of typhus. The Board especially oversaw quarantines, designed to restrict the almost yearly outbreaks of disease that afflicted the city. Samuel Choppin was elected as the Board's first president. (Samuel Paul Choppin [1828–1880] was a prominent Confederate surgeon who had been educated in Paris. He was a strong advocate of the "germ" theory of yellow fever and supported the use of carbolic acid to disinfect clothing, bedding, and the streets.)

In 1866, the New Orleans Board of Health consisted of a number of Dr. Tebault's associates and friends, including Professor Warren Stone. Tebault was appointed as Health Officer for the 2nd District of New Orleans. As such, he was responsible for investigating health-related matters in the city. In an 1866 report by the *New Orleans Daily News* on the weekly meeting of the Board of Health, Dr. Tebault's work was noted:

> The report of Dr. Tebault, health officer of the Second District, was read. It stated that two distilleries had been permitted to resume, on terms similar to those imposed on others previously permitted to do so. They are not to empty anything into the gutter, not to allow any drippings in the distillery, and are to carry all their refuse by night to the nuisance wharf and empty it into the river.... He had visited bakeries in his District, and had found nothing objectionable except that the bread was not cooked enough, and this he had ordered to be done.... He had found some 10,000 pounds of tainted and rotten meats in a store, and had it transferred to a soap boiler under a bond of $5,000 that it should be used for no other purpose than soap-making.[33]

The 1898 Louisiana Constitutional Convention would eventually establish a Department of Health with the purpose of working towards improvements in sanitation and overseeing efforts to eradicate disease epidemics in the state. Before that time, however, Drs. Tebault, Chaillé, and others worked towards the same objectives in unofficial capacities. Dr. Chaillé was a spokesman for the establishment of community sewage and drainage systems, street paving, pure water supplies and mosquito control in New Orleans. He was also involved in the establishment of the National Board of Health.

The concept of separate drainage systems for sewage and rainwater was an important public health development in

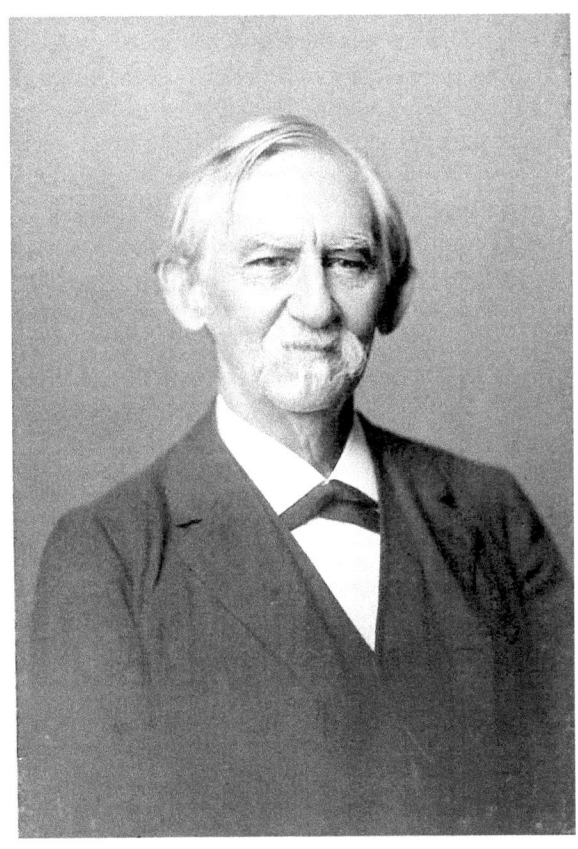

Dr. Chaillé headed the 1879 Yellow Fever Commission to Cuba. He became a nationally renowned expert in sanitation, and his work eventually led to the formation of a National Board of Health. Drs. Tebault and Chaillé were friends who met one another in Macon, Georgia, during the last year of the war. Dr. Chaillé also served as Jefferson Davis's physician and was with him at his death in 1889. Image reproduced with permission from the Rudolph Matas Library of the Health Sciences, Tulane University.

New Orleans. Through the 1870s private cesspools and privies were still being used to deal with wastes. Frequent flooding from the Mississippi and Lake Pontchartrain created severe health issues. Canals designed to provide drainage from the city would quickly become filled with feculent matter, garbage, and dead animals. The 1878 yellow fever epidemic in New Orleans highlighted concerns over sanitation, with approximately 20 percent of the population of New Orleans fleeing the city in panic.[34] Quarantining those sections of the city where yellow fever outbreaks occurred was still considered of critical importance in curtailing an epidemic.

The growing trend of urbanization in the mid-19th century strained the ability of most cities to effectively remove and treat sewage, garbage and other waste. Most of the growing population in New Orleans and other cities came from rural farm areas, and these newcomers were used to throwing out their garbage and "night spoil" into a yard or onto the streets, which theoretically would be washed away with the rains. Adding to the dilemma in New Orleans was the fear of contracting rabies from feral dogs during the warmer months. Dogs were mostly considered as domesticated animals that had to earn their keep—many an old dog would be turned loose on the street, as a result, and it was not uncommon to see packs of such dogs roaming the streets seeking handouts, garbage and other sources of food. While the dogs were generally tolerated by the public who regarded them as a noisy nuisance, the threat of rabies was something else altogether. Rabies season was thought to begin in June, at which time poisoned sausages would be used to clean the streets of the potential menace. Thus, in addition to overflowing privies, garbage, and other malodorous wastes, the decaying carcasses of dogs and cats added to the harshness of smells and unsanitary conditions experienced in New Orleans and other cities in the 19th century.

In Dr. Tebault's 1889 report on the city's drainage system he noted the many positive effects on health that resulted from improved sanitation while the city was under military rule.[35]

> ... Now from the sanitary officers of the city we learn that diseases and mortality have been chiefly diminished in connection with the abatement of those local conditions that are recognized as the <u>localizing causes</u>. These causes, in the language of Dr. E.H. Barton, consisted mainly in—
>
> 1. Bad air.
> 2. Offensive privies, cemeteries, various manufactories, stables, slaughter houses, filthy streets, etc.
> 3. Bad water, stagnant water, bad drainage.
>
> These were the causes of disease first noticed and officially controlled by the military government under the national forces.
>
> <u>The Appliances and Means of Sanitary Reform</u>—1. The streets, the courts, the market places, and all the private and public premises of the city have been cleansed and kept in a state of unusual cleanliness by an absolute authority.
>
> 2. The drainage of the city was a matter of constant official concern, and the steam drainage works kept in great activity night and day. As all the drainage is superficial by gutters, ditches, and canals, the mechanical appliances for drainage located at the junctions of canals and bayous leading towards Pontchartrain maintain an important relation to civic purity and the public health. Some of the water lifting machines exhaust from the canals and basins at the rate of more than 100,000 cubic feet per minute, raising the sewage from the lowest levels of the town and sending it forward toward Lake Pontchartrain by way of the bayous. During the frequent rain falls when the water floods the gutters and covers whole streets, cleaners are seen at work with hoes and stiff brooms, adding the effectiveness of their arms to the process of cleaning by water-flushing.
>
> 3. The water supply, which is wholly from the river, was, from the beginning of the military government, a matter of first rate importance. Though the river surface is higher than the plane of the city, the supply depends mainly upon steam pumps and reservoirs. The pumps were ordered to be kept in the highest activity, and the water company was held accountable for any failure in its works.

4. Street cleaning was literally a cleansing. The faithful broom was, immediately, and all night long, as constantly as night returned, succeeded by a flushing stream of water from the hydrants, filling and flushing gutters and the pavement joints, and aided by the sleepless sweepers, thus rendering the Augean work complete. So clean a city had never before been seen upon the continent.

5. Scavenging and domiciliary hygiene were enforced by order of the Provost-Marshal. Privies and garbage, stables and butcheries, damp and unventilated quarters, and the haunts of vice and debauchery, were all brought under police control. The privies in populous streets and those connected with places of public resort were sometimes cleaned as frequently as twice each week. All animals for the markets were impounded at the outskirts of the city, and the cattle boats were there scrubbed and cleansed before proceeding down to the commercial levees. And, as an illustration of the salutary exercise of authority over improper habitations, the writer would mention that he saw all the tenements upon the first floor of an entire block vacated by peremptory orders in a single day.

6. The destitute were supplied with wholesome food at the expense of the city. Such were the leading features of the sanitary government of the Crescent City under military rule. The errors of that government, and the criticisms it may have provoked, were neither the cause nor consequence of the protection it gave to life and health. *All the acts that related directly to the public health can be repeated in any city and by any enlightened civil government.*

Quarantine—Perhaps there has never been a more enlightened and faithful exercise of regulations in the nature of quarantine than has been witnessed at New Orleans the past four years. Yellow fever and small pox were the only infections feared or guarded against. All the exotic and transportable causes or fomites of these maladies were detained at the quarantine anchorage sixty five miles down the river near Fort Philip. Shall we be told that it was by this very application, of a judicious and inviolable quarantine, that the city escaped the epidemic visitations of disease. We have seen that small pox appeared as a widespread epidemic, and that it was checked by a house to house visitation of a medical police armed with vaccine virus.

Yellow Fever—This disease did not become epidemic in the city. Nearly three and a half years have passed without so many as a score of sporadic cases occurring in the streets, where that enemy and pest of the city had been wont to destroy its thousand victims every year, and sometimes to kill no less than five thousand in a single month![36]

In addition to Dr. Tebault's report, Dr. Chaillé had been giving considerable thought to what additional laws could be enacted to reduce illness and clean up the city. He created a list in his notebook of the sanitary laws he thought might benefit New Orleans:

Sanitary Laws Required:
Drainage of Land between River & Lake
Sewage of City, with Utilization of Miss. River
Sewage Conveyance forthwith into sewers of Feces, Urine, Filth
Cleansing of every privy in April & every 3 mos.
Elevation of every lot before a house is built
Elevation of every House 3 ft. above ground, well ventilated & enclosed
Paving every street
Public baths
Prohibit internments within city limits
Paint Houses outside to reflect & radiate heat
Prohibit stench bearing manufacturers.[37]

Chemical cleaning of the city's streets was used to sanitize the city. Carbolic acid was one of the first antiseptics and was in common use in hospitals after the war. It was a rather logical leap to assume that the same chemical might also disinfect the city. The acid was sprayed onto the city's streets in attempts to eliminate yellow fever and other contagions, but residents soon complained of its odor and ill effects. The *New Orleans Bulletin* underscored the problem in a front-page article in September 1875: "The action of the Board of Health in throwing in the gutters large quantities of carbolic acid is severely condemned by many prominent physicians, and the results have been pronounced pernicious."[38] Two weeks later a meeting of physicians was held to openly discuss the matter. The meeting's purpose was to address the following questions:

1. Is carbolic acid a disinfectant?
2. Is it an antiseptic?
3. Is it a poison?
4. Is it possible to disinfect the atmosphere of the city either by carbolic acid or any other substance?[39]

Dr. Tebault was one of the physicians in attendance and stated that the Board of Health was using a mixture of chlorine and coal mixed with carbolic acid. Dr. Warren Brickell had given Dr. Tebault his opinion in writing, which Tebault read. (Dr. Daniel Warren Brickell [1824–1881] was an obstetrician, an associate editor of the *New Orleans Medical News*, and Editor of the *Southern Journal of Medicine*.) "Dr. Brickell, in his letter, stated that he had analyzed the acid used by the Board of Health, and found it to be evil acid, which was a compound of coal, and that it does not contain ten percent of the genuine carbolic acid."[40]

Dr. Tebault then recalled that yellow fever had been discovered in 1867 aboard the brig *Valparaiso*, which had been quarantined. The Board of Health sprayed the ship with carbolic acid, and two weeks later a shipmate was stricken with yellow fever and died, thus suggesting that the acid disinfection was not having any effect on the disease. Dr. Tebault cited numerous examples of the "fatal results" of carbolic acid.

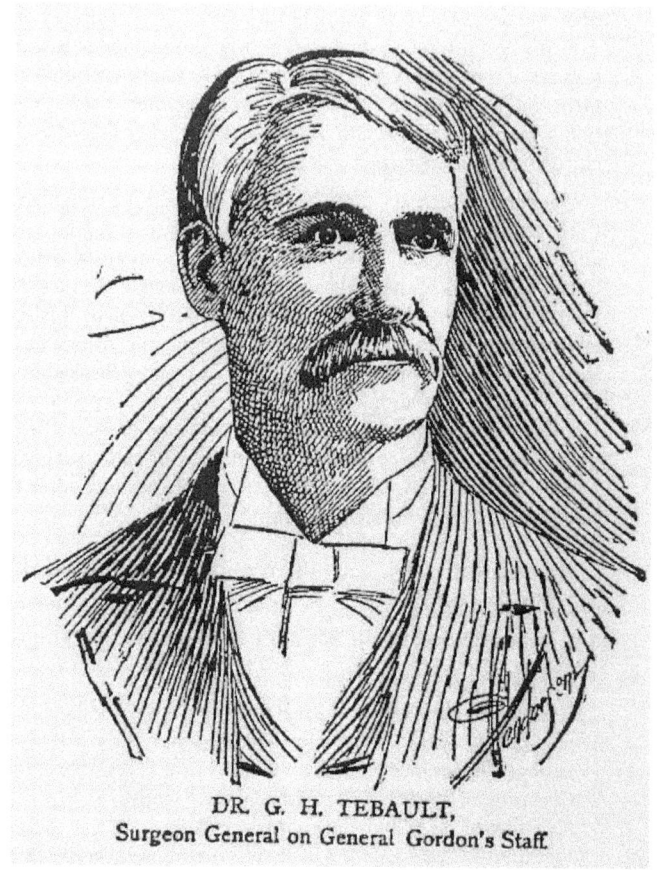

DR. G. H. TEBAULT,
Surgeon General on General Gordon's Staff.

In 1895 the *Galveston Daily News* published biographies of the "Commanders, Adjutants and Brigadier Generals" of the United Confederate Veterans. Dr. Tebault had been promoted to Brigadier General while serving as Surgeon General of the UCV, May 22, 1895, 10.

While the scourge of yellow fever was still not understood, the efforts of Drs. Tebault and Chaillé inadvertently did much to eliminate mosquitoes as well as contaminated water and arrest the outbreaks of yellow fever, malaria, typhoid and other endemic diseases.

Modified Inoculations vs. Vaccinations

After the war, Dr. Tebault continued to promote the concept of modified inoculations as an alternative to vaccinations. During most of the 19th century, the term "vaccination" was used to refer to the use of cowpox as an inoculant, while "inoculation" applied to the use of weakened variola matter from an infected person to give an individual immunity with a more localized, milder form of smallpox resulting in less scarring and low mortality.[41] Inoculation with weakened smallpox matter sounds unsafe, but it typically was successful, and in the 18th century parents had to balance the risk against the immunity it could provide when considering treating their children as well as themselves. In addition to safety, however, the problem with inoculations was that the inoculated individual might still be infectious and could pass on a more virulent form of the disease to others. Dr. Tebault disputed those concerns. His modified inoculations consisted of using variola material from the pustule of a smallpox victim mixed with an equal quantity of milk, which in his mind weakened the smallpox and made the procedure safe. This was not a new idea, as Dr. Tebault appeared to have learned about the procedure from others. At the time, many physicians believed that the cow's system somehow modified the variolous contagion sufficiently to make it safe for humans. So, it seemed logical that mixing human variolous matter with milk or cream from a cow might accomplish the same result of weakening the infection and creating immunity.

Dr. Tebault published his experience on modified inoculations in the first post-war issue of the *New Orleans Medical and Surgical Journal*.[42] In that article, he cited the works of others, including Dr. M. Brachet of Lyons, France, and Drs. M. Thiele of Kassen, M. Robert of Marseilles, and M. Bouchacourt of Lyons; their investigations of inoculation with a mixture of milk and variolous pus were mentioned in an 1854 journal discussing successful experiments on 21 children.[43] Dr. Tebault describes his use of modified inoculations and states their success: "[I]mmunity never failed to follow successfully modified inoculation…. I cannot speak so favorably of vaccination, for I have seen small-pox itself occur again and again under exactly such circumstances, and, in spite of the unquestionable purity of the virus used." He concludes his description with four conclusions:

"1st. We hope to have demonstrated that its operation is equally benign with vaccination—in fact that their action is identical, and resting this statement on an experience of fully five hundred cases.

"2nd. That the disease so ingrafted, like vaccinia, is not communicable by contact.

"3rd. That the immunity it confers would seem to be more lasting, and otherwise superior to that responding to vaccination.

"4th. That simultaneously with the occurrence of small-pox, we are supplied with a seemingly all-potent means for its arrestation."[44]

In 1883, Dr. Tebault published an additional article where he urged the medical community to consider modified inoculations over vaccinations:

> The practice of inoculation proper gives only a very mild crop of eruptions, and in careful hands is to the patient operated on a safe remedy; that this practice introduces the small-pox poison in such small quantity that it does not seriously disturb the patient, whereas to take the small-pox in the usual way is to overwhelm the system with a tremendous or poisonous dose of the distemper…. By admixture of the small-pox lymph with milk attenuates and lessens still more the small-pox virus, and it can be thus diluted at will so as to command the most perfect and assured safety, not only to the individual operated on, but to everybody with whom he comes into contact, and so, like vaccinia, causing no

effluvium of a contagious character.... Vaccination is not without danger, as many a grave will tell, and the fact of the absolute necessity of its frequency to assure protection, adds to the danger to both life and limb inseparable from its proper practice.... Vaccination requires fully a week to succeed, and small-pox may overtake such patient within two weeks of such operation, and take possession of him by arresting the vaccination and causing it to dry up.... Modified vaccination succeeds in two days and will defy small-pox after three days, and this celerity is a most valuable and important factor in favor of its practice and the security it affords.[45]

Others took Dr. Tebault's advice and utilized the rather dangerous procedure. One such case was described in the *Gaillard's Medical Journal*, in 1883:

On June 4th, of this year, I was called to see Etienne A.'s daughter, aged 12 years. On entering the room of the patient I observed an extensive eruption on her face; on further examination I found both the anterior and posterior surfaces of nearly the entire body in the same condition. After carefully examining my patient and closely questioning the mother, I gained such information as to lead me to suspect I had a case of variola, discrete in form, to treat.

As to the cause of this one case (only) having made its appearance in this locality was due to the following reasons, I judge, i.e., the patient herself had not gone off of the place, but a number of visiting friends from a plantation some miles below on the river (which had been visited by small-pox some weeks previous) came to spend a short time with patient's family. In all probability some of these persons themselves had been subjects of the disease, and, owing to their poverty, could not well afford to destroy the clothing, etc., and carried the malady as it were by "fomites" to this house. My treatment for this case was in accordance with the general plans and rules laid down by eminent authors for mild forms of the trouble.

On noticing carefully the patient I observed that the eruption was of three days' standing, and a few of the pustules looked as though they contained a sufficient quantity of pus to justify me in trying Dr. C.H. Tebault's (of New Orleans, La.) plan, that of modified inoculation (it seemed somewhat early, but I tried it nevertheless), which I proceeded to do at once on six members of the family and two in an adjoining house. I did not see my patient again until the 8th, then in company with Drs. Charles Hamlin and Z.T. Gallion, who agreed in diagnosis with me: "An undoubted case of variola, mild in form."

On examining the inoculated parties, found one who had the appearance of taking, but being in doubt we reinoculated this one as well as the others.... I am pleased to state, that after I had paid my first visit to my patient, I spoke to my worthy friend and confrere, Dr. Charles Hamlin, and told him I feared I had a case of variola to treat very near us, and that to be on the safe side (knowing the liability of the household to take the disease) I had tried Dr. Tebault's mode, that of "modified inoculation," on several cases. He remarked, "Well, you did exactly what was right; there is nothing like trying it, for those in the house with the case are more than apt to take small-pox, so give it a trial, and let's see what it will do." So I did, and the result was a success. Should it be my lot again to be called to treat small-pox, I will use every endeavor to institute Dr. Tebault's plan of inoculation. If I cannot get oil, milk (condensed) or milk of any kind, I truly believe common warm water will answer every purpose as well, and with equal success.

Let those of the profession who are in the dark give it a fair test when an opportunity offers itself and report the result, for we never know what can be done until we do try.[46]

As previously described, Dr. Joseph Jones questioned the safety of Dr. Tebault's modified inoculations, as he felt that the patients thus inoculated could infect others with more virulent infections. Smallpox inoculations, which had also become popular in Europe during the 18th century, fell out of favor to the more benign and safer vaccinations introduced by Edward Jenner in 1798. Dr. Tebault was forced to use inoculation when on Hatchie Island, as there was no other alternative open to him and doing nothing would have meant that other soldiers would have surely been infected with smallpox.

4

Reconstruction

"A conflict of the past that should teach us lessons for the future."
(The above is an inscription on the base of the Battle of
Liberty Place monument, commemorating the
overthrow of carpetbag rule in New Orleans.)

The Civil War resulted in a changed society. The world's largest slave-based economy had been destroyed, leaving the South in economic and political ruin. Due to the demise of slavery, the sugar trade collapsed, bankrupting many who had prospered in the business. Many white women in both the North and South had to learn to fend for themselves and their families during the war, and if their husbands were crippled or killed, after the war as well. Women were forced to learn new skills. In the country, they managed farms, purchased equipment, tended to livestock, and planted and harvested crops. In the cities, they became involved in nursing care and entered formerly male-dominated offices. Men coming home were unused to having women managing farms and working in businesses, and no doubt there were many new stresses on relationships as a result.

Returning Confederate veterans also had to cope with the fact that many of their former enemies were now in positions of power, wealth and influence. To put into proper perspective the events that were to plague New Orleans and much of the South during the long years of Reconstruction, one needs to understand the mindset of the returning Confederate veterans. As the war had dragged on, many Confederates began to realize that they might lose the war. They started to encounter black soldiers, a sight that led to racial vigilantism such as at Fort Pillow and the Battle of the Crater where blacks were slaughtered in rage, even as many of them tried to surrender. This anger would carry over from the war into the Reconstruction years as many southern whites felt persecuted and unfairly taxed and put upon.

The purpose of Reconstruction was to control the self-governance and readmission into Congress of the eleven seceding states, to address the status of the former leaders of the Confederacy, and to tackle the issue of the legal status of freedmen and their right to vote as citizens. While he wanted to avoid subjugation and punishment of the South, President Abraham Lincoln had devised no concrete plan for Reconstruction after the war. When asked by Maine Congressman James G. Blaine what his policy on Reconstruction after the war would be, Lincoln responded rather obliquely: "The pilots on our Western rivers steer from point to point as they call it—setting the course of the boat no farther than they can see, and that is all I propose to myself in this great problem."[1] (James G. Blaine was a Republican Congressman from the state of Maine. He voted in favor of the dissolution of the South's state governments that President Andrew Johnson had installed to replace them with harsher military rule. He also voted to impeach Johnson.)

After the assassination of President Lincoln, President Andrew Johnson tried to follow Lincoln's policies and declared that the goals of national unity and the abolishment of slavery had been accomplished. With the partnership of Louisiana Governor James Wells, President Johnson was intent on restoring the antebellum status without the formalities of slavery rather than truly reconstructing southern society along the lines of many Republicans in Congress intent upon retribution and punishment. Johnson's more benevolent approach was to restore confidence among whites in the South that the outcome of the devastating war would not significantly change their way of life. His lenient policies towards the South infuriated so-called Radical Republicans led by Massachusetts Senator Charles Sumner and Pennsylvania Congressman Thaddeus Stevens, who demanded vengeance on those who had subjected the country to incredible economic and human loss. Radical Republicans, while not formerly organized, were self-described "conservatives" who distrusted former Confederates, wanted harsh policies for the former rebels, and strongly advocated civil and voting rights for freedmen.[2] Ending slavery was not enough—the Radical Republicans proposed confiscating plantations and distributing 40 acres of land to each adult freedman. President Johnson dismissed such drastic proposals and argued that southern states merely had to agree to pledge loyalty to the Union, and they would be allowed to elect and send representatives to Congress.

Thaddeus Stevens was irate. In an address given in Lancaster, Pennsylvania, in September 1865, Stevens commented:

> Under "restoration" every rebel State will send rebels to Congress, and they, with their allies in the North, will control Congress and occupy the White House. Then restoration of laws and ancient constitutions will be sure to follow, our public debt will be repudiated, or the rebel national debt will be added to ours, and the people be crushed beneath heavy burdens. Let us forget all parties, and build on the broad platform of "reconstructing" the government out of the conquered territory converted into new and free States, and admitted into the Union by the sovereign power of Congress, with another plank—THE PROPERTY OF THE REBELS SHALL PAY OUR NATIONAL DEBT, and indemnify freedmen and loyal sufferers—and that under no circumstances will we suffer the nation's debt to be repudiated, or the interest scaled below the contract rates; nor permit any part of the rebel debt to be assumed by the nation.[3]

Stevens was correct in his prediction of old guard rebels returning to power. In October 1865, the Democratic Party in Louisiana held a State Convention in New Orleans where they adopted a platform that clearly indicated their support of President Johnson's policies of reconciliation:

> First, Resolved, That we emphatically approve of the views of President Johnson with regard to the reorganization of the State Governments of the South.
> Resolved, That we hold this to be a Government of White People, made and to be perpetuated for the exclusive political benefit of the White Race, and in accordance with the constant adjudication of the United States Supreme Court, that the people of African descent cannot be considered as citizens of the United States, and that there can in no event nor under any circumstances be any equality between the White and other Races.[4]

Many former Confederate officers and politicians were given power by their states, and dismaying Republicans worried that Congress might now refuse to enact black suffrage. Southern "Rebel Legislatures" immediately began to pass what were termed "Black Codes" depriving freedmen of most of their rights and essentially continuing slavery under a different name. These Codes were quickly adopted by all the southern states and reaffirmed the inferiority of former slaves and refused to accept them as equals to whites. Certain rights, such as the rights to marry and own property, were allowed.[5] In December 1865 the southern-elected representatives arrived in Washington. Among these men were the Confederate Vice President, members of Jefferson Davis' Cabinet, Confederate Generals and former Confederate Congressmen. As a result of the Republican sweep of the Congressional elections, however, Congress refused to reseat the southern legislators, who were all members of the Democratic party. Congress then passed legislation that overruled the Black Codes. While Johnson vetoed the bills, the Republican-controlled Congress was able to overrule him.

In an effort to forever end slavery and provide citizenship to freedmen, Congress went on to adopt three Constitutional amendments. The 13th Amendment abolished slavery and was ratified in 1865. Lincoln's Emancipation Proclamation had been a wartime measure that many abolitionists feared would not stand up in the courts after the war. Thus, the 13th Amendment established the end of slavery as a legal and constitutional requirement. The 14th Amendment guaranteed citizenship to all persons born or naturalized in the United States and was bitterly contested by southern legislatures. All the southern state legislatures, with the one exception of Tennessee, refused to ratify the 14th Amendment. This led to the Reconstruction Acts in 1867 imposing military rule until new state governments could be put into place that would ratify the Amendment. The Reconstruction Acts created five military districts, each commanded by a general who served as the acting governor of the region. These generals reported to the Secretary of War regarding any matters relating to military duties but were independent in their authority over civilian issues. Congress additionally required that each southern state draft a new constitution that would be approved by Congress, and before reinstatement, each state would be required to ratify the 14th Amendment. These state constitutional conventions thus overthrew the old order of the southern states. The Reconstruction Acts suspended voting rights for Confederate officials and officers, and the required conventions to draft new constitutions supportive of the Union were controlled by freedmen, northerners ("carpetbaggers"), and southerners sympathetic to the Union ("scalawags").[6]

The 14th Amendment was finally ratified in 1868. Following that success, the 15th Amendment was drafted to assure that the right to vote could not be denied because of "race, color, or previous condition of servitude" and was passed in 1870—the Amendment did not actually grant rights but instead prohibited discrimination. The Reconstruction Acts established biracial state governments, raised taxes, disenfranchised former Confederates, and created integrated public schools and charitable organizations. While these appear on the surface to be well-intentioned and noble accomplishments, the Acts initiated a decade of crime and oppressiveness led by the Radical Republicans in Congress and northern carpetbaggers who moved into the southern states and took advantage of the recently freed black population who were largely illiterate and naive regarding political graft.

It is generally agreed that Reconstruction ran from 1865 until 1877, but in Louisiana, Reconstruction policies had actually begun to be implemented before the end of the war as Confederate states were conquered by the Union Army. Louisiana had been the first state to be subjected to Reconstruction after its fall in May 1862. During the war, the military ruled the state. In 1862 General Benjamin Butler freed some slaves and enlisted some of them in Federal regiments. He closed all breweries and distilleries in New Orleans to retaliate against civilians, who showed the occupying Federals little respect. Famously, Butler invoked an order that women showing any disrespect for Federal soldiers or the flag were to be treated as prostitutes. Largely due to the hatred he spawned in New Orleans, General Nathaniel Banks was ordered to the city in December to replace Butler. As Banks arrived, slaves from plantations in rural parishes around New Orleans were pouring into the city to seek refuge. These "contrabands" were in great need of shelter, food and clothing, and Banks subsequently established a system to enlist them for work. Banks issued General Order No. 12, which stated:

> The public interest peremptorily demands that all persons without other means of support be required to maintain themselves by labor. Negroes are not exempt from this law. Those who leave their employers will be compelled to support themselves and families by labor upon the public works.... To secure the objects both of capital and labor the sequestration commission is hereby authorized and directed, upon conference with planters and other parties, to provide and establish a yearly system of negro labor, which shall provide for the food, clothing, proper treatment, and just compensation for the negroes, at fixed rates or an equitable portion of the yearly crop, as may be deemed advisable.[7]

While they were required to agree to a one-year contract, the former slaves could choose where they worked, and they were to receive compensation. Banks's order prohibited corporal punishment and limited the number of hours they could be expected to work. His order also provided for them to enlist in the state militia. His system, however well intentioned, met with considerable criticism from both freedmen who found the contracts little more than slave labor as well as employers, many of whom felt that slaves could only be controlled by the threat of corporal punishment.[8]

A requirement of the Federal occupation of New Orleans and Louisiana was the convening of a state convention to revise and amend the existing state constitution, which had called for the dissolution of the Union. In April 1864 the convention was convened. The resulting new constitution abolished and prohibited slavery; established legislative, executive and judicial branches of the state government; required an oath of allegiance to the United States for all members and officers of the General Assembly; and provided for the education of "all children of the State, between the ages of six and eighteen years, by maintenance of free public schools by taxation or otherwise." The convention, however, added an unusual resolution: "That when this Convention adjourns, it shall be at the call of the president [of the convention], whose duty it shall be to reconvoke the Convention for any cause...."[9] That loophole would later lead to much discontent and bloodshed.

Political Chicanery

During Reconstruction, Louisiana had five different governors—James Madison Wells, Henry C. Warmoth, P.B.S. Pinchback, William P. Kellogg and Stephen B. Packard. Each governor's reign was beset by threats of impeachment or replacement, assassination and death threats, and armed insurrection.

Elected in 1865, Governor Wells was a conservative Democrat who supported black suffrage and was considered to be a scalawag by most southern Democrats. The other Louisiana elections that year had ensured that the state's legislature would be controlled by former Confederates. Democrats considered scalawags like Wells to be radicals supporting the Republican agenda. Wells had formerly been a wealthy Louisiana plantation and slave owner but had become a staunch Unionist. He and other "radicals" supported the idea of enfranchising blacks and disenfranchising former Rebels as a way of ensuring the Republican platform.[10] The way they would implement this idea came from the loophole in the 1864 Constitution; they planned to call for a new Constitutional Convention where they could rewrite the 1864 Constitution according to Republican ideals.

On May 17, 1865, General Grant had appointed one of his wartime favorites, General Philip H. Sheridan, to be in charge of the Military District of the Southwest covering the states of Louisiana and Texas. Sheridan strongly supported the civil rights of freedmen and the registration of black voters and considered Governor Wells to be an obstructionist who only supported issues beneficial to himself: "I say now, unequivocally, that Governor Wells is a political trickster and a dishonest man. I have seen him myself, when I first came to this command, turn out all the Union men who had supported the Government, and put in their stead rebel soldiers who had not yet doffed their gray uniform."[11] Sheridan subsequently removed Wells from office in 1867 for refusing to prevent violence and protect freedmen.[12]

Governor Warmoth was elected in 1868 as a Republican with the strong support of blacks. During his corrupt reign, however, Warmoth took a more moderate approach to civil liberties, and his strong endorsement of Democrat John McEnery in the 1872 gubernatorial elections led to impeachment charges from former Republican supporters. He left office only 35 days before the end of his term.[13]

Pinckney Benton Stewart Pinchback was Warmoth's Lieutenant Governor and succeeded him as Governor for the 35 days left in his term, notably as the first black governor ever to hold such office.[14]

Republican William P. Kellogg was the next governor elected in 1872, also with significant controversy. The Louisiana State Democratic Convention was held in New Orleans on June 3, 1872, with Democrat John D. McEnery selected to run against the Republican Kellogg for the Governor's seat. During the 1872 election, Warmoth surprisingly switched parties and threw his support to the Democratic candidate. John McEnery had commanded the 4th Louisiana Battalion at Vicksburg and had a reputation of being a race-baiting orator who supported the Black Codes and rejected ratification of the 14th Amendment. His Republican opponent for governor, William Pitt Kellogg, appeared to win the election, but Democrats

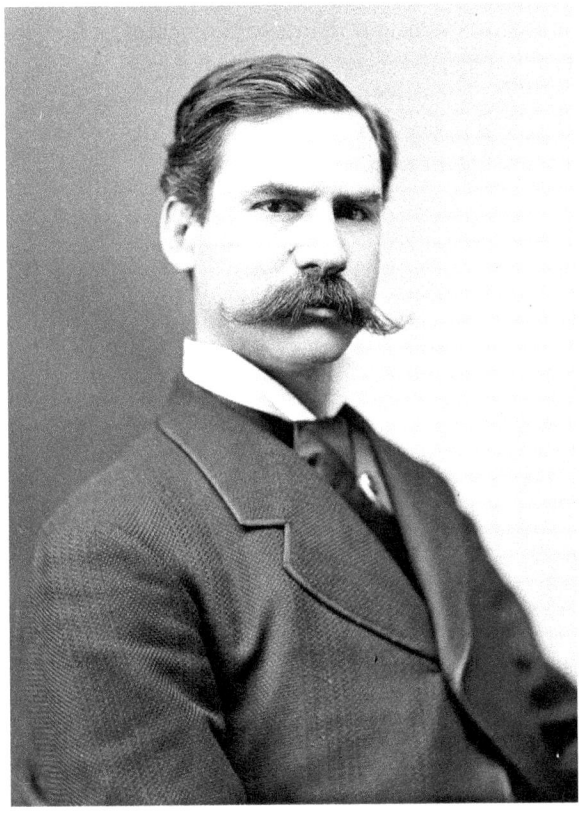

Warmoth, a Republican, was the first governor of Louisiana elected during Reconstruction. He was later impeached due to corruption but left office before his trial. He was responsible for creating a State Returning Board to certify election results, and this Board was used in the 1872 gubernatorial election to certify the Democrat candidate. President Grant's supporters established their own Returning Board, however, that certified the Republican candidate as legitimate. The result was chaotic, with two separate and competing governments in Louisiana for the next two years. Library of Congress, Prints & Photographs Division, Civil War Photographs, LC-DIG-cwpbh-03726.

disputed the election results, claiming fraud. The State Returning Board, under pressure from President Grant, named the Republican Kellogg the winner. In protest, Warmoth and McEnery established a rump government to oppose Kellogg, with several parishes recognizing theirs as the true government. As a result, there were two rival governments in Louisiana—both Kellogg and McEnery were inaugurated on the same day in January 1873. Most southern whites viewed the McEnery administration as the true government of the state, while Washington viewed the Kellogg administration as the legitimate one.

In December 1872 the Republican House of Representatives voted to impeach Warmoth for trying to throw the election, forcing him to resign. This led to the swearing in of Lieutenant Governor Pinckney Benton Stewart Pinchback, who would become the first black governor in the United States but would serve for only 35 days until the end of Warmoth's term. E.H. Durell, the U.S. District Judge, issued an order recognizing the Republican Returning Board and its decision to find Kellogg the victor and enjoining McEnery for trying to exercise any functions as Governor. (A native of New Hampshire, Edward Henry Durrell [1810–1887] was a federal judge for the Eastern District of Louisiana. He strongly supported the Civil Rights Act of 1866 and was the first judge to seat a jury that included both blacks and whites.)

President Grant intervened on December 3 and sent a telegram to Pinchback: "You are to enforce the decrees and mandates of the United States courts, no matter by whom resisted, and General Emory will furnish you with all necessary troops for that purpose."[15]

Even northern states took umbrage regarding the overturn of the New Orleans election by the Returning Board. The *Cincinnati Enquirer* described and underscored the story as one for which other states should be concerned:

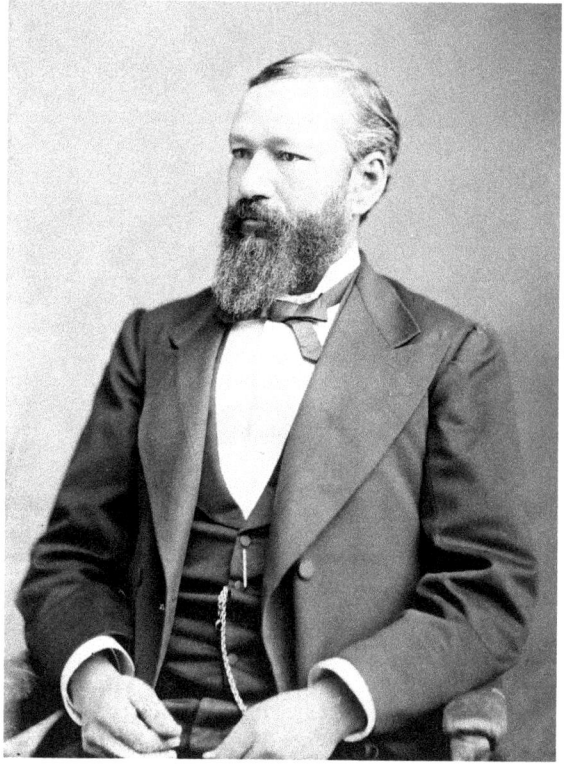

Governor Warmoth chose P.B.S. Pinchback as his Lieutenant Governor. When Warmoth left office unexpectedly, Pinchback became governor to serve out Warmoth's remaining term of 35 days. He thus became Louisiana's first and only black governor. Library of Congress, Prints & Photographs Division, Civil War Photographs, LC-BH826-3467.

> The right of the people of Louisiana to elect a State Government has been nullified by the act of a corrupt judge, executed by a squad of Federal soldiers. Her whole election machinery has been overturned and her offices filled with a robber crew, many of whom were candidates to those offices to which they pretend to be elected but were defeated by the people. This mock government could not exist by itself a day in Louisiana. It would be hooted out of existence by the voice of public opinion but for the fact that it is under the protectorate of Federal bayonets, which stand between it and those whose rights and authority it has usurped…. It is well known that as soon as the result of the election was made manifest that it involved a change in the State administration and

United States Senator, a secret caucus of the leaders of the defected party, mainly United States Government office holders, was held in the Custom House in New Orleans. The principal leader in it were Durrell, a United States District Judge; Kellogg, a United States Senator and candidate for Governor, who was bested, together with Norton, Durrell's Assignee in Bankruptcy for the State, by which he amassed a large fortune, and Billings, a lawyer who is Norton's partner and shares in his bankruptcy proceeds.... Now, as between these parties, it was agreed that Durrell, as judge, was to issue the necessary processes from the United States Court for the enthronement of the Kellogg Government. Billings and Norton were to be chosen for seats in the United States Senate.... It was necessary to bring in the Negro Pinchback on account of his control of the colored vote. That was to be done by a money consideration, the price of which was to be estimated in greenbacks. The first part of the agreement was fulfilled, but when it came to the election of United States Senator, Pinchback could not resist the glittering temptations. He flew his bargain and broke the slate. So he comes to in place of Norton as Senator.... The people of Louisiana are, therefore without any remedy for their terrible grievances except in the public opinion of the country and the influence it may upon the affairs of the Government.[16]

(Pinckney Benton Stewart Pinchback was later elected to the House of Representatives in 1874, and in 1876 to the U.S. Senate, but Democrats contested both elections. As Democrats dominated Congress at the time, they would eventually seat Democratic candidates.) Later, Democratic efforts to impeach Kellogg were rejected by the then-Republican–controlled legislature.[17]

Stephen B. Packard (1839–1922), a former Captain in the Union Army and a Maine carpetbagger, was appointed by now President Grant as the United States Marshall in New Orleans.[18] Packard had directed Republican Kellogg's candidacy and had supported Warmoth's impeachment. In 1876 Packard ran for governor of Louisiana, and in yet another disputed election both he and his Democratic opponent claimed victory and again set up two separate governments. Members of the White League made an unsuccessful assassination attempt on Packard's life.[19] All of the political and racial turmoil during the Reconstruction period left Louisiana, and New Orleans in particular, struggling to recover from the economic and social devastation left by the war.

Reconstruction was initiated against a background of an economy in ruins. Farms lacked animals and equipment, the transportation infrastructure lay in ruins, the economy was devastated with worthless Confederate dollars, 25 percent of southern white men were dead, and cities were flooded with an influx of new freedmen. On September 27 and 28, 1867, elections were held in Louisiana for the required constitutional convention. This was the first time blacks voted in Louisiana. Forty-nine white and an equal number of black delegates were elected, only two being registered Democrats. Among other provisions, they drafted a constitution that disqualified most former Confederates from public office, established interracial schools, and outlawed segregation. The new constitution also established a minimum wage and a progressive income tax. Louisiana was readmitted into the Union on June 25, 1868.[20] The state's new puppet regime included native southerners, many of whom had returned to the South following the war, and northerners—all Republicans supportive of the Reconstruction policies. People who had previously held power were angered when new elections skewed in favor of Republicans were held. New Republican lawmakers were elected by a coalition of white Unionists, former slaves and northerners who had recently settled in the South ("carpetbaggers").

Most in the North viewed the newly appointed southern Congressmen and Senators as being of high character and intelligence.

> The representation of the Southern States being complete in both Houses before the close of the first session of the Forty-first Congress, an impartial estimate could be made of the strength and capacity of the men who were opprobriously designated in the South either as carpetbaggers or scalawags. It was

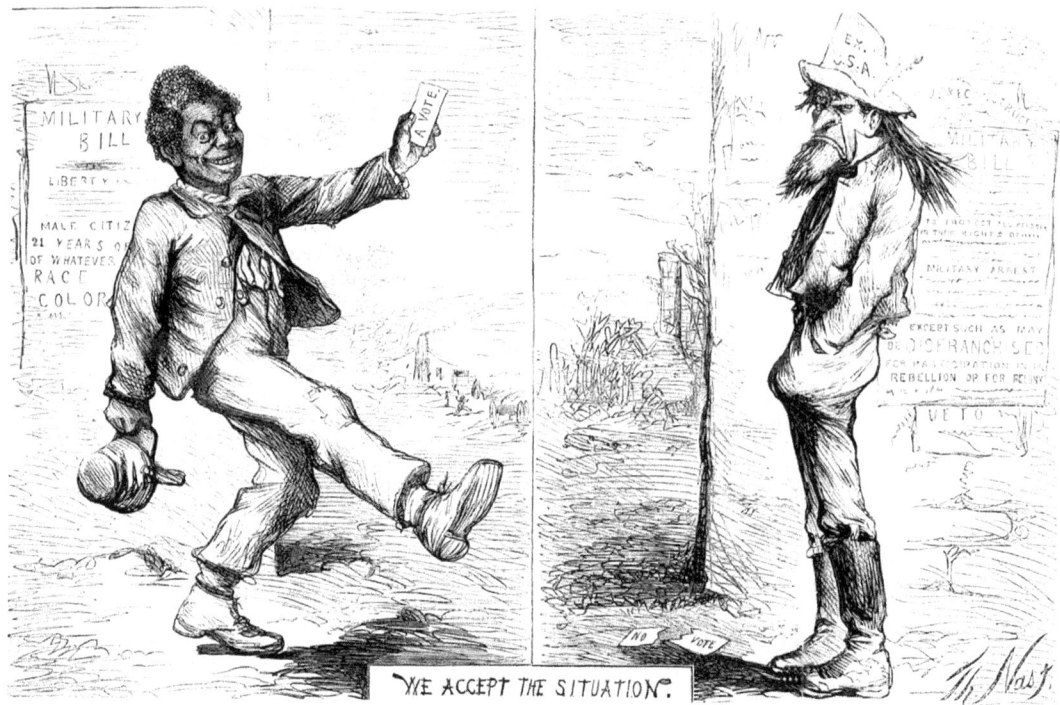

"WE ACCEPT THE SITUATION."

While blacks were given the vote, former Confederates were not allowed to run for office, and Confederate officers were initially disenfranchised. The above cartoon from 1867 shows a gleeful black voter while the disgruntled former Confederate has no vote; the broadside behind the Confederate is a "Military Bill ... to protect all persons in their rights of.... except as may be disfranchised for participation in the Rebellion or for felony..." (*Harper's Weekly*, April 13, 1867, 240).

soon ascertained that the unstinted abuse heaped upon them as a class was unjust and often malicious. The large proportion, and notably those who remained in Congress beyond two years, were men of character and respectability, in many cases indeed of decided cleverness.... [But] they were doomed to a hopeless struggle against the influence, the traditions, the hatred of a large majority of the white men of the South.[21]

Former Confederates, like Dr. Tebault, were outraged that their city and state were now being run by northern carpetbaggers and scalawags. To add to their indignity, Republicans also now commanded the positions of tax collectors and assessors, judges and constables, local police forces and state militia. A number of these positions of authority were held by former slaves, many of whom were still illiterate.

Governor Wells had been concerned about the growing power of former Confederates in Louisiana. In 1866 the state legislature had mandated new municipal elections over Wells's veto, which resulted in the return to power in New Orleans of Mayor John F. Monroe, the Confederate mayor who had refused to take an oath of allegiance to the Union following the occupation of the city. In all the county elections, Confederate supporters replaced officeholders who were supportive of the Union. The Legislature also passed an act that added a residence qualification to the police in an effort to remove from the force former Union soldiers. Governor Wells supported the reconvening of the Convention of 1864 in the hope of supporting black suffrage and disenfranchising the rebels. Louisiana Democrats, who had been inching their way back into positions of power, were outraged, and Mayor Monroe determined to prevent the Convention from meeting, which was scheduled for July 30, 1866.

New Orleans Riots

An incident occurring in distant Memphis, Tennessee, would help set the stage for what was about to happen in New Orleans. On May 1, 1866, a traffic accident between two hacks—one driven by a black man and the other by a white man—led to three days of race riots during which 46 blacks and 2 whites were killed, 75 people were injured, 5 women were raped, and numerous churches and schools were burned.[22] Those riots highlighted the impotence of the federal government and the Freedmen's Bureau to assist blacks, and the complicity of municipal government authorities, largely northern Republicans, to prevent violence. Those in Louisiana must have noted the general lack of repercussions for the Memphis riots. (Congress established the Bureau of Refugees, Freedmen, and Abandoned Lands, commonly known as the Freedmen's Bureau, on March 3, 1865. The Bureau's mission was primarily to provide relief and food for former slaves, and its agents were largely northerners. As such, the Bureau was generally despised by southerners who considered it to be part of the federal occupation of the South.)

General Sheridan had been called to Texas at the time that the Convention of 1864 was to be reconvened. On a hot and muggy July 30, 1866, a meeting of 300 to 400 blacks supporting the Convention milled around Mechanics Institute. Proudly marching in column to join them were 200 black Union veterans. A mob of armed whites led by the local police quickly formed and attacked the marchers, in what is commonly referred to as the New Orleans Massacre. The resulting riot left 38 dead and 46 wounded, and negative reactions to it contributed to the Radical Republican takeover of the House of Representatives and Senate in 1866.[23]

In his memoirs, Sheridan detailed his report of the riot, which he found to be disgusting:

> HEADQUARTERS MILITARY DIVISION OF THE GULF,
> NEW ORLEANS, La., August 6, 1866.
>
> HIS EXCELLENCY ANDREW JOHNSON,
> President of the United States:
>
> I have the honor to make the following reply to your dispatch of August 4. A very large number of colored people marched in procession on Friday night, July twenty-seven (27), and were addressed from the steps of the City Hall by Dr. Dostie, ex-governor Hahn, and others. [Anthony Paul Dostie was a dentist in New Orleans who had supported the Union during the war and returned to New Orleans following its occupation by Federal forces. He was a staunch support of equal rights for blacks and whites and was considered by many southerners to be a scalawag. During the 1866 New Orleans Massacre, he was specifically targeted and brutally shot and stabbed to death.] The speech of Dostie was intemperate in language and sentiment. The speeches of the others, so far as I can learn, were characterized by moderation....
>
> In front of Mechanics Institute, where the meeting was held, there were assembled some colored men, women and children, perhaps eighteen (18) or twenty (20), and in the Institute a number of colored men, probably one hundred fifty (150). Among those outside and inside there might have been a pistol in the possession of every tenth (10) man.
>
> About one (1) P.M. a procession of say from sixty (60) to one hundred and thirty (130) colored men marched up Burgundy Street and across Canal Street toward the convention, carrying an American flag. These men had about one pistol to every ten men and canes and clubs in addition. While cross-

ing Canal Street a row occurred. There were many spectators on the street and their manner and tone toward the procession unfriendly. A shot was fired by whom I am not able to state but believe it to have been by a policeman or some colored man in the procession. This led to other shots and a rush after the procession. On arrival at the front of the Institute there was some throwing of brickbats by both sides. The police who had been held well in hand were vigorously marched to the scene of disorder. The procession entered the Institute with the flag about six 6 or eight 8 remaining outside. A row occurred between a policeman and one of these colored men and a shot was again fired by one of the parties which led to an indiscriminate fire on the building through the windows by the policemen. This had been going on for a short time when a white flag was displayed from the windows of the Institute whereupon the firing ceased and the police rushed into the building.

From the testimony of wounded men and others who were [in] the building the policemen opened an indiscriminate fire upon the audience until they had emptied their revolvers, when they retired, and those inside barricaded the doors. The door was broken in, and the firing again commenced, when many of the colored and white people either escaped throughout the door or were passed out by the policemen inside; but as they came out the policemen who formed the circle nearest the building fired upon them, and they were again fired upon by the citizens that formed the outer circle. Many of those wounded and taken prisoners, and others who were prisoners and not wounded, were fired upon by their captors and by citizens. The wounded were stabbed while lying on the ground, and their heads beaten with brickbats. In the yard of the building, whither some of the colored men had escaped and partially secreted themselves, they were fired upon and killed or wounded by policemen. Some were killed and wounded several squares from the scene. Members of the convention were wounded by the police while in their hands as prisoners, some of them mortally.

The immediate cause of this terrible affair was the assemblage of this Convention; the remote cause was the bitter and antagonistic feeling which has been growing in this community since the advent of the present Mayor, who, in the organization of his police force selected many desperate men, and some of them known murderers. People of clear views were overawed by want of confidence in the Mayor, and fear of the thugs, many of which he had selected for his police force. I have frequently been spoken to by prominent citizens on this subject and have heard them express fear and want of confidence in Mayor Monroe. Ever since the intimation of this last convention movement I must condemn the course of several of the city papers for supporting by their articles, the bitter feeling of bad men. As to the merciless manner in which the convention was broken up I feel obliged to confess strong repugnance.

It is useless to disguise the hostility that exists on the part of a great many here toward Northern men, and this unfortunate affair has so precipitated matters that there is now a test of what shall be the status of Northern men—whether they can live here without being in constant dread or not, whether they can be protected in life and property, and have justice in the courts. If this matter is permitted to pass over without a thorough and determined prosecution of those engaged in it, we may look out for frequent scenes of the same kind, not only here but in other places. No steps have as yet been taken by the civil authorities to arrest citizens who were engaged in this massacre, or policemen who perpetrated such cruelties. The members of the convention have been indicted by the grand jury, and many of them arrested and held to bail. As to whether the civil authorities can mete out ample justice to the guilty parties on both sides, I must say it is my opinion unequivocally that they cannot. Judge Abell, whose course I have closely watched for nearly a year, I now consider one of the most dangerous men that we have here to the peace and quiet of the city. [Judge Edmund Abell of the First District Court, a member of the 1864 Convention, had openly questioned the validity of reconvening the convention.] The leading men of the convention—King Cutler, Hahn, and others—have been political agitators and are bad men. [King Cutler and Michael Hahn were among the leaders of the reconvened convention, but also had been strong advocates of secession before the war. As such they were viewed by Sheridan as opportunists.] I regret to say that the course of Governor Wells has been vacillating, and that during the late trouble he has shown very little of the man.

P. H. Sheridan, Major-General Commanding.[24]

In a city simmering with pro-white and Democratic sentiments, Paul Dostie and a small group of whites had planned to start the convention standing before a largely black audience where they would describe a "new world" where blacks were equal to whites. And,

4. Reconstruction

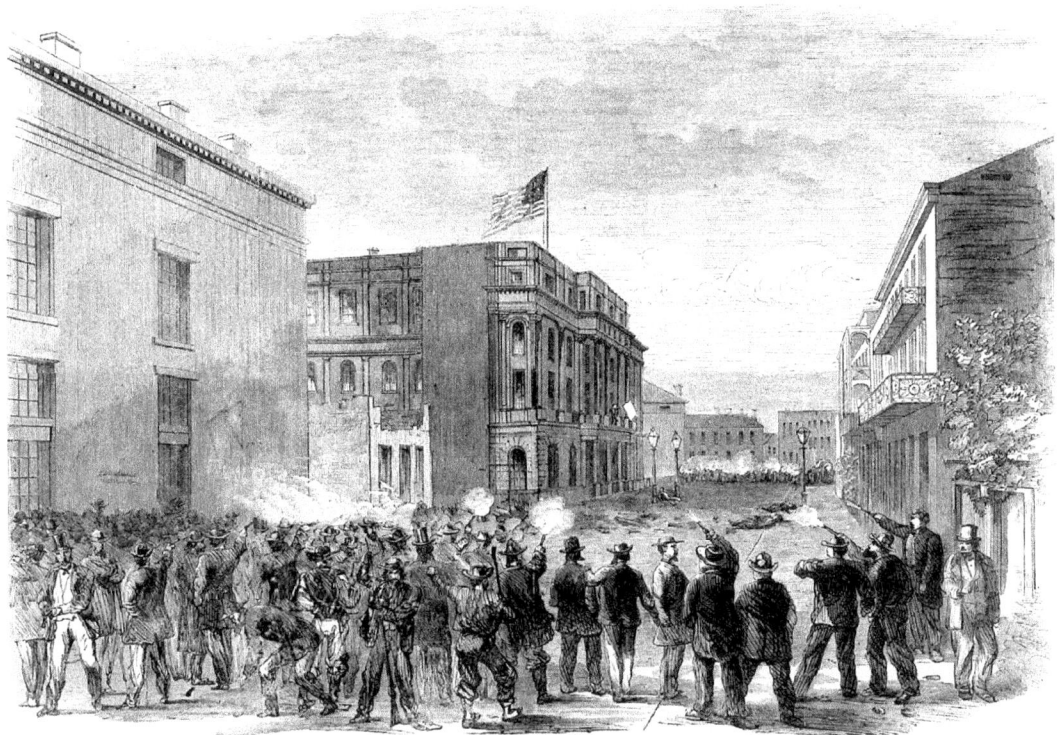

THE RIOT IN NEW ORLEANS—SIEGE AND ASSAULT OF THE CONVENTION BY THE POLICE AND CITIZENS.—Sketched by Theodore R. Davis.
[See Page 535.]

New Orleans Riot. In 1866 approximately 300 to 400 blacks met at the Mechanics Institute in New Orleans to reconvene a state Constitutional Convention. A mob of armed whites and local policemen attacked the group, leaving 38 dead and 46 wounded. The incident created an uproar in the North, helping the rise in power of the Radical Republicans who were hell-bent on retribution. Public domain—copied from *Harper's Weekly*, August 25, 1866, 536.

whites would either have to accept that new southern order or go elsewhere.[25] The results were predictable.

The 1866 New Orleans Massacre created uproar in the North and intensified opposition to President Johnson's policy of Reconstruction. *Harper's Weekly* described the riot as an affront: "The rebel flag was again unfurled. The men who had bravely resisted it for four years were murdered under its encouragement."[26] The riot came at a time when Radical Republicans were gaining strength, and as a result they swept both houses of Congress in the 1866 elections, demanding retribution. In December, Congress passed laws forcing Reconstruction and giving powers of governing to military commanders. Meanwhile, President Johnson learned through some of his Cabinet members that Edwin Stanton, President Lincoln's Secretary of War, was undermining him and criticizing his administrative capabilities. Stanton was also a supporter of the Radical Republicans' hardline towards Reconstruction. Johnson wanted to dismiss Stanton but was limited in doing so by the Tenure of Office Act. The Act had been enacted in 1867 over Johnson's veto and restricted the power of the President of the United States to remove certain office-holders without the approval of the Senate. Johnson challenged the Act and tried to dismiss Stanton. Stanton refused to resign, had his would-be successor arrested, and barricaded himself in his office with armed guards. Johnson further riled his opponents by removing three well-known figures from their positions as military governors—George Thomas, Philip Sheridan and Daniel Sickles. (General George Henry Thomas was a Virginian who had served with distinction in the Union army during the war and was appointed the commander of the Military Division of the Pacific headquartered in San Francisco in 1869; Daniel Edgar Sickles had been a rather colorful and incompetent major general during the war and was appointed the commander of the Second Military District that included North and South Carolina.)

The House of Representatives subsequently impeached Johnson, lacking only one vote for his forced removal from office.[27] Stanton immediately resigned from office after the unsuccessful impeachment vote.

The Black Codes

In the South, freedmen suddenly found themselves citizens rather than property, a cultural change for which neither blacks nor whites were ready. In Louisiana, South Carolina and Mississippi, the number of slaves outnumbered the white population in the 1860 census; such a large number of freedmen moving into cities such as New Orleans created difficulties never before seen, and ones for which there were no easy solutions. Between 1860 and 1870 New Orleans experienced a 109.6 percent growth in the black population compared to 2.5 percent for whites.[28] Having spent generations away from their cultural ancestry and lacking education and literacy, blacks struggled with their newfound freedom. Even the concept of legal marriage was new to them, as well as the more general notion of family as owners oftentimes sold and separated children and spouses. Abolitionists who had fought loudly for slaves' freedom now were too sanguine about the prospects of their transition into a free society with no job skills, land, or resources. And, former supporters of slavery were adamant in their efforts to suppress and obstruct such a transition by enacting Black Codes and Jim Crow laws and forming the White League and the Ku Klux Klan.

(The Black Codes were laws enacted in southern states after the war, which limited the civil rights and liberties of blacks. Their purpose was to emphasize the inferiority of the

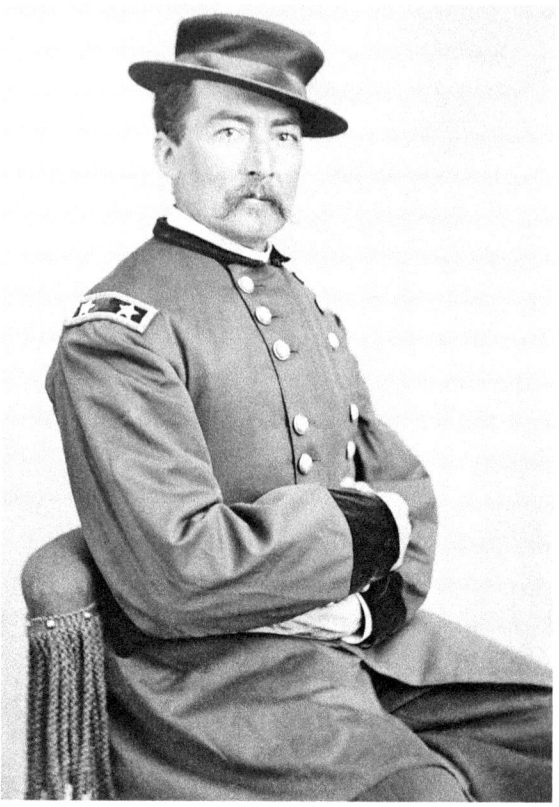

President Grant appointed Union General Sheridan to become the Commander of the Military District of the Southwest. He was patrolling the Mexican–Texas border in 1866 when the New Orleans Massacre occurred. Sheridan subsequently returned to New Orleans and became the military governor of the Fifth Military District, which included Texas and Louisiana. Credit: Library of Congress, Prints & Photographs Division, Civil War Photographs LC-BH82-4012 A.

freed slaves as being unequal to whites and guaranteeing sources of cheap labor to planters. The Jim Crow laws were enacted in southern states and localities, which promulgated the practice of segregation and systemized a number of social, educational and economic disadvantages for blacks. The White League was a white paramilitary group started in 1874 and organized to remove Republicans from office and intimidate blacks from voting. It was often described as "the military arm of the Democratic Party." The group successfully reduced Republican voting and contributed to the Democrats' taking control of the Louisiana Legislature in 1876 through acts of violence and intimidation. Unlike the secretive Ku Klux Klan and the Knights of the White Camellia, the White League sought publicity and its members were generally well-known. The Ku Klux Klan (KKK) was a secret society founded in 1865 by former Confederates to advocate white supremacy. It was an effective vigilante group that used threats and violence against blacks and Republicans. In 1870 the Federal government passed laws to prosecute Klan crimes, which had the effect of suppressing its activities, leading to the formation of the White League in its place. Director D.W. Griffith's 1915 epic movie, *The Birth of a Nation*, glorified the Klan and renewed interest in the group, leading to its resurrection in 1921 as a fraternal organization. Its popularity rose again in the 1950s for opposing desegregation.)

Now with unaccustomed freedom and rights, some former slaves were thrust into positions of authority in local and state governments by carpetbaggers and Union agents intent on punishing the old Confederate guard. Most of these freedmen were illiterate and unsuited for such positions, although it must have provided a sense of justice to many.

An example of the Black Codes was an ordinance passed in July 1865 in the Town of Opelousas located approximately 130 miles northwest of New Orleans:

Whereas the relations formerly subsisting between master and slave have become changed by the action of the controlling authorities; and whereas it is necessary to provide for the proper policing and government of the recently emancipated negroes or freedmen, in their new relations to the municipal authorities;

Sect. 1. Be it therefore ordained by the Board of Police of the Town of Opelousas: that no negro or freedman shall be allowed to come within the limits of the Town of Opelousas without special permission from his employer specifying the object of his visit and the time necessary for the accomplishment of the same. Whoever shall violate this provision shall suffer imprisonment and two days' work on the public streets, or shall pay a fine of two dollars and fifty cents.

Sect. 2. Be it further ordained that every negro or freedman who shall be found on the streets of Opelousas after 10 o'clock at night without a written pass or permit from his employer, shall be imprisoned and compelled to work five days on the public streets, or pay a fine of five dollars.

Sect. 3. No negro or freedman shall be permitted to rent or keep a house within the limits of the town under any circumstances, and any one thus offending shall be ejected, and compelled to find an employer or leave the town within twenty-four hours. The lessor or furnisher of the house leased or kept as above shall pay a fine of ten dollars for each offence.

Sect. 4. No negro or freedman shall reside within the limits of the Town of Opelousas who is not in the regular service of some white person or former owner, who shall be held responsible for the conduct of said freedman. But said employer or former owner may permit said freedman to hire his time, by special permission in writing, which permission shall not extend over twenty-four hours at any one time. Any one violating the provisions of this section shall be imprisoned and compelled to work for two days in the public streets, or pay a fine of five dollars.

Sect. 5. No public meetings or congregations of negroes or freedmen shall be allowed within the limits of the Town of Opelousas, under any circumstances or for any purpose, without the permission of the Mayor or President of the Board. This prohibition is not intended, however, to prevent freedmen from attending the usual church services conducted by established ministers of religion. Every freedman violating this law shall be imprisoned and made to work five days on the public streets.

Sect. 6. No negro or freedman shall be permitted to preach, exhort, or otherwise declaim to congregations of colored people without a special permission from the Mayor or President of the Board of Police, under the penalty of a fine of ten dollars or twenty days' work on the public streets.

Sect. 7. No freedman who is not in the military service shall be allowed to carry firearms or any kind of weapons within the limits of the Town of Opelousas, without the special permission of his employer, in writing, and approved by the Mayor or President of the Board of Police. Any one thus offending shall forfeit his weapons and shall be imprisoned and made to work five days on the public streets or pay a fine of five dollars in lieu of said work.

Sect. 8. No freedman shall sell, barter or exchange any articles or merchandise of traffic within the limits of Opelousas, without permission from his employer or the Mayor or President of the Board, under the penalty of the forfeiture of said articles, and imprisonment and one day's labor, or a fine of one dollar in lieu of said work.

Sect. 9. Any freedman found drunk within the limits of the Town shall be imprisoned and made to labor five days on the public streets, or pay five dollars in lieu of said labor.

Sect. 10. Any freedman not residing in Opelousas, who shall be found within its corporate limits after the hour of 3 o'clock P.M., on Sunday, without a special written permission from his employer or the Mayor, shall be arrested and imprisoned and made to work two days on the public streets, or pay two dollars in lieu of said work.

Sect. 11. All the foregoing provisions apply to freedmen and freedwomen, or both sexes.

Sect. 12. It shall be the special duty of the Mayor or President of the Board to see that all the provisions of this ordinance are faithfully executed.

Sect. 13. Be it further ordained, that this ordinance is to take effect from and after its first publication.

Ordained the 3rd day of July, 1865.

(Signed) E.D. ESTILLETTE, President of the Board of Police.[29]

The white people of Opelousas were obviously not opening their arms to freedmen, and one of the punishments for violating the rules was to be enslaved and work for five days for the city.

The Crescent City White League

In 1874 the black Republican candidates for sheriff and parish judge in one of the New Orleans parishes were both illiterate and could neither read or write. "Yet they have complete power over the parish taxes, roads, bridges, and all county matters."[30] Whites were not used to tolerating free blacks, and many were fearful of black crimes against whites, especially women.[31] Newspapers stirred up such fears with belligerent reporting:

A BLACK LEAGUE
Information reached us yesterday of a determined effort on the part of the colored people now in our city to seize the occasion of the coming Fourth of July for a grand coup on the white people to enforce their "civil rights," if need be, at the point of the bayonet.[32]

The so-called Black Leagues were actually the Union Leagues that had originally sprung up in the North to promote pro-Union matters. As such, Union Leagues were also known as Loyal Leagues and supported the Republican Party.[33] During Reconstruction, a number of Union Leagues were established in the South, and all-black Leagues became known as Black Leagues with most of their leaders coming from the North. The clubs sought to organize blacks to unite politically and support Republican candidates.[34]

The southern white population had greatly feared a slave revolt in the antebellum South. In 1822 a plot by slaves to seize Charleston had been uncovered. The conspiracy had involved as many as 8,000 slaves in the area.[35] In 1831 Nat Turner had led a rebellion of slaves that resulted in the deaths of 60 whites. In addition to these two well-known cases, there were numerous other rebellious attempts by slaves throughout the South, leaving whites fearful and blaming Northern abolitionists for inciting rebellion. Now, in post-war Reconstruction, southern whites feared a well-organized and armed rebellion of former slaves stirred up by northern carpetbaggers and scalawags. Many pro-Democrat southern newspapers almost continually roused white fear and indignation in their articles: "While we have been willing, and always have been, to give the Negro everything he needs and should have to make him happy, free and contented, we are not and never will be in favor of his ruling the State of Louisiana any longer and we swear by the Eternal Spirit that rules the universe we will battle against it to the day of our death if it costs us a prison or gallows."[36]

On July 1 the *Times-Picayune* ran yet another incendiary article, alarming its white readers with stories of organized blacks with violent intent:

> It has been well known for some time that there was a movement among the negroes to secure practically all the nominations for their race; and those who have become acquainted with the nature of the proceedings at club-rooms know that that the temper towards the whites has been of increasing animosity.... Is there anything foolish, considering all these facts—knowing that the negroes are thoroughly organized on political as well as military basis; that they are drilling nightly in different parts of town; that, above all, their bearing is becoming more aggressive as the campaign thickens—is there anything foolish, we ask, in supposing that the time has come for us to take measures of protection?[37]

The fears spread by such editorializing hastened the formation of the White Leagues in many southern states. In Louisiana the *Lafayette Advertiser* printed an announcement for whites to join together and form a White League:

> TO THE WHITE PEOPLE OF THE PARISH OF LAFAYETTE
>
> Fellow Citizens,
>
> Since the termination of the war between the States, the negroes, banded together under the leadership of carpetbaggers and bad men, have acted and voted as a <u>unit</u> in all our State and parish elections.... Our brothers of other parishes throughout the State, believing that the time has arrived to make an effort to change the current of events and rid the State of the present polluted Government, and knowing that to combat successfully a political organization, a counter political organization is necessary, have at last raised the white banner in opposition of the black banner. They invite all who belong to the Caucasian race to join them in the supreme effort and perhaps the last struggle at the ballot box, to restore our beloved Louisiana to her former prosperity, and her sons to their once proud and fair name. They have formed what is called the White League that is a political party composed of white men, the main object of which is to reform the abuses of our State Government and to place the same under the influence and control of the white people. The two banners, white and black, are now unfurled. Each banner indicates the principles and objects of their followers.[38]

A number of White Leagues were formed throughout the state of Louisiana, but the principle club was the Crescent City White League in New Orleans. A member of the League testified to a Congressional Committee investigating conditions in the South: "The leaders of the organization have to this day shown themselves moderate, liberal-minded, fair men, denouncing all violence and advocating nothing but peaceful measures in all emergencies. In Iberia Parish, of which alone I speak, they control the people, keep them orderly and fair in their behavior, and in consequence of this there was no violence or intimidation practiced toward republicans, black or white, within my knowledge, on account of their policies."[39] Another member of the Crescent City League testified that the name "White League" was adopted in contrast to the "Black League."[40] The Constitution of the Crescent

City White League stated the club's objectives in noble-sounding terms: "The object of this club is to assist in restoring an honest and intelligent government to the State of Louisiana; to drive incompetent and corrupt men from office; and by a union with all other good citizens, the better to maintain and defend the Constitution of the United States and of the State, with all laws made in pursuance thereof; and to maintain and protect and enforce our rights, and the rights of citizens thereunder."[41]

This benign view of the White League's purpose was not shared by the House of Representatives, which published a report following its committee investigating the 1876 Election in Louisiana[42]:

> The White League commanded by Fred N. Ogden was and is an association consisting entirely of white men, all democrats, and all united for the express purpose of asserting the supremacy of the white race in political matters and in the change of government. [Fred N. Ogden, a former Confederate General and attorney, was the head of the Crescent City White League in New Orleans.] They are adroitly organized into clubs whose open and printed constitution is on its face legitimate. But that constitution when dissected shows what its inner purpose is. Certain officers of a civil character are named all innocent and harmless but the constitution also provides for the appointment of such other officers as the president of the club may think proper, and such officers when appointed are to be obeyed and respected and each member takes an oath to render full obedience to such officers. Under this clause each of these clubs has a complete military organization; every able-bodied member is regularly enrolled by companies, battalions, brigades, and divisions—all the paraphernalia of staff departments exist; and the whole force, by a system of private signals known only to the initiated, can be paraded, handled, and thrown into order of battle on short notice.... The pretense set up by Mr. Ogden in his testimony that the organization was intended only to defend the white people of New Orleans from danger from the Blacks is shown to be shallow and dishonest from the known fact that of the 190,000 population of the city, 150,000 are white and not exceeding 40,000 colored, and we will not insult the high reputation nor courage of the white citizens of New Orleans by supposing that they suffer under intimidation when they have in their favor such overwhelming odds of numbers and with almost sole possession of proper arms. The White League in September 1874 extended to nearly all the parishes in the State and acted secretly and solidly as a branch of the democratic party.[43]

This report incorrectly cited the 1870 census data with misleading conclusions. New Orleans was the ninth most populous city in the 1870 census. Table 6 shows the population of both whites and blacks in the decade from 1860 to 1870.

Table 6: New Orleans Population, 1860–1870

	Total Population	*Whites*	*Blacks*
1860	168,405	144,331 (86%)	24,074 (14%)
1870	191,148	140,653 (71%)	50,495 (26%)

These data show the white population slightly decreasing over the decade while the black population almost doubled. The population of white men in the age bracket 15–40 years, however, dramatically declined. In 1860 there were 1,537 more males than females, while in 1870 there were 10,860 more females than males. Of these 10,860 females, 72 percent were black.[44] Thus, the data cited in the Congressional report failed to recognize the decrease in young white males and the doubling of young blacks in the city.

The White League was not a secret society and published the names of their members. While Dr. Tebault and his brothers were not members, they did take up arms with members of the Crescent City White League to serve in one of its companies at the Battle of Liberty Place, which would take place in September 1874. It is important to understand the underlying tensions that led to that armed conflict that took place in the heart of the city.

Governor Henry C. Warmoth was the first governor of Louisiana elected after the war, and he took full advantage of the military rule by openly campaigning for black votes with the promise of civil equality. When all the southern-elected Representatives were refused seats by Congress, Warmoth returned to New Orleans where he successfully ran for Governor in a special election following the resignation of Joshua Baker. At the time, Warmoth was considered by many in Louisiana to be a "carpetbagger." In his four years as governor, Warmoth would earn the reputation of being notoriously corrupt. Once elected, many of

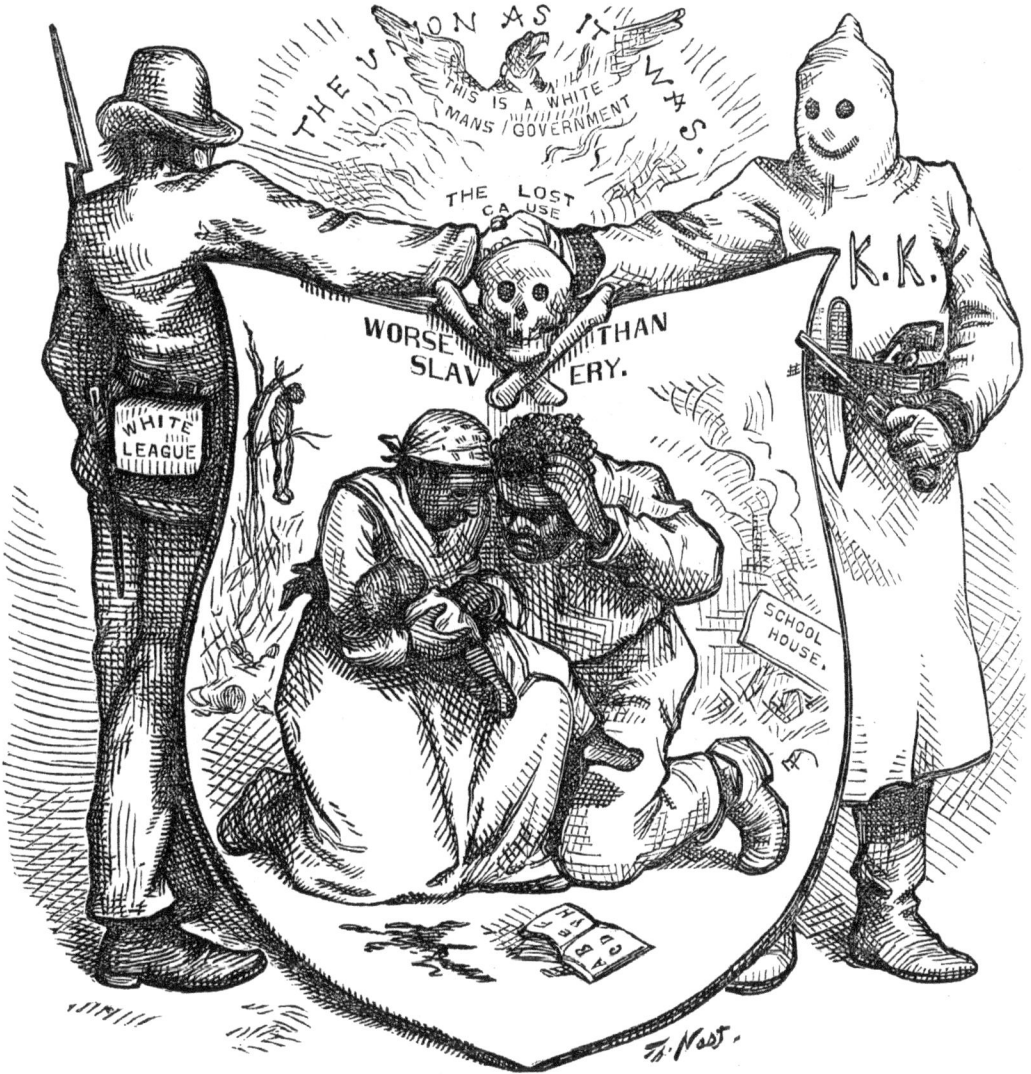

The Union As It Was, The Lost Cause Worse Than Slavery. The above cartoon by Thomas Nash shows the White League and Ku Klux Klan joining hands with the Lost Cause. Just below the eagle is the phrase: "This Is a White Man's Government" (*Harper's Weekly*, October 24, 1874, 878).

his Democratic opponents continued to reject the legitimacy of a government that was supported by black votes. Warmoth was also accused of buying the election. During his reign, Louisiana's bonded indebtedness would rise from $6 million to $25 million. Warmoth established the State Returning Board to supervise election returns, granting the board the extraordinary power to overthrow elections in the event of perceived fraud, a power that could also be used nefariously to shape the political landscape. He required "exacting retribution" from the recently developed Louisiana railroads that left him a wealthy man.

In the first page of his autobiography, Warmoth began defensively with the following statement: "Lies, unmitigated lies, notorious and malicious lies, have been printed and broadcast, and willing and eager readers have been glad to believe them."[45] Without question Warmoth profited from his term as governor, and he was accused of leveraging conflicts of interest, insider trading and other nefarious transactions. But these accusations obscure the true objections to his election. First, he rode to power on the backs of black votes. Second, Warmoth tried to push aside the old regime and traditions. And, finally, he controlled the Metropolitan Police and Militia, appointing James Longstreet in charge. Longstreet had been a key Confederate General whom General Robert E. Lee had dubbed his "old warhorse." Longstreet's decision to join the Republican Party after the war and to endorse General Grant's candidacy for President in 1868 earned him the disdain of many southerners. Following the war, Longstreet moved to New Orleans. Many still blamed him for Lee's defeat at Gettysburg, and such southern bitterness shadowed him until his death in 1903. Longstreet was also a Republican and friend of President Grant, causing many of his former Confederate associates to call him a scalawag.[46] Longstreet at the time was a rising star of the Republican party and felt that the time had come for southerners to accept the new political realities of black suffrage.[47] The Metropolitan Police force was 500 strong and served more as a militia subject to the governor's command. Many former black soldiers joined the force, which wore prominent red and black uniforms.

The small town of Colfax, Louisiana, located about 200 miles northwest of New Orleans, is the parish seat for Grant Parish. Prior to the war, the area was known as Calhoun's Landing, after Meredith Calhoun, who built his plantation along the Red River. In 1873 Colfax was only a tiny hamlet centered around a one-story, rectangular courthouse that represented the symbol of control of the parish. Calhoun was a Republican who supported McEnery and who encouraged freedmen to set up quarters on his 17,000-acre plantation.[48] As a result, many whites viewed Colfax as a black man's town.

In support of the Republican Kellogg's government, about 150 black men moved to defend the county seat in Colfax, digging trenches to protect the courthouse from possible attack by those sympathetic to the Democratic McEnery government. Newspapers were quick to sensationalize the takeover of the courthouse as a first step towards a race war where no white women or children would be safe. The *Daily Picayune* was among the leaders of such lurid reporting and on April 8, 1873, ran the following headline:

THE RIOT IN GRANT PARISH
FEARFUL ATROCITIES OF THE NEGROES
  No Respect Shown to the Dead
  A band of negroes were a short time ago organized in the parish of Grant, and … have seized and taken possession of the Court House in Colfax and driven all the white men from that place. They broke into the house of Judge W.R. Rutland and other white people and plundered them. In Mr. Rutland's house was the body of a dead child, embalmed and in a coffin. This the ruffians actually carried away and threw upon the banks of the river.[49]

As Easter Sunday, April 13, 1873, approached, the courthouse's black defenders were drilling, stockpiling ammunition, fabricating makeshift cannons out of stovepipes, and preparing for the inevitable attack. On Easter Sunday morning, 165 armed whites, many of them former Confederate soldiers, approached Colfax. These men were on a mission, with "fear and outrage at the prospect of a Negro revolt. These men had come to fight for civilization itself—to save themselves—from ruin and their women from rape."[50] The men had prepared themselves with army-style organization of infantry, cavalry and scouts. About 150 black men and an equal number of women and children anxiously awaited. They had no chance. When the fighting began, the defenders quickly discovered that the trenches had been dug too shallow to offer them any real protection, and they were quickly driven back into the courthouse, which was set afire. The Colfax massacre left 150 black bodies in its wake, many of them having been executed after surrendering, reminiscent of the Fort Pillow massacre. The Colfax massacre is considered to be the largest single incident of racial bloodshed during Reconstruction.[51] The ringleaders of the massacre were never punished. Southern newspapers referred to the incident as a "Negro Riot." The *Daily Picayune* reported falsely on April 16 that detachments of whites had been fired on as the defenders displayed white flags:

> The Whites have taken Colfax, and there is not a negro to be found for miles around.... The negroes had strongly entrenched themselves in the Court-House, built breastworks three and four feet high. There were, it was said, about 400 men, armed and equipped thoroughly, and they improvised two cannons from gas pipe.... On Sunday, at about 12 O'clock, about 150 white men, who had gathered from surrounding parishes, made an attack on the breastworks, and a brisk fight was kept up until somewhere near 3 O'clock. The breastworks were then stormed and captured, the negroes taking refuge in the Court-House, the doors of which were barricaded.
>
> After some further fighting, the negroes threw out a flag of truce, and several detachments of men advanced on it, when they were fired on by the besieged party, wounding several, one of whom was Capt. Hadnot, who was shot in the bowels, and it is feared, fatally wounded.[52]

Two days later the *Daily Picayune* summarized their rather biased version of the Colfax "riot":

> The Whites, before the fight took place, endeavored to avoid bloodshed.... Whilst the negroes were in possession of the town of Colfax, they committed many cruel acts against the people of their own color. They sent different bodies of armed men to the plantations throughout the whole parish to compel the negroes to come into town and assist the revolutionists in defending the same. When resistance was made the leaders of the mutiny and their followers did not hesitate to resort to violence. Indeed, many of the poor, inoffensive field laborers were unmercifully beaten.[53]

The Colfax massacre again agitated northern sentiments and, at the same time, encouraged the creation and growth of white paramilitary groups such as the White Leagues; as a result of Colfax, thousands of whites would join White Leagues in 1874. And, the paramilitary technique of racially oriented killings would go unpunished in Louisiana and other southern states, encouraging white supremacists.

The Democratic Party in Louisiana voiced a concern shared by many whites in 1874:

> We the white people of Louisiana, embracing the Democratic party, the Conservatives party, the White Man's party, the Liberal party, the Reform party, and all others opposed to the Kellogg usurpation, do solemnly resolve and declare that the government now existing in Louisiana originated in and has been maintained by force and fraud in opposition to the will of a large majority of the voters of the State, in opposition to the principles of the Constitution of the United States and in violation of every principle of justice and liberty.
>
> That the dominant faction of the Radical party in the State has, by false and fraudulent represen-

tations, inflamed the passions and prejudices of the negroes, as a race, against the whites, and has therefore made it necessary for the white people to unite and act together in self defense and for the preservation of white civilization.

That the white people of Louisiana have no desire to deprive the colored people of any rights to which they are entitled, but we are convinced that reform is imperatively demanded, and can be effected only by electing to office white men of known capacity and integrity; and we believe that large number of colored citizens will vote with us, to secure a government which must be beneficial alike to both races.[54]

While the White League platform preached that they had no desire to deprive blacks of their rights, that policy in practice was much different. Dr. R.I. Cromwell, a black leader originally from Wisconsin, wrote a letter to the *New Orleans Tribune*, a black newspaper, instructing black voters not to vote for former Confederates who now professed to be supporters of black rights:

They should have nothing to do in reconstructing a State they attempted to destroy, wishing as they did at that time that you and me and all the black race be kept in bondage. Remember the Vice President of the Confederate States who said that the cornerstone of the Confederate Government was negro slavery. And yet these men, the very ones, now come to us—black men—and tell us that they are our best friends—the low debauchee, the overseer of plantations who once dared prowled around your cabins to destroy your families, the old master (so-called) now comes to tell you that he is your best friend, vote for a Southerner whom you know!... And will you be deceived by these old foxy fellows? You must remember how often they have deceived you.... We must take hold of this reconstruction matter, elect as many of our own race as we can, join in with our Southern loyalists, choose good men from among them. But be sure to vote for no Southern man that was a rebel or secessionist.[55]

After refusing to admit defeat in the 1873 election, John McEnery and former Governor Warmoth spent time in Washington diplomatically trying in vain to receive recognition as the State's duly elected governor. Warmoth later recalled in his autobiography: "In our efforts to induce Congress to recognize the McEnery Government, we had great difficulty in keeping the violent element in our State in order. The outrage upon the people was so stupendous and the establishment and maintenance of the Kellogg Government by force aroused such bitter resentment that it is to the credit of the masses of the people of Louisiana that they bore it as well as they did. But unfortunately we had one element that we could not control; that was some of the fiery newspaper editors."[56]

At the same time McEnery was in Washington, shipments of arms were arriving in New Orleans to outfit the White League. Governor Kellogg and his municipal police made every effort to block these shipments and confiscate the arms based on the League's stated purpose of opposition to the sitting government. On September 12 the steamer *Mississippi* arrived carrying crates of weapons and ammunition consigned to the White League. As soon as the steamship arrived, the Municipal Police ordered the shipment seized. Many whites viewed Kellogg's actions as further intimidation by the Republican puppet government and a direct intrusion on their Second Amendment rights. Consequently, a mass meeting was called for the morning of Monday, September 14, 1874, to demonstrate against the sitting government and demand Kellogg's resignation. The meeting was to take place at the Henry Clay Statue on Canal Street. Several thousand white citizens showed up, giving the McEnery followers confidence that the public was on their side.[57] The public gathering at the Clay Statue was meant as a show of support. Once they felt that the public was on their side, they could then take more direct action. Their plan was to forcefully obtain possession of the government by occupying the offices and capturing the State officials.

The Honorable R.H. Marr addressed the crowd with a resolution demanding that Kellogg abdicate his role as governor. (R.H. Marr was one of the defense attorneys for the nine paramilitaries charged in the federal case against those involved in the Colfax Massacre.)

Whereas, at a general election held in Louisiana on the 4th day of November, 1872, John McEnery was elected Governor by a majority of nearly ten thousand over his opponent, William Pitt Kellogg, and D.B. Penn, Lieutenant Governor, by a majority of fifteen thousand over his opponent, C.C. Antoine; and, whereas, by fraud and violence, these defeated candidates seized the Executive chair, … And whereas, by false and infamous representations of the motive of our people, he has received the promise of aid from the Federal army, placed at the orders of the Attorney General of the United States, and subject to the calls of United States supervisors, for the purpose of overawing our State and controlling the election; and, whereas, in the language of the call for this meeting, "one of our dearest rights have been trampled upon," until at last, in the supreme height of its insolence, this mockery of a republican government has even dared to deny that right so solemnly guaranteed by the Constitution of the United States, which declares "that the right of the people to bear arms shall never be infringed." Be it resolved, that we reaffirm solemnly the resolutions adopted by the white people of Louisiana, in convention assembled at Baton Rouge, on August 24, 1874:

That the white people of Louisiana have no right to deprive the colored people of their rights.

That W.P. Kellogg is a mere usurper, and we denounce him as such.

That his government is arbitrary, unjust and oppressive, and can only maintain itself through Federal interference….

Therefore, in the name of the citizens of New Orleans, in mass meeting assembled, and of the people of the State of Louisiana, whose franchise has been wrested from them by fraud and violence, and all of whose rights and liberties have been outraged and trampled upon—

We demand of William Pitt Kellogg his immediate abdication.[58]

Once the group's leaders felt the public was behind them, their

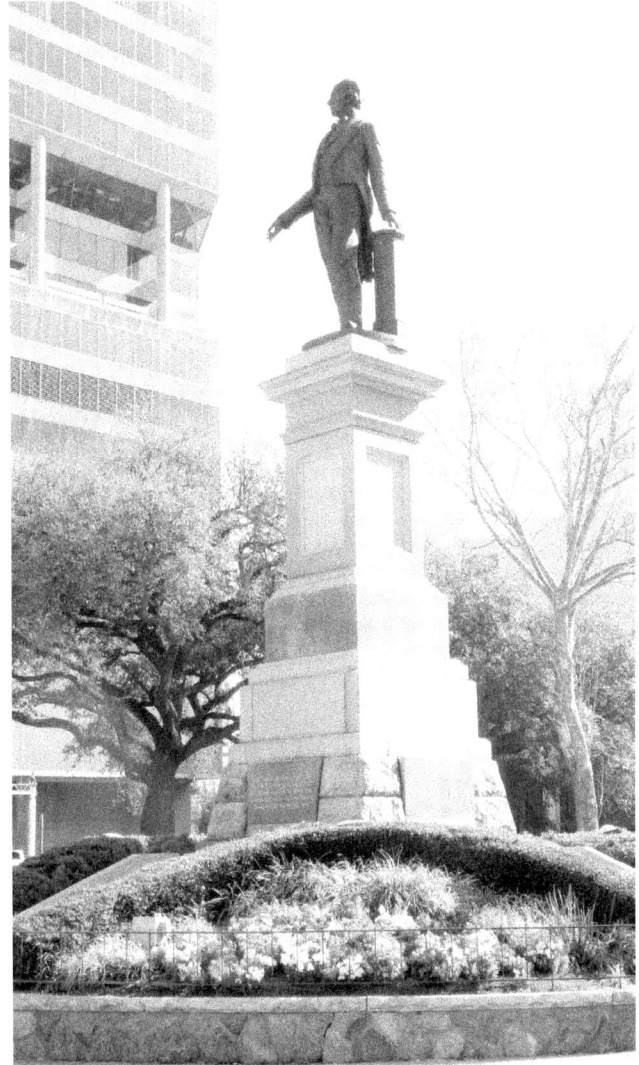

The Henry Clay statue was originally erected on Canal Street where Judge Marr and members of the Crescent City White League met in 1874 prior to the Battle of Liberty Place. In 1900 the statue was relocated to Lafayette Square, its current home and the locale where Dr. Tebault lived. Photograph by author.

strategy was to erect barricades in the streets in a defensive posture that would draw out Major General James Longstreet and his Metropolitan Police from the State House, leaving it unprotected and easily taken. Many viewed the Metropolitan Police with contempt as the governor's paid soldiers, guarding the State House and spending little time pursuing crime in the city. At the end of the demonstration, Marr asked the assembled mob to go home to arm themselves and return at 2:30 for instructions. Meanwhile, the White Leagues had already started assembling elsewhere in the city by Companies. Dr. Tebault arrived as a Private in Company D of the Crescent City White League under the command of Captain Archibald Mitchell. His brother William Grantland Tebault joined Company E, and his other brother, B. Rutledge Tebault, joined arms with Company B. All these Companies formed the right wing under the commands of Captains Edward Flood, F.M. Andress, and C.H. Allen.[59] The men were additionally supported by one 12-pound artillery piece. The center extended from Tchoupitoulas Street to Camp Street under the commands of Captains George Dupree, Thomas McIntyre and A.B. Phillips. On the left were the commands of Major Gustave LeGardeur and Captains O.M. Tennison and Charles Vautier. Additionally, sharpshooters were positioned on top of roofs and in the upper floors of buildings lining Canal Street.

They also erected barricades from wagons, mattresses, streetcars, bales of cotton and anything else that could be found that would afford protection to the guards who waited behind them.

The Battle of Liberty Place

Accounts of robberies and the rapes of white women by blacks ignited open hostilities. Unsubstantiated rumors of the Republican administration providing weapons to blacks created fear and anger in the white community. The White League in New Orleans had begun to buy shipments of arms under the pretense of defending themselves, one such shipment having been confiscated, which led to the morning meeting at the Henry Clay statue on Canal Street on September 14.

At around 4 PM that afternoon, 500 Metropolitan Police led by General Longstreet stationed themselves in front of the Custom House where Kellogg had taken refuge. A few minutes later the police opened fire on an approaching mob with two 12-pound Napoleon cannons and a Gatling gun. Meanwhile some of the White League men attacked the flanks of the police, forcing them back to the Custom House in a disorganized panic. What remained of the Metropolitan Police force retreated to Jackson Square. The battle had lasted only 15 minutes with a loss of 16 White League men killed and another 45 wounded, and 11 Metropolitan Police killed and 60 wounded.[60] The next morning the White League captured the State House and police headquarters.

The White League had carefully prepared assault plans but had not anticipated the need for a medical staff. Around 7 PM on the day of the battle, Dr. Samuel Choppin asked Drs. Tebault, Samuel Logan and Howard Smith to set up a medical corps. Dr. Tebault was appointed as Medical Purveyor. Dr. Logan was put in charge of the ambulance corps. City druggists contributed chloroform, bandages, opium, sponges, and other medical supplies.[61] Later, Dr. Tebault wrote a letter to the editors of the *Times-Picayune* on September 16 in response to an article in the paper erroneously attributing his namesake as supporting the Kellogg forces during the battle:

4. Reconstruction

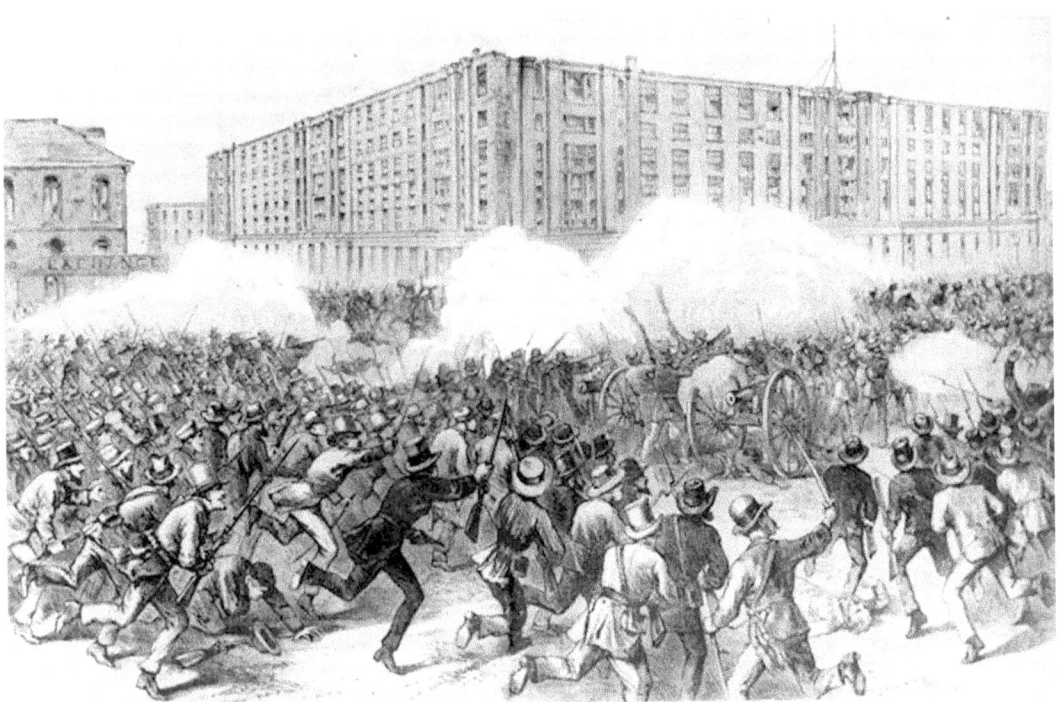

The Battle of Liberty Place. On September 14, 1874, approximately 5,000 members of the Crescent City White League and their supporters fought against the outnumbered New Orleans Metropolitan Police, led by former Confederate General James Longstreet. The object of the rioters was to forcibly remove from office Republican Governor John McEnery, who was appointed after the contested 1872 election and whom they considered to be illegitimate. Public domain—copied from *Frank Leslie's Illustrated Newspaper*, December 31, 1874.

New Orleans, Sept. 16, 1874

To the Editor of the Picayune:

In your issue of this evening, I observe that you mention the name of Tebault as belonging to one of Kellogg's wounded policemen. Permit me to state that the name mentioned has never served in any such position, nor has it ever faltered in its uncompromising opposition to Kellogg. In proof of this, two bearing that name—B. Rutledge Tebault of Company B, and William G. Tebault, of Company E, of the Crescent City White League—were where the fighting was hottest and cannons to be taken at the point of the bayonet.

C.H. Tebault, M.D.
Late Asst. Med. Purveyor State Forces.[62]

A short-lived celebration followed the Battle of Liberty Place, as the confrontation was called. On September 16, the *Picayune* ran a tribute to the dead "martyrs" of the White League:

HONORS TO THE DEAD
Who Gave Up their Lives in Defense of Our Common Liberties
Tears which Embalm the Memory of Martyrs
Yesterday evening was a time when the true citizens of New Orleans had their hearts stirred with the proudest and most triumphant emotions that the higher nature of men can feel, and it was a time, too, when many hearts were clouded with the deepest sorrow that dims the luster of victory in the midst of tears....

Three days later, the *Picayune* published a rather histrionic congratulatory article under the headline:

> "A Free People." At 9 o'clock this morning Louisiana leaped from bondage into the full strength and splendor of freedom. Borne down, repressed, tortured and despoiled for six long, weary years, the jest of spectators and the spoil of thieves her great arm has at last been lifted, and with one tremendous blow the fetters have been stricken from her limbs. For this one day, if never again she breathes the air of liberty. Her persecutors are scattered. The scurvy horde of robbers, paid ruffians and brutal task masters are vanished. There is no one who dares to brave the indignation of a great people roused at last. The *Picayune* congratulates the noble State in which for nearly half a century its destinies have been cast. If at any time in the past it has seemed lacking in sympathy, it has been because we differed in opinion as to the wisest method of achieving the commonly desired end. We may do so again. But with freedom the emancipation of our people, with the gallant assertion of the people's rights and the glorious manifestations of our brethren's courage, the *Picayune's* heart beats in unison, and swells in honest, unaffected pride. We congratulate New Orleans as the author of the grand blow which as freed the State—we congratulate Louisiana on the long, sweet breath of freedom she inspires today![63]

The celebration would not be a long one. On September 15, 1874, President Grant issued Proclamation 220—Law and Order in the State of Louisiana:

> Whereas it has been satisfactorily represented to me that turbulent and disorderly persons have combined together with force and arms to overthrow the State government of Louisiana and to resist the laws and constituted authorities of said State: and
>
> Whereas it is provided in the Constitution of the United States that the United States shall protect every State in this Union, on application of the legislature, or of the executive when the legislature can not be convened, against domestic violence; and
>
> Whereas it is provided in the laws of the United States that in all cases of insurrection in any State or of obstruction to the laws thereof it shall be lawful for the President of the United States, on application of the legislature of such State, or of the executive when the legislature can not be convened, to call forth the militia of any other State or States, or to employ such part of the land and naval forces as shall be judged necessary, for the purpose of suppressing such insurrection or causing the laws to be duly executed; and
>
> Whereas the legislature of said State is not now in session and can not be convened in time to meet the present emergency, and the executive of said State, under section 4 of Article IV of the Constitution of the United States and the laws passed in pursuance thereof, has therefore made application to me for such part of the military force of the United States as may be necessary and adequate to protect said State and the citizens thereof against domestic violence and to enforce the due execution of the laws; and
>
> Whereas it is required that whenever it may be necessary, in the judgment of the President, to use the military force for the purpose aforesaid, he shall forthwith, by proclamation, command such insurgents to disperse and retire peaceably to their respective homes within a limited time.
>
> Now, therefore, I, Ulysses S. Grant, President of the United States, do hereby make proclamation and command said turbulent and disorderly persons to disperse and retire peaceably to their respective abodes within five days from this date, and hereafter to submit themselves to the laws and constituted authorities of said State; and I invoke the aid and cooperation of all good citizens thereof to uphold law and preserve the public peace.
>
> In witness whereof I have hereunto set my hand and caused the seal of the United States to be affixed.
>
> Done at the city of Washington, this 15th day of September, A.D. 1874, and of the Independence of the United States the ninety-ninth.
>
> U.S. GRANT.[64]

Federal military units began to arrive in New Orleans to ensure order. The support of the Federal Government gave confidence to Governor Kellogg who returned peacefully to his office on September 19 after the White Leagues notified him that the insurrection was over.

On September 20, 1874, the *Daily Picayune* published a retrospective of the event:

> We take it that every good citizen of New Orleans will devote part of this day to the events of the week just passed. It was difficult at first to estimate them properly, and even now they seem too vast for measurement. We can think of them though we can never forget them. They are so tragic and glorious and tremendous.... In five minutes the Kellogg administration had collapsed, and so far as its unaided resources were concerned, was a thing forever obliterated. Then came the Government of the people with joy and hope and gladness for its consecration and strength and safety as its promise.... Next day the United States Army stepped in, and now the situation is completed. A Government which could not summon fifty followers on Thursday morning is thrust by United States bayonets into the place of one that had fifty thousand soldiers at its back.
>
> But we have shown the world three all important truths...:
> 1. That we were not seeking to deprive the colored people of their rights.
> 2. That we were not in rebellion against the United States authority.
> 3. That the Kellogg Government had not the ghost of support independent of the U.S. army; that it was not republican in any essential respect, and that the people, white or colored, extended no hand to prop or save it.[65]

To Dr. Tebault and many whites in Louisiana, the Battle of Liberty Place was a repercussion of what they considered to be the unjust Reconstruction policies imposed upon Louisiana. To them, there was reason to celebrate the battle and honor those whites who had died defending the nobility of their cause.

Another opinion piece written in 1924 on the 50th anniversary of the Battle of Liberty Place reaffirmed the importance of the battle:

> On the surface, it would seem that the movement which had resulted in the battle of September 14th, was a failure. But really it was far from such. Although Kellogg remained in power, it was with the clear understanding on all sides that the days of the radical government in Louisiana were numbered. Kellogg learned to pay more deference to the wishes of the people unhappily under his charge. The whole of the United States was interested in the situation which had culminated in so violent an outburst. Thoughtful men everywhere felt that the conditions must indeed have been unendurable which called for a remedy so drastic. Even the Republican leaders began to see that they could no longer carry with safety the load of the "carpetbag" administration. Unquestionably, the results of the congressional elections, which took place six weeks later, were influenced to a considerable degree by what had taken place in Louisiana. The Democrats won a majority of 87 in the House of Representatives—the first time in over twenty years that they had found themselves in control of either branch of Congress.[66]

The Battle of Liberty Place served to shock "the Grant Administration out of the paralysis that had marked its attitude towards Louisiana."[67] Many Republicans now began to sense the futility of certain Reconstruction policies and to understand the brutal determination of its opponents. To succeed, Reconstruction relied upon the active support of white southerners, a factor that Liberty Place had shown to be ineffective. Threats and terrorist acts by the White Leagues, the Ku Klux Klan, and the Knights of the White Camellia had been effective in discouraging white southern Republicans.

The Presidential election of 1876 between Republican Rutherford B. Hayes and Democrat Samuel J. Tilden was to become one of the most controversial and bitterly disputed elections in American history. Early election returns favored Tilden, but as the night grew long Hayes appeared to have won 165 electoral votes and Tilden 184, just one vote shy of a majority. The outcome hung on the 20 electoral votes held by three southern states—Louisiana, South Carolina and Florida—that were still under military rule. In these states the Republican Party controlled the votes.[68] A bipartisan commission was appointed to review the election results, and in a compromise the Republicans on the commission agreed to concessions in return for agreement by the Democrats to award the entire 20 votes to Hayes. The main concessions were the withdrawal of federal troops from the South and the Republican acceptance of locally elected Democratic governments in southern states.[69] The Democrat Tilden and his supporters protested and threatened to march on Washington with force.[70] Tilden appeared to have won the popular vote in those states. Many northern Republicans, however, understood that Reconstruction was failing and supported such a compromise. The result was the Compromise of 1877—in return for the southern votes, the Republicans would withdraw most troops from the South, appoint at least one Democrat to the President's Cabinet, allow the southern states to elect their own governors, and finally bring an end to Reconstruction.[71]

President Hayes wanted to restore good will between Republicans and the southern Democrats in Congress declaring, "the party of Lincoln and Grant was no longer hostile to the South."[72] But in Louisiana, such optimism would be swallowed by conflicting economic and cultural realities. The policies of Reconstruction had punished New Orleans longer than any other Southern city, and the resulting wounds would require decades to heal. The city's economy had declined sharply the last few years of Federal oversight, and most citizens sought a return to normalcy by bringing back many of the old traditions.

On September 14, 1891, the cornerstone of a monument to the Battle of Liberty Place was erected with much fanfare in front of a large crowd of proud onlookers "in honor of those who fell in defense of civil liberty and home rule in that heroic and successful struggle of the 14th of September 1874."[73] In his book, *The Battle of Liberty Place*, Stuart Landry summarizes the effect the conflict had on American opinion:

> The White Leaguers accepted the situation, and it seemed that all their efforts were useless and their splendid victory unavailing. But it was far from such.... The struggle of the people in Louisiana against inefficient and corrupt government, instituted by fraud and kept in power by Federal bayonets, won the admiration and sympathy of much of the press as well as many of the people in the North.... The Battle of Liberty Place in 1874 changed the tide of opinion, brought the end of Reconstruction in the South, and started the Southern people on their way to the great prosperity which they now enjoy.... It was a glorious victory, but as with many other great battles, what was the use?[74]

(Landry is the great-great-grandson of one of the participants.)

The Battle of Liberty Place monument consisted of a stone obelisk mounted onto an engraved plinth and was located on what was considered to have been neutral ground near the foot of Canal Street. In the later part of the 20th century, many residents, especially blacks, became vocal in their objections to the monument as a symbol of racism, and the obelisk was the site of numerous protests and rallies by both white supremacists and those who wished the monument torn down. White supremacist David Duke, who lives just outside of New Orleans, referred to the monument as a symbol of pride and used it for some of his rallies, while others frequently vandalized it as an unwanted emblem of racism.[75] In 1974 the city took the conciliatory measure of adding a base recognizing the sacrifices on both sides with an inscription: "In honor of those Americans on both sides of the conflict who died in the Battle of Liberty Place" with the names of members of the Metropolitan Police who also had died in the struggle. The inscription ends with "A conflict of the past that should teach us lessons for the future." In 1993 the monument was relocated to a much less prominent position next to railroad tracks and behind a parking garage. The monument was finally removed in 2017 under the cover of darkness and placed into storage as it once again served as an unwelcome lightening rod for violence and discord.

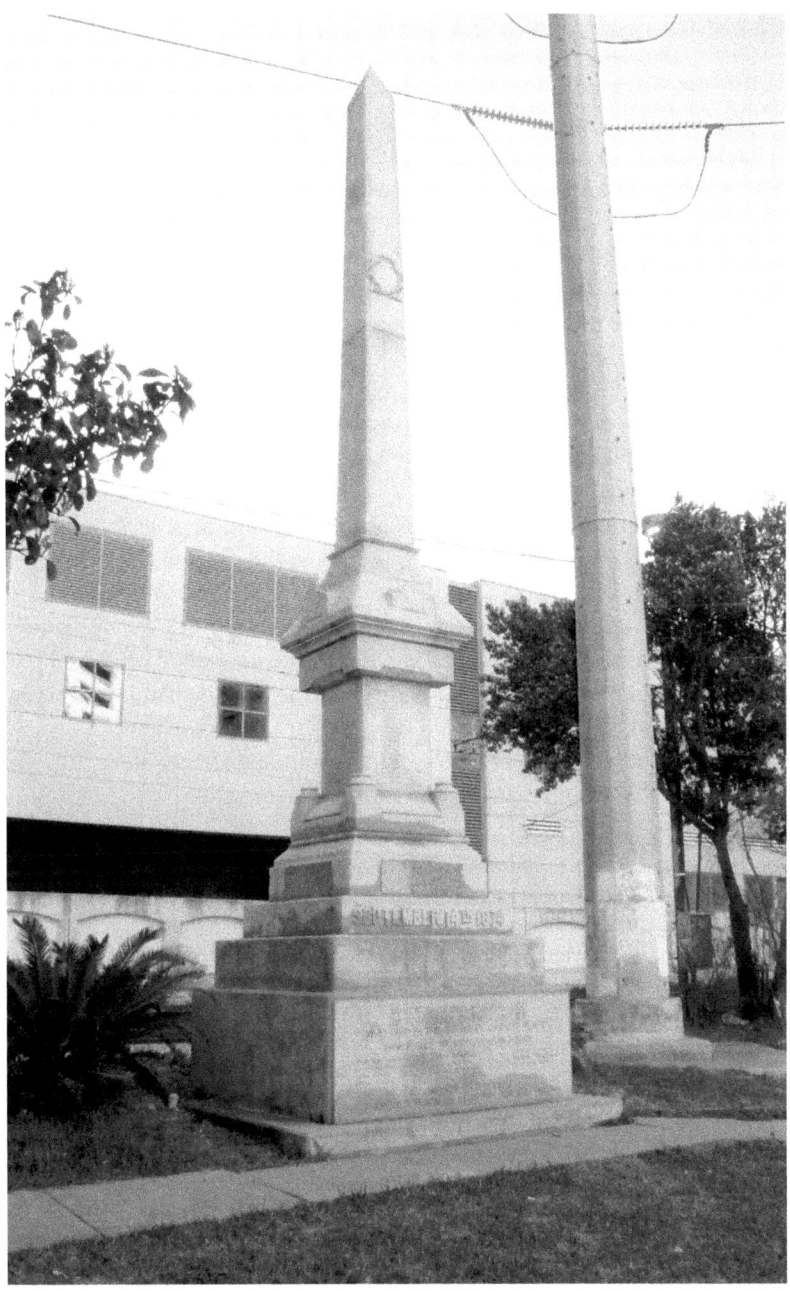

In 1891 the city erected the Battle of Liberty Place Monument on Canal Street, a white marble obelisk commemorating the white men who had died during the fight. In 1932 an inscription was added: "…the national election of November 1876 recognized white supremacy in the South…." In 1993 the original inscriptions were replaced with a more inclusive statement: "In honor of those Americans on both sides who died in the Battle of Liberty Place," and added a list of the names of the Metropolitan Police who had also died; below those names was engraved: "A conflict of the past that should teach us lessons for the future." Because the monument had become a catalyst for white supremacist groups and protesters, the monument was moved to a less conspicuous place near a parking garage in 1993, where the above photograph was taken. It was finally removed and placed into storage in 2017 (author's collection).

The Real Estate and Direct Taxpayers' Union

Following the Battle of Liberty Place and the Compromise of 1877, Reconstruction gradually dissipated and southern states began to slowly exercise control of their own governments. Racial issues became less important as a Democratic party issue and began to be replaced by the punishing taxation imposed on the South by Radical Republicans in Congress intent on making the former rebels pay for the economic cost of the war. New Orleans had been profoundly in debt before Reconstruction, but post–Reconstruction debt soured to all-time highs. City taxes became significant additions to the already burdensome state taxes—New Orleans property holders were forced to pay the city approximately $5 for every $100 of assessed value.[76]

Land in the South had largely been untaxed before the war. Poll taxes, and taxes on slaves and commercial activities provided most of the revenues needed by each state. (A poll tax requires an individual to pay a levy in order to vote. During Reconstruction, many southern states used the tax to restrict black votes by levying high poll taxes on anyone whose father or grandfather had not voted prior to the abolition of slavery.) The new property taxes forced many landowners to sell their land as they lacked the cash with which to pay. During Reconstruction vast tracts of land were turned over to the states for failure to pay the taxes. In 1874 Stephen Duncan, the largest cotton producer in the South before the war, lost seven of his Louisiana plantations that were auctioned off.[77] Many blacks had hoped that such auctions would enable them to buy inexpensive land, which did occur in some southern states such as Georgia.

At a Republican meeting in Raleigh, North Carolina, a former slave, Abraham Galloway, voiced his strong opinion regarding the new property taxes:

> Mr. President, Ladies and Gentlemen: It is with much embarrassment that I address you this evening, being a young man scarcely out of my teens. The great issue, it seeing to me, which agitates the wounds of the American people is the reconstruction of the so-called Confederate States; and, it is the design of the Republican party to reconstruct these States on such a basis that this Union can never be again disturbed by rebellion or a rebellious spirit.... When Congress conveyed to the negro the right to vote, it also conveyed to him the same right to hold office, if we are capable, and I am perfectly willing to vote for any man upon the Republican platform, let him be black or white, let him be Yankee or Southerner, Dutchman or Irishman.... Now, what we want to establish is a free school system in North Carolina. And how are we going to get that? By taxation. I know we have got a pretty heavy tax now. But I want to see these men in North-Carolina who own twenty acres of land that pay as much taxes, as a man that owns five or six hundred, I want to see that stopped. I want to see the man who owns one or two thousand acres of land taxed a dollar on the acre; and if they can't pay the taxes, sell their property to the highest bidder let the Sheriff sell it. And then we negroes shall become land holders. I would say to the poor white men of North Carolina, it behooves you as well as the negro, to participate in the reconstruction of the Commonwealth of North-Carolina. Only look around us. Poverty stares us in the face. Why? Because the Northern people have the money! And I tell you they will never send it down here until you are reconstructed, and when you do that peace and harmony will prevail, and there will be no longer any talk about negro insurrection, and the man who talks that is not only an enemy to the negro, but an enemy to the Commonwealth of North Carolina.[78]

Abraham Galloway was a former North Carolina slave whose father was the white son of the plantation's owner. Galloway had escaped to Pennsylvania and later served as a spy for General Benjamin Butler, gathering intelligence regarding the locations of Confederate forces.[79]

Dr. Tebault became President of the Central Executive Council of the Real Estate and Direct Taxpayers' Union, which he helped organize in 1878. This Union, and similar organizations in other parishes, had the mission of fighting for the reduction of taxes. In his position as President, Tebault was vocal about his feeling regarding the post-war South: "The people of New Orleans during the Reconstruction era of rapine and misrule, not to say anarchy ... were made to pay in taxes on an excessive assessment, in one single decade, in round numbers, the stupendous sum of $110,000,000. But even this was not enough, for a bonded debt had also been contracted in addition, in principal and interest, of more than $103,000,000 more. The mind of man becomes confused and dazed in contemplating this prodigious further spoliation of our people, with nothing to show for this wholesale robbery."[80]

In his writings, Tebault focused on the severe tax rates and what he believed to be the unconstitutionality of such taxation.

> This City ... in these ten years [1865–1874] has had a tax contribution extorted from her, on the part of the State and City together, equivalent to her present combined wealth, real and personal.... Do not these facts plead with all the eloquence of truth for mercy and actual reform—that reform, which does not pause in right doing, to ascertain who are the holders of this fraudulent or illegal debt?... How much of our resources have been consumed by these penalties, it is probably impossible to discover. Many properties have passed into other hands through the rigorous and merciless application of this Act; and among these, notably, the properties of widows and orphans and others too reduced in circumstances to contest its constitutionality.... <u>This City cannot recuperate with a tax for all purposes, of State and City, exceeding one and one half percent.</u>[81]

In arguing the unconstitutionality of the taxes, Dr. Tebault refers to the Premium Bond Act 105 that was passed on March 28, 1874, known locally as the Premium Bond "Scheme." It provided harsh penalties for delinquent taxes and for the taking of property if such fines were left unpaid, ranging from 25 percent for taxes unpaid from the previous year (1874) to 150 percent for taxes that had been unpaid five years earlier (1869). Administrative costs were added to these penalties, further inflating the penalties. Dr. Tebault also argued that the Act provided enormous profits to a small number of individuals charged with the Act's supervision. "This is simply preposterous, and I do not think our suffering tax-payers, our working classes, our merchants, bankers, and business men generally, will seriously undertake to make slaves of themselves for the balance of their natural lives, in order to pay with such 'enormous profit' an illegally incurred debt." He referenced a Supreme Court decision that taxes or bonds could not be used by a state or city to benefit private individuals or enterprises. On February 1, 1875, the Supreme Court agreed with a Circuit Court ruling:

> To lay with one hand the power of the government on the property of the citizen and with the other to bestow it upon favored individuals to aid private enterprises and build up private fortunes is none the less a robbery because it is done under the forms of law and is called taxation. This is not legislation. It is a decree under legislative form. Nor is it taxation. A tax, says Webster's Dictionary, is a rate or sum of money assessed on the person or property of a citizen by government for the use of the nation or State. Taxes are burdens or charges imposed by the Legislature upon persons or property to raise money for public purposes.[82]

In November 1875, Dr. Tebault appeared before the Republican State Central Executive Committee with a resolution proposing a maximum tax of 1 percent local and 0.5 percent for the state, making the maximum tax to be paid throughout the state 1.5 percent. He also proposed a Constitutional Convention to set that taxation rate and to prevent "any city, town or parish or county thereof, from contracting any debt or loan, for any purpose or purposes whatever, unless the same be first submitted to the people and receive the approval of three-fourths of the voters of this State."[83] The Republican-dominated Committee opposed Dr. Tebault's resolution. Dr. Tebault commented that "he wished to see a better feeling exist between political parties."[84] In response to that observation, a member of the Committee asserted that it was Republicans, especially "colored Republicans," who were being harassed in New Orleans by Democrats.

Dr. Tebault, undaunted, would continue his fight as President of the Taxpayers' Union to push for a Constitutional Convention to lower the Reconstruction taxes. When the New Orleans Pacific Railway pushed for bonds to support their building of the road, Dr. Tebault was there fighting them and again pushing for a convention to limit the state's debt burden.

A meeting of the Real Estate and Direct Taxpayers' Union on February 16, 1878, was disrupted by a mob of egg-throwing Republicans supported by the police. A Republican-leaning newspaper described the event:

> It was evident from the first that this crowd had come together for the purpose of having a little fun, and before the proceedings were concluded it was plain that they were bound to have their fun, no matter who were made victims.... Dr. Tebault then stepped to the front and began to read a series of propositions, which he desired to submit to the assembly. Then arose a violent tumult on the part of the audience; yells were heard on every side, and eggs and other missiles came hurtling through the air, aimed apparently at the sacred person of the President of the R.E. and T.P. Union. Nevertheless, the Doctor was not to be intimidated, and persisted in his remarks to the end maintaining a dauntless front.[85]

The Union had passed a resolution asking the State Legislature to reduce police salaries, which had not gone unnoticed by the police. Dr. Tebault and other administrators of the Union protested the disturbance of their meeting at the Mayor's office with a threat to take up arms to protect themselves. The *Times-Picayune* described the meeting:

SATURDAY NIGHT'S DISTURBANCE. A Call on the Mayor by Members of the Property Holders Union, The Proceeding's at Clay Statue Indignantly Denounced, An Investigation Ordered.

Yesterday afternoon a delegation composed of Drs. C.H. Tebault and D.W. Brickell, and Messrs. F. Leibrook and T.O. Sally, entered the Mayor's parlor. [Dr. Daniel Warren Brickell (1824–1881) founded the New Orleans School of Medicine and was active in public affairs, being an active member of the White League.] There were present the Mayor, Administrator of Police and Chief Boylan, these officials being then engaged in a consultation as to the arrangements to be made apropos of the Papal ceremonies to be held on Wednesday. Dr. Tebault approached the Mayor and stated that he desired to read a communication which the delegation proposed to submit. Dr. Tebault then read a short communication addressed to the Mayor and Administrators, in which the event which transpired at the meeting in Canal street, Saturday night, were recited, and an investigation was demanded into the conduct of the police on that occasion. Members of the delegation then expressed themselves on the subject in the most energetic manner and insisted that the disturbance at the meeting was an outrage on the rights of citizens, and had the aspect of being in accordance with some preconcerted scheme. Dr. Brickell intimated that he had reason to believe that there was "a power behind the throne" which had instigated the disturbance, but he declined, for private reasons, to give his authority for the statement, or to particularize as to his meaning. Sufficient quiet having been restored, the Mayor requested the gentlemen to be seated, and, read the following communications: Mayoralty of New Orleans, February 18, 1878 To: T.N. Boylan, Chief of Police: You will make an immediate and thorough investigation of the causes which led to the disturbance of the meeting on Canal street on Saturday evening last; also, as far as possible, the parties engaged therein. I also wish to ascertain by what means—and through whose influence, the place of meeting was changed from Lafayette Square to corner of Canal and Royal. Yours. Ed. Pilsbury, Mayor.

(Thomas N. Boylan was named Chief of Police following the September 1874 Battle of Liberty Place and served until 1882; Edward Pilsbury was the 38th Mayor of New Orleans and served from December 19, 1876 to November 18, 1878.)

4. Reconstruction

Police Orders, New Orleans. Feb. 17, 11 A. M.

Capt. J.B. Kelly, Commanding Third Precinct: You will make a thorough investigation of the disgraceful affair which took place on the corner of Canal and Royal streets, last night, whilst a public meeting was being conducted.... It is possible that you tolerated such conduct and allowed peaceable citizens to be disturbed and assaulted without any arrest being made, or even a report being made to this office on the subject. You will furnish me with the names of all your detail at that point, and you will make affidavit and make arrest of all whom you can find out were guilty of throwing missiles of any kind on the gallery of A.B. Griswold & Co. whilst the meeting was going on. Every effort must be made to ascertain the names of such parties. In short, I want a full report of this matter, and of your action in the disturbance.

T. N. Boylan, Chief of Police.

The Mayor stated that no one lamented the disturbance more than him—he had not anticipated any interruption to the meeting and regretted that it had occurred. If the events could have been foreseen he would have caused such a disposition of police to have been made as to have fully protected the assemblage. He remarked that it was at the request of the parties having charge of the arrangements that permission had been granted to them to hold the meeting at the corner of Royal and Canal streets instead of in Lafayette Square. Mr. Boylan stated that he was in possession of the names of the policemen who were on the beat at the time, and he was desirous of obtaining all the information, in regard to their conduct. He, together with the Mayor and the Administrator of Police, expressed their intention to cause the fullest investigation to be made into the circumstances of the affair.

The members of the delegation commented very severely on the conduct of the police, and indicated their opinion that the movement was incited by parties who were interested in breaking up the meeting. Dr. Tebault stated that it was proposed to hold a mass meeting in Lafayette Square on Saturday night, and that if the city authorities would not guarantee protection, measures would be taken by the parties concerned to protect themselves. The Mayor said that such steps would be taken as to insure the safety of the speakers and prevent a repetition of the scenes of Saturday night. The delegation then withdrew. It is understood that the investigation will be opened at the next meeting of the Police Board.[86]

While the incident was further investigated with public hearings, no arrests were made. Dr. Tebault, however, was earning the contempt of the Republican-led police force as well as Republican-leaning newspapers. One such newspaper disapprovingly commented on Dr. Tebault's push for a Constitutional Convention: "a series of resolutions passed by the fanatic Dr. Tebault.... The right of a people to petition for a redress of grievances is undisputed but if this terrific demand for a Constitutional Convention has been so prevalent among the masses, why have they not expressed themselves in the way and manner in which their sentiments and wishes are universally known: by petition and remonstrance?"[87] Another editor criticized: "With the exception of a mass meeting in New Orleans headed by Dr. Tebault, who ought to be an inmate of an insane Asylum so far as his politics are indications of his sanity, there have been no demonstration of any such demands by the people anywhere in the State."[88] Still another newspaper insultingly remarked:

Our own, our beloved Tebault has breathed out his presence like an exhalation on an equinoctial, and for a decade of long, yearning days, we shall know him no more. The labyrinths of Lafayette Square shall echo not to his firm and strident voice; the halls of the frisky legislator shall be cold with absence of his smile.... Like Spartans from the arena—like Catiline from the Senate, he has departed. Where now is Property? Where Repudiation? Where all the noble and inherent principles so patriotically and enthusiastically laid down from Griswold's gallery, amid the fiery hiss of flying eggs, and the lurid volley of carrots? Ha! Thinkest all dead? Never! Tebault will never desert Property and Principle, Repudiation and the Rag Baby. He will again, again be in our midst, as the *Pic* rapturously remarks, with renewed vigor and smoothed front, waiting from time to time, as eggs happen to fluctuate, to impart to thirsty ears the only true way to insolvency and happiness.[89]

(*Pic* refers to the *Times-Picayune*, a Democrat-leaning newspaper in New Orleans.)

In spite of all the negative rhetoric from Republican-leaning newspapers, the Real Estate and Direct Taxpayers' Union was ultimately successful in limiting the burdensome taxation policies of Reconstruction. The 1898 Constitutional Convention would finally put the issue to rest by writing into the new state constitution the limitations Dr. Tebault proposed. His tireless efforts, which began as an almost hopeless dream, had been ratified by the people of Louisiana.

Louisiana State Lottery

In addition to fighting the punitive taxation policies of Reconstruction, Dr. Tebault, as President of the Real Estate and Direct Taxpayers' Union, also launched his opposition to the Louisiana State Lottery in 1878. Dr. Tebault's argument that city taxes or bonds should not be used to benefit private individuals also applied to the Lottery, as its formation was the result of bribes and extortion, and ultimately a few individuals would line their pockets with vast sums.

The Louisiana State Lottery was originally proposed as a means of increasing the state revenues. Under the proposed charter, the State of Louisiana would grant the Lottery Company a 25-year term, and, in turn, the Lottery would pay the state of Louisiana $40,000 per year. The Lottery would also be given an effective monopoly, as no other lottery company would be allowed. Opposition to the bill was raised on grounds of the immorality of gambling, the monopoly that was proposed, and the fact that the Lottery would be exempt from taxation. Governor Warmoth vetoed the bill establishing the Lottery but was overridden by the Republican state legislature, which at the time was largely controlled by northern carpetbaggers and legislators who were bribed by the Lottery Company's backers. It was Warmoth's veto that ultimately led to his impeachment, a political effort led by the Lottery's supporters. Warmoth's successor, Pinckney Benton Stewart Pinchback, was an opportunist who had also taken bribes from the Lottery supporters. The Louisiana Lottery Company was granted its charter in 1868 and was ready for business by year's end. Act 25 of the 1868 State Legislature authorized the lottery's incorporation and granted it a 25-year charter, with an annual fee of $40,000 paid to the State.[90]

Initially, the Louisiana Lottery Company benefited from being the only legitimate lottery in the country. Lottery tickets were sold by mail throughout the United States and even in foreign countries. In an effort to legitimize its workings, former Confederate generals P.G.T. Beauregard and Jubal Early were paid handsomely to help supervise the drawings. (General Pierre Gustave Toutant Beauregard was one of Lee's prominent generals during the war. He became rich from his sponsorship of the lottery; General Jubal Anderson Early served under Thomas "Stonewall" Jackson and Robert E. Lee during the war. His writings published in the *Southern Historical Society* helped establish the tenets of the Lost Cause. He was an unrepentant rebel until his death in 1894.)

While General Beauregard was not a big lottery supporter, he was also not opposed to it and felt that it could add significantly to the wealth of the state if properly conducted. He agreed to lend his name and support to the lottery under the provision that he would choose his associate, Jubal Early, and that they had the authority to stop the drawings at once if any fraud was detected and report the matter to the state's Attorney General. Of course, it was almost impossible for either Beauregard or Early to detect any fraud, as their role was to oversee the actual drawings themselves—how much money was allocated as a prize and to whom it would be paid was not under their scrutiny. The Company benefited greatly from Beauregard's and Early's participation. The Lottery Company continued to control the state legislature through bribery and extortion. It not only was able to prevent the chartering of a competitive lottery in 1874, but it also ensured that no lottery tickets from another state could be sold in Louisiana. Charles T. Howard was the company's managing director, and he exercised control over many politicians and legislators. Howard (1832–1885) was born in Baltimore and had arrived in New Orleans in 1852. After the war, Howard claimed to have been a Confederate soldier and sought membership in the Society of the Army of Tennessee; his application was dismissed after it was discovered that Howard had never served. In 1866 he was appointed as agent for the Kentucky Lottery, which desired to expand their operations into Louisiana. Howard applied to the Louisiana Legislature to form a state lottery, but his application was rejected. Two years later, after bribing key state officials, he was finally granted the go-ahead. Wanting complete control in the new enterprise, Howard refused to relinquish control to his employer, the company that ran the Kentucky lottery. Thus, the Louisiana Lottery Company came into existence in 1868 with much controversy and Howard as its President. He and his friends, whom he had appointed to the Board of Directors, received 50 percent of all profits and liberally "greased" the palms of key legislators to ensure the Lottery's success.[91]

An amusing legend of corruption relates to the Metairie Cemetery, where Charles Howard, Dr. Tebault, and General Beauregard are now buried. The Metairie Racecourse had been a renowned one-mile track constructed in 1838 just outside New Orleans. It was the exclusive club of its time and had hosted a number of famous races. During the war, part of the racecourse was used as Camp Walker, a camp to house and train Confederate soldiers. Now, after the war, it was in the process of being restored to its prior glory. In 1871 Charles Howard was asked to lend his support to the effort by the founders of the Metairie Jockey Club, its new name. In return for his support, Howard would become a member of what was planned as an exclusive club of influential and wealthy men. Such a club membership perfectly fit Howard's agenda, as he aspired to become a leader of New Orleans society. The old Creole families, however, viewed Howard with mistrust and disdain. They balked at

Howard organized the Louisiana State Lottery Company in 1868. Noted for its bribery of lawmakers and corrupt practices, the lottery sold tickets throughout the country by mail until the U.S. Postal Service finally banned the practice in 1890. Former Confederate generals P.G.T. Beauregard and Jubal Early were hired by Howard to draw numbers and add credibility to the lottery. Public domain—copied from *Times-Picayune*, 1888.

his corrupt ties to northern Republicans, and most opposed the corruption of the Lottery Company. As a result, the old-guard members of the new club blackballed Howard. When Howard heard, he was furious and was quoted as saying: "Black-balled me, have they? I never forgive an insult. I'll turn their damn racetrack into a cemetery."[92] The Metairie Jockey Club struggled in its efforts; the war had destroyed much of the wealth of Louisiana as well as many of its young men leaving a changed society. By 1872, the Club was ready to sell, and Howard got his wish. He built the Metairie Cemetery around the one-mile track oval, and Howard's tomb is centrally located and one of the largest tombs in the cemetery.[93] The veracity of this story can be debated, but the legend has survived because it is quite plausible based on Howard's character. And, the Metairie Cemetery's crypts and memorials today remain arranged on a one-mile oval.

The growing power and success of the corrupt Lottery Company stimulated new opposition, and in 1876 three bills were unsuccessfully introduced to the state legislature that would (1) repeal the company's charter; (2) repeal the 1874 acts that guaranteed the company's monopoly; and (3) investigate the charges of bribery of the legislators who originally granted the company its charter.[94] Another bill to repeal the company's charter was introduced in 1877 but again defeated. The Governor of Louisiana at the time was Governor Nicholls, who had happily accepted donations from the lottery during the election but later showed no allegiance to it after he was secure in office. Many of the Governor's friends were opponents to the Lottery Company, and consequently, the company planned to undermine the Governor's political power and ensure their continued status.

Dr. Tebault's active opposition to the Lottery added to the building furor over the corrupt organization leading to a Constitutional Convention in 1879. As a result of the Convention, a compromise solution was enacted that recognized the original 25-year charter of the Louisiana Lottery Company but removed its monopoly by allowing competing lottery organizations to participate as long as they paid the state $40,000 per year. The annual payments would be used for supporting the Charity Hospital as well as public schools. Dr. Tebault may have influenced the support of Charity Hospital where he was on staff. He ran as a delegate along with James Nugent for the Convention of 1879, but they both lost to two Republican-backed candidates, John Phelps and James McConnell. Dr. Tebault and Nugent filed a claim of voter fraud with the Committee on Contested Elections based on apparent miscounts at one of the polls, where different results were tallied after each re-count. After examination of the facts, the Committee, which included former Republican Governor Warmoth, found in favor of the Republican candidates.[95] Whether the results had been fixed or not will never be known. Dr. Tebault would later become a delegate to the 1898 Constitutional Convention. But, in 1879, Republicans would exercise complete control of the Convention.

The Louisiana Lottery Company sold many of its tickets outside Louisiana and brought much wealth back to the state of Louisiana, but only to a few men. Before it ultimately went out of business, it had attempted to bribe the state by offering an annual fee of $1,250,000, a testament to the huge sums of money that annually went through the lottery and lined the pockets of its founders, managers and political supporters.

The period of Reconstruction came to an official end with the inauguration of Rutherford B. Hayes in 1877 and the Compromise of 1877. Now "home rule" would be used to resolve the social and political conflicts of southern states, including the issue of black suffrage. New state constitutions were created, the salaries of state officials were reduced, local and state property taxes were slashed, and the states' abilities to incur bonded debt were severely limited, to name a few outcomes of the now "reconstructed" South.[96]

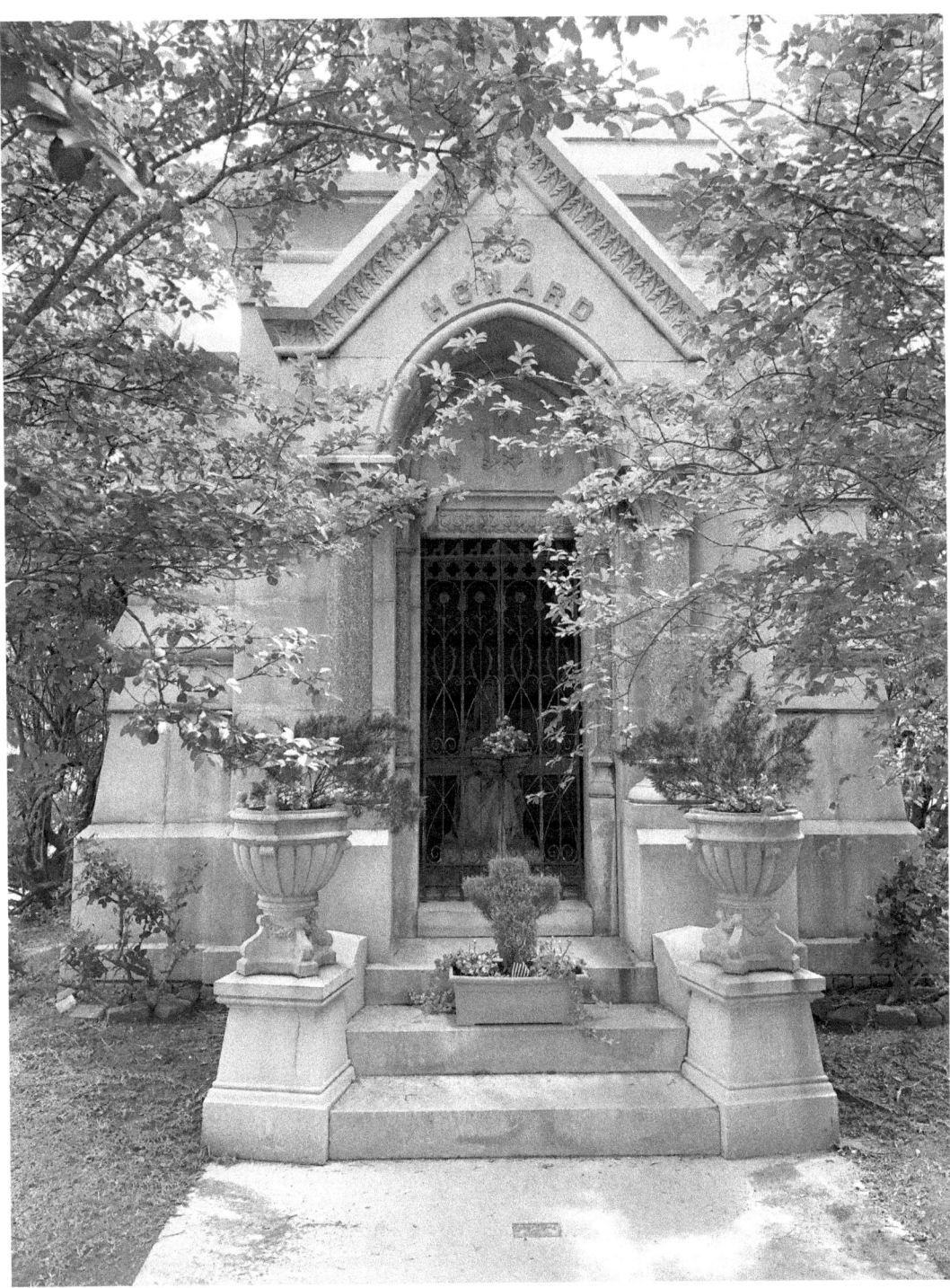

Howard used some of his fortune from the lottery to create Metairie Cemetery on the grounds of the former Metairie Jockey Club. Legend has it that he was blackballed from the club as it was being reinstated following the war, and in retribution he made good on his threat to turn it into a cemetery, with his tomb prominently located at its center. Howard died in 1885 from a carriage accident at the age of 53 (author's collection).

Louisiana State Constitutional Convention of 1898

Former Governor Warmoth was again able to use his political clout to get the unpopular Governor Foster re-elected in 1896 with fraudulent counts. The election had been yet another contentious one full of racism, fraud, and hot emotions. In 1896 the question of a State Constitutional Convention that would be used to disenfranchise ignorant and otherwise "unreliable voters" was put to the ballot. Many blacks and poor whites were unable to vote at the time due to recently passed voter registration laws. These "organic" laws required literacy or property requirements in order to vote, although they also included "grandfather clauses" that would enable poor whites who had previously voted to participate in elections.

The Convention opened in January with an address by the Honorable Ernest B. Kruttschnitt, the President-elect of the Convention. (Ernest B. Kruttschnitt [1852–1906] was a lawyer who served as president of the New Orleans School Board for several years. He played a significant role in denying blacks the right to vote and crafted revisions to the State Convention of 1898 that allowed nonunanimous jury verdicts for criminal trials that ensured that white jurors could override any resistance from black jurors.)

> We are all aware that this convention has been called by the people of the State of Louisiana principally to deal with one question, and we know that but for the existence of that one question this assemblage would not be sitting here today. We know that this convention has been called together by the people of the State to eliminate from the electorate the mass of corrupt and illiterate voters who have during the last quarter of a century degraded our politics.... Only a few years back it might have been considered impolite to say what I am now saying, but there are men standing high today in the councils of the nation who have seen the doors of the White House barred to them by the ignorant and corrupt delegations of Southern negroes, and we know that they cannot but feel a sympathy with us in our aspirations and efforts. (Applause.)
>
> My fellow delegates, let us not be misunderstood! Let us say to the large class of the people of Louisiana who will be disfranchised under any of the proposed limitations of the suffrage, that what we seek to do is undertaken in spirit, not of hostility to any particular men, or set of men, but in the belief that the State should see to the protection of the weaker classes; should guard them against the machinations of those who would use them only to further their own base ends; should see to it that they be not allowed to harm themselves. We owe it to the ignorant, we owe it to the weak, to protect them just as we would protect a little child and prevent it from injuring itself with sharpened tools placed in its hands....
>
> Next to the suffrage question is the question of education, and it requires no argument to prove that we owe it to all of our citizens to say that no man in the future shall complain that he has been deprived of the right to vote because of the poverty of himself or his parents. (Applause.) The State owes it to all that proper educational facilities should be afforded, by which every man shall have the power to educate himself if he so desires, and therefore, gentlemen, I think that the question of public education may rightly be considered a corollary of the suffrage questions....
>
> May this hall where, thirty-two years ago, the negro first entered upon the unequal contest for supremacy, and which has been reddened with his blood, now witness the evolution of our organic law which will establish the relations between the races upon an everlasting foundation of right and justice. (Applause.)[97]

William Jennings Bryan addressed the Convention on March 17, 1898, regarding the Science of Government. (William Jennings Bryan [1860–1925] was a prominent Democrat from Nebraska who was the party's nominee for President on three separate occasions. He perhaps is most famously known for his opposition to Darwinism in the 1925 Scopes Trial just prior to his death.)

> You meet to make your laws. You meet to frame your Constitution and the people of Nebraska have no right to interfere as you have no right to interfere in the local affairs of our State, and yet we are

grouped together in a nation that is greater than any State, and as citizens of sister States we are interested alike in those things that promote the welfare of a nation as a whole and in those things that advance the interests of each State individually.

Let me therefore invite your attention to one fundamental principle. It was the foundation of the political philosophy of Thomas Jefferson, and it was the guiding principle of the public career of Andrew Jackson, and it must be the foundation of all government that is Democratic in form, because no Democratic government can be erected upon any other foundation. What is this principle? I find it in the language of Jefferson expressed in these words: "Equal rights to all and special privileges to none." (Applause)....

My friends the people will bear any sort of legislation no matter how hard it is provided they feel that it is just and impartial, but they won't submit to the least injury if they feel that they are being singled out and that others are being given advantages over them.... But on the other hand, it compels the government to enact such laws as may be necessary for the protection of the weaker members of society against the stronger members, and you will pardon me if I express it as my opinion that the restraining power of government is needed more today than ever before in all the history of the world (applause) and that our government will be a failure unless we proceed to enact such legislation as shall protect the humblest citizen in all the land from injury at the hands of the strongest citizens of all the land. (Applause.)[98]

The Convention also attracted the interest and concerns of both blacks and whites in northern states. Booker T. Washington wrote an open letter to the delegation appealing for fairness (Booker Taliaferro Washington [1856–1915] was a prominent leader of the black community who lived in Alabama. He rallied blacks with the goal of promoting the community's economic development through education and entrepreneurship, rather than advocating direct attacks on the oppressive Black Codes and Jim Crow laws.):

> The Negro agrees with you that it is necessary to the salvation of the South that restriction be put upon the ballot. I know that you have two serious problems before you; ignorant and corrupt government on the one hand, and on the other, a way to restrict the ballot so that control will be in the hands of the intelligent, without regard to race. With the sincerest sympathy with you in your efforts to find a way out of the difficulty, I want to suggest that no State in the South can make a law that will provide an opportunity or temptation for an ignorant white man to vote and withhold the same opportunity from an ignorant colored man, without injuring both men. No State can make a law that can thus be executed, without dwarfing for all time the morals of the white man in the South. Any law that controls the ballot, that is not absolutely just and fair to both races, will work more permanent injury to the whites than to the blacks....
>
> I beg of you, further, that in the degree that you close the ballot-box against the ignorant, that you open the school house. More than half of the people of your State are Negroes. No State can prosper when a large percentage of its citizenship is in ignorance and poverty and has no interest in government....
>
> The highest test of the civilization of any race is in its willingness to extend a helping hand to the less fortunate. A race, like an individual, lifts itself up by lifting others up. Surely no people ever had a greater chance to exhibit the highest Christian fortitude and magnanimity than is now presented to the people of Louisiana.... It is along this line that I pray God the thoughts and activities of your Convention be guided.[99]

Washington's well-intentioned entreaty to the conventioneers to live up to the Convention's stated principles would mostly be ignored. Prior to 1898 most blacks had been disenfranchised from voting, but the Convention and resulting legislation made voting even more difficult for them. Black voter registration fell from 44 percent to only 4 percent by 1900.[100] The Articles of the Convention relating to Suffrage and Elections were quite specific:

> Art 197. Every male citizen of this State and of the United States native born or naturalized, not less than twenty one years of age, and posseting the following qualifications shall be an elector and shall be entitled to vote at any election in this State by the people, except as may be herein otherwise provided:

Sec 1. He shall have been an actual bona fide resident of this State for two years, of the parish one year, and of the precinct in which he offers to vote six months next preceding the election; provided that removal from one precinct to another in the same parish shall not operate to deprive any person of the right to vote in the precinct from which he has removed, until six months after such removal.

Sec 2. He shall have been at the time he offers to vote, legally enrolled as a registered voter on his personal application, in accordance with the provisions of this Constitution and the laws enacted thereunder....

Sec 3. He shall be able to read and write and shall demonstrate his ability to do so when he applies for registration, by making, under oath administered by the registration officer or his deputy, written application therefor, in the English language, or in his mother tongue, which application shall contain the essential facts necessary to show that he is entitled to register and vote, and shall be entirely written, dated and signed by him, in the presence of the registration officer or his deputy, without assistance or suggestion from any person or any memorandum whatever, except the form of application hereinafter set forth; provided however that if the applicant be unable to write his application in the English language, he shall have the right, if he so demands to write the same in his mother tongue from the dictation of an interpreter; and if the applicant is unable to write his application by reason of physical disability, the same shall be written at his dictation by the registration officer or his deputy, upon his oath of such disability. The application for registration, above provided for, shall be a copy of the following form with the proper names, dates, and numbers substituted for the blanks appearing therein to-wit:

I am a citizen of the State of Louisiana. My name is _____. I was born in the State (or country) of _____, Parish (or county) of _____, on the day of _____, in the year _____. I am now _____ years, _____ months, and _____ days of age. I have resided in this State since _____, in this parish since _____, and in Precinct No. ____, of Ward No.____, of this parish since _____, and I am not disfranchised by any provision of the Constitution of this State.

Sec 4. If he be not able to read and write as provided by Section three of this article, then he shall be entitled to register and vote if he shall, at the time he offers to register, be the bona fide owner of property assessed to him in this State at a valuation of not less than three hundred dollars on the assessment roll of the current year in which he offers to register, or on the roll of the preceding year, if the roll of the current year shall not then have been completed and filed, and on which, if such property be personal only, all taxes due shall have been paid....

Sec 5. No male person who was on January 1st, 1867, or at any date prior thereto, entitled to vote under the Constitution or statutes of any State of the United States, wherein he then resided, and no son or grandson of any such person not less than twenty-one years of age at the date of the adoption of this Constitution, and no male person of foreign birth who was naturalized prior to the first day of January 1898, shall be denied the right to register and vote in this State by reason of his failure to possess the educational or property qualifications prescribed by this Constitution; provided, he shall have resided in this State for five years next preceding the date at which he shall apply for registration, and shall have registered in accordance with the terms of this article prior to September 1, 1898, and no person shall be entitled to register under this section after said date....

Art 202. The following persons shall not be permitted to register, vote or hold any office or appointment of honor, trust or profit in this State, to wit: Those who have been convicted of any crime punishable by imprisonment in the penitentiary, and not afterwards pardoned with express restoration of franchise; those who are inmates of any charitable institution, except the Soldiers Home; those actually confined in any public prison; all interdicted persons and all persons notoriously insane or idiotic whether interdicted or not.[101]

The results of the Convention were almost the exact opposite of its noble, stated purposes. Ernest Kruttschnitt had opened the assembly with the promise of "establishing the relations between the races upon an everlasting foundation of rights and justice." William Jennings Bryan had addressed the conventioneers with a quote from Thomas Jefferson regarding the principle of "equal rights to all and special privileges to none." Based on that principle, he suggested that the government needed to enact laws "as may be necessary for the protection of the weaker members of society." The reality was further disenfranchisement and persecution of blacks in Louisiana.

Even so, there were some rather impressive accomplishments of the Convention. Dr. Tebault was an elected delegate to the Convention, serving as a Democrat on three different committees: Health, Quarantine and State Medicine; Internal Improvements; and Pensions for Confederate Veterans. He chaired the Health, Quarantine and State Medicine committee, and the Convention passed laws that established Boards of Health for each parish and for the State. His committee added the provision that the General Assembly shall protect "the people from unqualified practitioners of medicine, and dentistry; protecting confidential communications made to medical men by their patients while under professional treatment and for the purpose of such treatment; for protecting the people against the sale of injurious or adulterated drugs, foods, and drinks, and against any and all adulterations of the general necessaries of life of whatever kinds and character."[102] These provisions protecting against adulterated drugs were enacted 32 years before the U.S. Congress passed the 1906 Pure Food and Drugs Act, which was the predecessor of the Food and Drug Administration (FDA).

It is also a testament to Dr. Tebault's legacy that he strongly supported and promoted public health overseen by boards of health. During his post-war years in New Orleans, Dr. Tebault was actively working towards sanitation and other health policies to reduce the impact of epidemics such as yellow fever. It is remarkable that his committee proposed, and the Convention passed, laws to protect the confidentiality of patients in 1898, not unlike the HIPA Act passed by Congress almost 100 years later. (The Health Insurance Portability and Accountability Act [HIPAA] was passed in 1996 and included patient privacy provisions that carefully control the confidentiality of patients' health information.)

The new Constitution Dr. Tebault helped draft also provided needed relief to Confederate veterans:

> Art 302. The Soldiers Home of the State of Louisiana known as Camp Nicholls shall be maintained by the State, and the General Assembly shall make an appropriation for each year based upon the number of inmates in said home on the first day of April of the year in which said appropriation is made, of one hundred and thirty dollars per capita for the maintenance and clothing of such inmates from which one dollar per month shall be allowed to each inmate for his personal use, and shall make such further appropriations for building, repairs, and incidentals, as may be absolutely necessary.
>
> Art 303. A pension not to exceed eight dollars per month shall be allowed to each Confederate soldier or sailor veteran, who possesses all of the following qualifications:
>
> 1st He shall have served honorably from the date of his enlistment until the close of the late Civil war, or until he was discharged or paroled in some military organization regularly mustered into the army or navy of the Confederate States, and shall have remained true to the Confederate States until the surrender.
>
> 2d He shall be in indigent circumstances and unable to earn a livelihood by his own labor or skill.
>
> 3d He shall not be salaried or otherwise provided for by the State of Louisiana or by any other State or Government....
>
> Art 304. The General Assembly shall appropriate not less than twelve hundred dollars per annum for the maintenance in New Orleans of a Memorial Hall or repository for the collection and preservation of relics and mementoes of the late Civil War and of other objects of interest, and shall be authorized to make suitable appropriations for the erection of monuments and markers on the battlefields of the country, commemorative of the services, upon the fields, of Louisiana soldiers and commands.[103]

Pensions for Confederate veterans lagged behind the care that the North provided Federal veterans, so these new enactments were important, especially given the aging population of the old soldiers. The concept of government-subsidized housing for veterans was not new—the U.S. Naval Home had been established in 1834 and the Old Soldiers' Home for army veterans in 1851.[104] President Lincoln liked to escape the heat and stress of the White House by staying at a summer cottage on a hill overlooking Washington on the Soldiers Home grounds.[105] But in the late 19th century there was an overwhelming need to care for aging and destitute Civil War veterans. The problem in the South was exasperated by the fact that the U.S. Government would not provide any financial support for Confederate homes. In fact, the use of funds to provide support for Confederate veterans was expressly forbidden by the 14th Amendment, which read: "Section 4. The validity of the public debt of the United States, authorized by law, including debts incurred for payment of pensions and bounties for services in suppressing insurrection or rebellion, shall not be questioned. But neither the United States nor any State shall assume or pay any debt or obligation incurred in aid of insurrection or rebellion against the United States, or any claim for the loss or emancipation of any slave; but all such debts, obligations and claims shall be held illegal and void." In contrast, Union soldiers enjoyed pensions and other benefits immediately following the war.[106] It was not until 1958 that Congress finally pardoned Confederate veterans and offered them benefits; at that time, there was only one surviving Confederate veteran.

The Health, Quarantine and State Medicine Committee, under Dr. Tebault's leadership, did much to provide comfort and support for the aging veterans of Louisiana.

Another positive result of the Convention was the establishment of a repository or museum of Confederate artifacts. To this day Memorial Hall in New Orleans preserves important artifacts, memorabilia and ephemera that add greatly to our understanding of the Confederate legacy. Louisiana residents donated much of the collection, and Frank T. Howard, the son of Charles T. Howard who infamously ran the lottery, donated the Romanesque building housing the museum in 1891 that is still in use today. (Frank Turner Howard was born in 1855 and became a prominent banker and financier who financially supported two public schools, the Howard Memorial Library and the Confederate Memorial Hall. He was an important philanthropist in New Orleans, and much of his wealth came from his father, C.T. Howard, who ran the corrupt Louisiana Lottery.)

While the Convention did much to support public health and the lives of Confederate veterans, these improvements were secondary to the main focus on suppressing black votes. Dr. Tebault proposed adding a resolution stating what he and many other white southerners still believed 33 years following the end of the Civil War:

Resolution No. 102. by Mr. Tebault—

Resolved. That the following history of the last three amendments to the Constitution of the United States, which was taken down by an experienced stenographer while being delivered in connection with a law lecture before the Tulane law class by a distinguished statesman, lawyer, and professor of the Tulane Law School, is deserving of preservation. The history is succinctly and briefly stated as follows:

There were no more amendments until the civil war. Mr. Lincoln issued his proclamation of 1863 as a war measure for the emancipation of the negroes. Nobody believed that he had the power to emancipate slaves, but he did it. As soon as we were subjugated, in 1865, they adopted what is called the Thirteenth Amendment. The adoption of this amendment ratified what had been done by Mr. Lincoln, and made constitutional what had been unconstitutional, and abolished slavery in the United States. That was the immediate result of our subjugation. In 1866 they adopted what is called the Fourteenth Amendment to the Constitution, which declares that all persons born or naturalized in the United States, etc. Why did they do it? It was to override the celebrated Dred Scott decision. In that case a free negro had instituted a suit in the courts of the United States in Missouri against a citizen of another State, claiming that he was a free man. The question was whether a free negro was a citizen of the United States. The Supreme Court of the United States decided that a free negro was not and never had been regarded as a citizen either of the colonies or of the State previous to the formation of the United

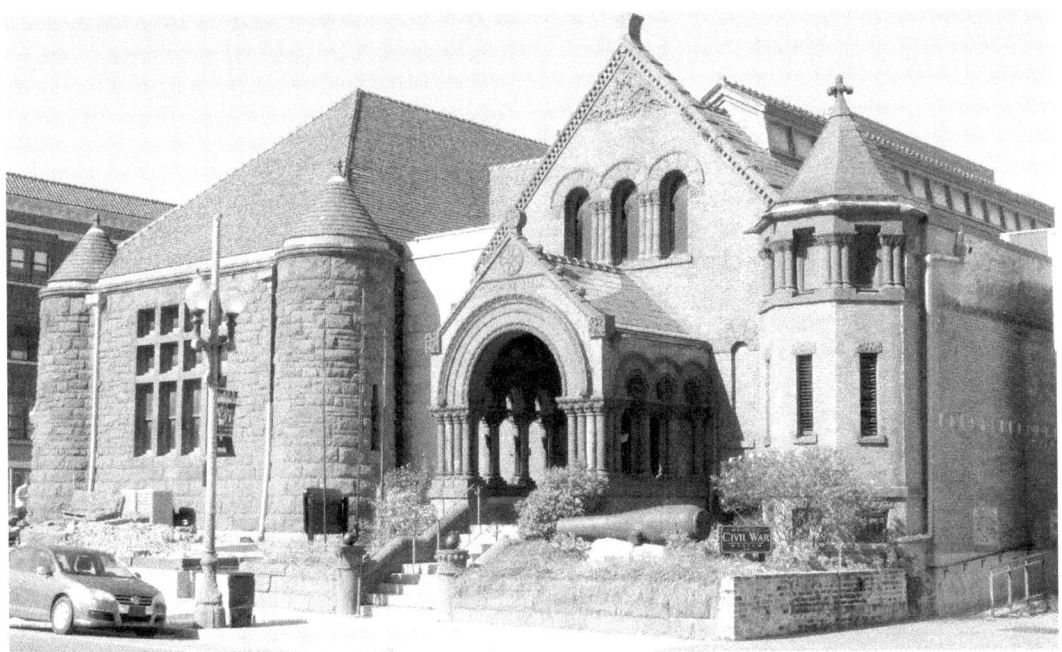

Memorial Hall was originally the Howard Library, built by Frank Howard in honor of his father, Charles T. Howard, who had made a fortune operating the lottery. In 1889 he agreed to finance an annex to the library to store Confederate relics and historical documents. Today the Hall is the home of the Confederate Memorial Hall Museum, housing an impressive historical collection that was largely donated by former Confederates and their families (author's collection).

States; and, therefore, never could be a citizen of the United States. The Chief Justice went into the history of the African race in this country.

Mr. Sumner and Mr. Seward, in the Senate, denounced this decision. The North rose up in arms. The Republican party, when it assembled to nominate a candidate, adopted as a part of its platform that the decision of the Supreme Court of the United States was not binding upon the country on such a question. And they would not recognize it.

Mr. Lincoln was elected upon that platform, and when he was elected the South thought that as the people of the North had prayed for half a century that the Supreme Court of the United States was the arbiter of this constitutional question; that as they had undertaken to repudiate this decision and elect a president on a platform which repudiated the authority of the United States Supreme Court; and that if there was ever a time to go to war that was the time, and they went to war upon it. That is the origin of the civil war. It was not that Mr. Lincoln was elected upon a free-soil platform, but a platform which repudiated a decision of the United States Supreme Court on this subject in contradiction to which they had contended for up to that time, simply because it was in favor of the South. Slaves were after that made citizens, in 1865–66.

Then came the last amendment: The right of citizens of the United States to vote shall not be denied, etc. They thought they had secured the predominance of the Republican Party in the South because the negroes in many of the States were in the majority. Note: "That the right shall not be abridged on account of race, color, or previous condition of servitude." The Supreme Court, when this article came up for consideration, said that this did not give anybody the right to vote. It is true negroes were citizens, but the State could discriminate as to what citizens should or should not vote for any other cause than race, color, or previous servitude. This did not secure to the negroes the right to vote, but merely secured to them that they should not be discriminated against on account of race, color, or servitude.

Resolved. That this valuable and instructive legal history be spread on the journal of this convention.[107]

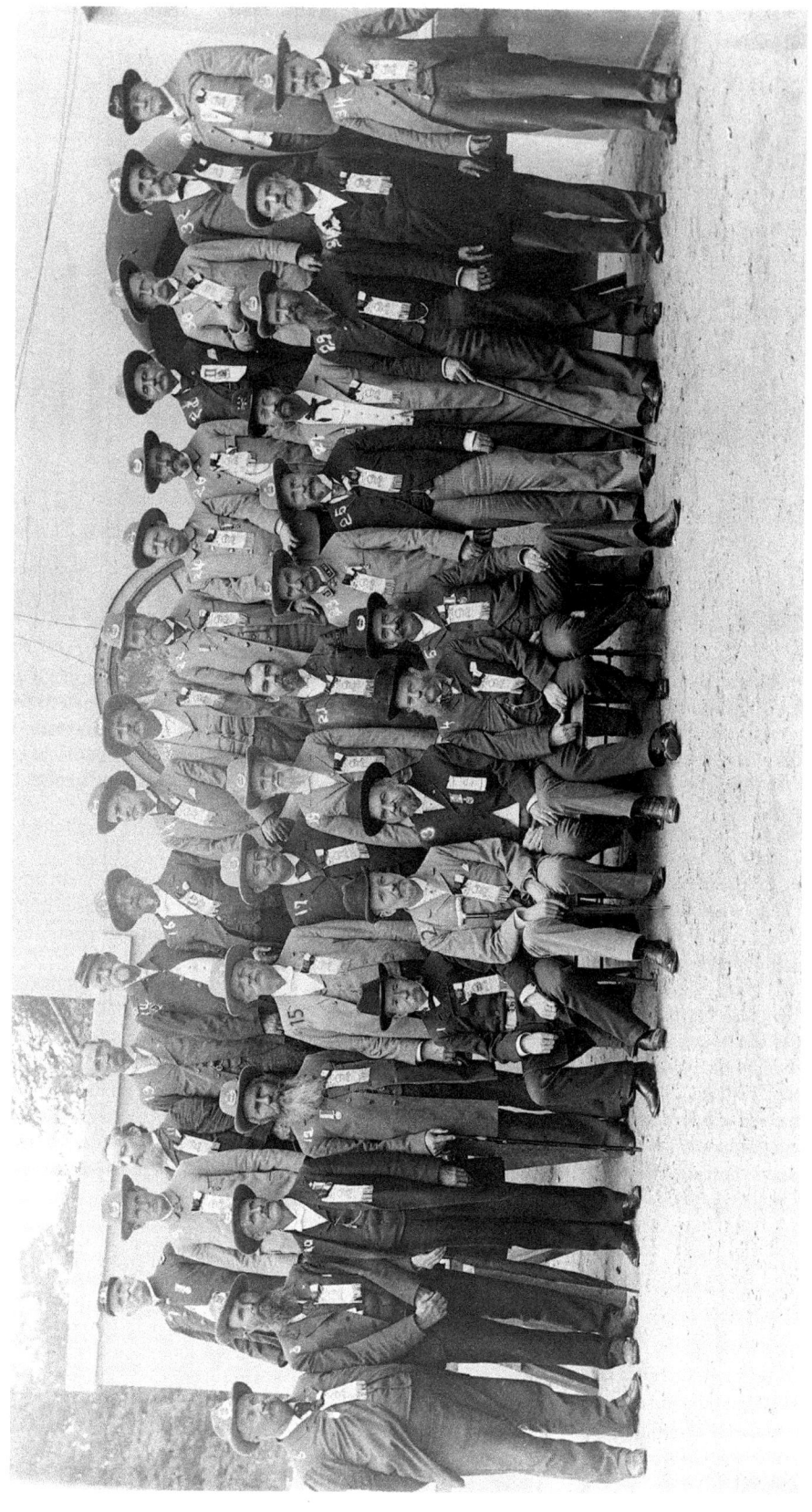

4. Reconstruction

His resolution was adopted. This "legal history" once again set the responsibility for the war with the North and attempted to establish that, while blacks could not be discriminated against, they still did not have the legal right to vote. These lasting sentiments would carry southern bitterness and racism well into the 20th century.

Jefferson Davis

Sixty thousand citizens loyal to the Confederacy crowded Memorial Hall in New Orleans over two humid days, May 27–28, 1893, to pay their respects to Jefferson Finis Davis whose remains lay in state. Davis had died in New Orleans four years earlier, and his body was in the process of being moved to Hollywood Cemetery in Richmond. Dr. Tebault was an esteemed member of Davis's guard of honor.

Figure 37 shows the 34 Louisiana men chosen for the honor to serve as escorts for the re-interment of Jefferson Davis, as his body was removed from Metairie Cemetery in New Orleans and transported to Hollywood Cemetery in Richmond, Virginia. Dr. Tebault is the distinguished-looking gentleman in the first row standing, third from the left.

On that muggy morning in May, a band of mounted Confederate veterans with a hearse and a couple of carriages carrying family members arrived at Metairie Cemetery and drew up in front of the mound forming the tumulus of the Army of Northern Virginia. Topped by a tall column supporting a statue of Thomas "Stonewall" Jackson, the tomb had been the temporary burial chamber of Davis's body. The year 1898 was a time following the difficult Reconstruction period when New Orleans was finally getting back on its economic feet, and when memories of the late war were gradually fading along with many of its thin-haired and graying Confederate participants. But, Davis's death in New Orleans

Opposite page: Jefferson Davis died in New Orleans in 1889 and was interned in Metairie Cemetery. In 1893 his body was moved to Hollywood Cemetery in Richmond, Virginia. Dr. Tebault was one of 34 former Confederates honored as escorts. Dr. Tebault is the distinguished-looking gentleman in the first row standing, third from the left. The numbers refer to the identities of the men in the photograph, which are listed below. Seated, left to right—1. General John Glynn, Jr. (commander of the Louisiana Division of the United Confederate Veterans); 2. Colonel W.R. Lyman (Adjutant General and Chief of Staff of the Louisiana Division of the UCV); 3. Colonel B.F. Eshleman (aide-de-camp of the Louisiana Division of the UCV); 4. Colonel M.T. Ducros; and 5. General W.J. Behan (Washington Artillery of New Orleans and twice elected Major General of the Louisiana Division of the UCV). First row, standing—6. H.T. Brown; 8. M.E. Shaddock (Chaplain); 10. Dr. Tebault; 12. Will Miller; 16. David Arent; 17. E. McCullom; 19. Thomas Clements; 21. Howell Carter; 23. J. Moore Wilson; 25. D.S. Sullivan; 27. Dr. G.H. Tichenor (the first Confederate surgeon to have used antiseptic techniques during the war, employing alcohol to clean wounds); 29. T.B. Finlay; 31. Colonel T.C. Standifer (Colonel of the 12th Louisiana volunteers); and 34. Charles Santana. Back row, standing—7. General John Baptiste Vinet; 9. Thomas Higgins (Sergeant in the 2nd Louisiana Infantry); 11. General Allen Barksdale (South Carolina 3rd Regiment); 13. John W. Watson; 14. Colonel L.J. Fremaux (8th Louisiana); 16. David Arent; 18. J.K. Renaud (member of the Orleans Cadets, the first volunteer company that left the state of Louisiana on April 11, 1861); 20. H. Dugas; 22. J.Y. Gilmore (one of the organizers of the Louisiana UCV); 24. Joseph Demoruelle (Commander of the New Orleans camp); 26. John T. Block (First Regiment of the Louisiana Volunteers); 28. E.I. Kursheedt (Lieutenant in the Washington Artillery); 30. Colonel Alex M. Haas; 32. T.J. Royster (sharpshooter in the 22nd Louisiana); and 33. T.W. Castleman (member of the Texas Cavalry and later the 1st Mississippi Cavalry. After the war he was appointed Commissioner of Confederate Records and also commanded the Louisiana Division of the UCV). Credit: American Civil War Museum, under the management of Virginia Museum of History & Culture.

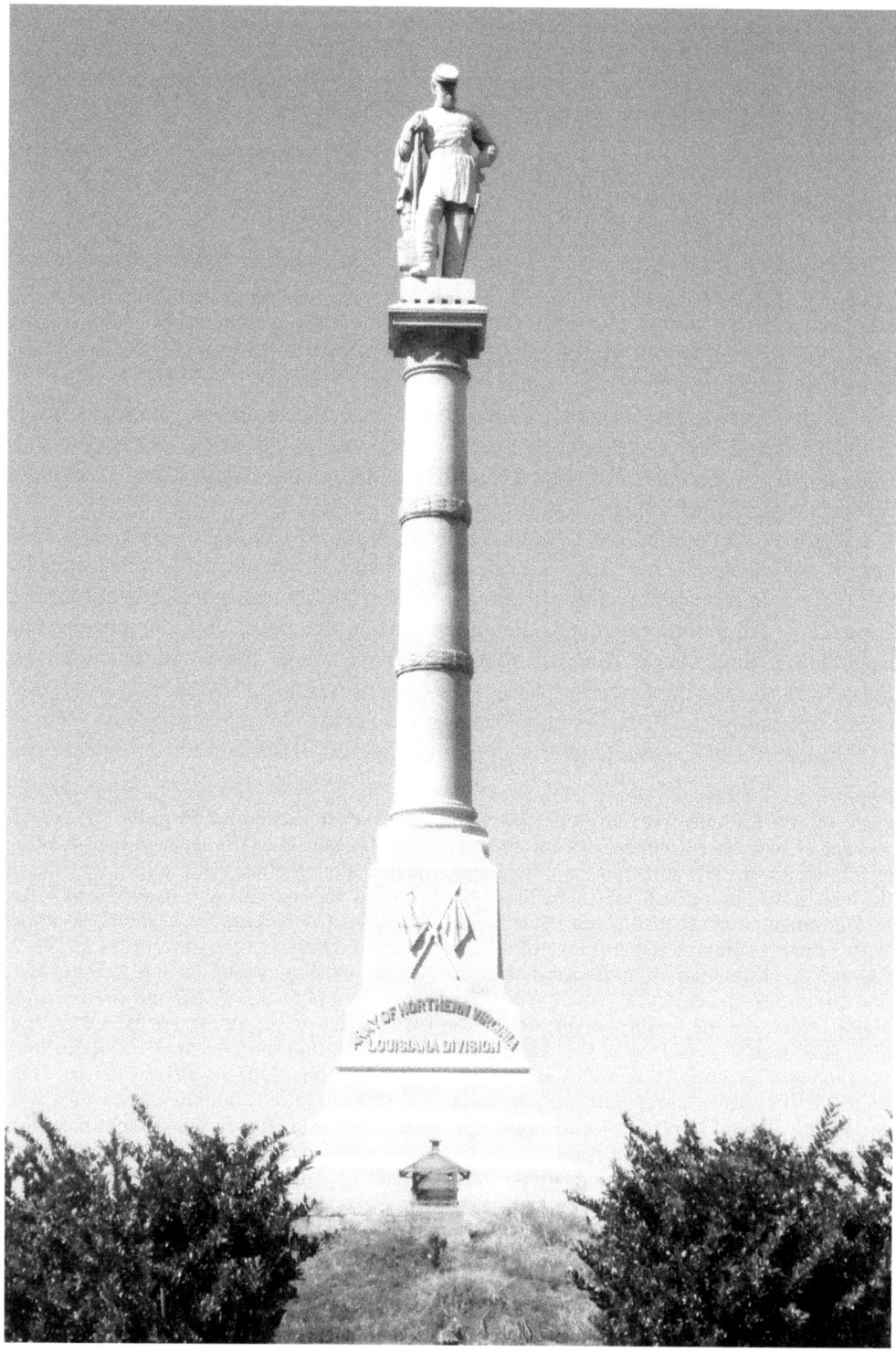

Tumulus of the Army of Northern Virginia. A 9-foot statue of General Thomas "Stonewall" Jackson stands atop a 38-foot column on top of the tumulus. Inside are 57 crypts that included the temporary resting place for Jefferson Davis (author's collection).

on December 6, 1889, had reignited southern feelings and sympathies. Twenty-eight years earlier, the *New York Times* offered Davis a complementary salute when it had erroneously reported a rumor of his death:

> The rebels may lose heart in losing DAVIS. He was not a great man; but his people believed him great, and with them the effect was morally the same. He had not genius. But he had that tenacity of purpose, that coolness of temper, that boldness of enterprise, and that practical knowledge of the fitness of means to his ends, which will always render a man, when clothed with power, a formidable leader. In many respects, Mr. DAVIS was the fittest man to lead the Confederate rebellion. He was experienced in national administration. He was thoroughly acquainted with the details of the military arm of the Government he was appointed to overthrow. He was a successful General in the field, and carried the popular enthusiasm with him when he went to war for his Confederacy. Who else among the Confederates combines such advantages?[108]

Davis had given his last public speech in Mississippi in 1888, a year before his death, where he encouraged putting aside all bitter feelings and coming together with their former enemies for the good of the country: "The past is dead; let it bury its dead, its hopes and its aspirations. Let me beseech you to lay aside all rancor, all bitter sectional feeling, and to make your places in the ranks of those who will bring about a consummation devoutly to be wished—a reunited country."[109]

On December 11, 1889, the day of Davis's funeral, schools were closed and the flower-draped caisson proceeded on a long march from City Hall where he had laid in state to the cemetery. An estimated 140,000 citizens had paid their last respects while the casket was in City Hall, and more would line the route of the funeral procession, moving from City Hall up St. Charles Avenue to Calliope Street, then to Camp and Canal to City Park Avenue, which ran out to Metairie Cemetery.[110] Marching behind the caisson were many surviving Confederates, including Dr. Tebault. Arriving at the cemetery, the procession was greeted by another 10,000 people gathered there to witness Davis's internment into the flower-covered tumulus. His casket was sealed inside the tomb with a marble tablet onto which was engraved his signature in gold lettering.

By contrast, four years later, the removal of Davis's body to Richmond was much less a spectacle, although thousands turned out in remembrance. Mr. Davis's remains were escorted from Metairie Cemetery to Memorial Hall in New Orleans where they laid in state for a day. His wife Varina and daughter, Winnie Davis, accompanied the remains. His casket resided on a simple

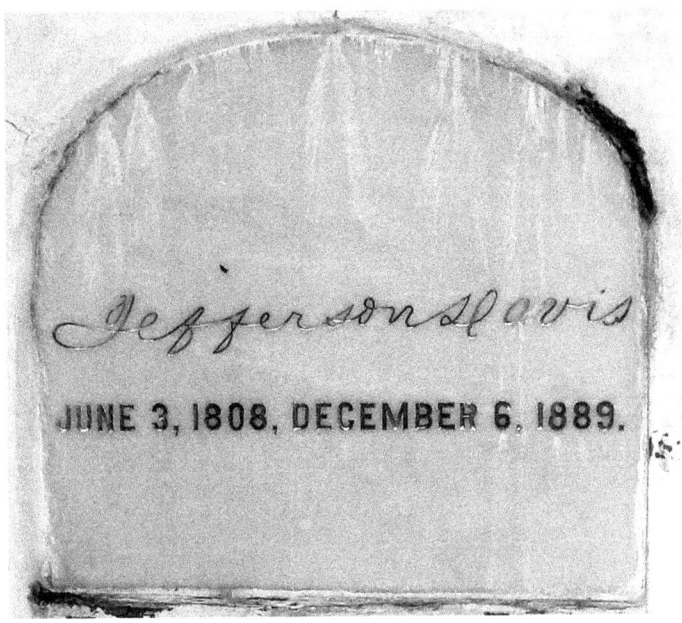

A marble tablet engraved with Davis's signature in gold lettering still guards the empty crypt where his casket was originally entombed in 1889 (author's collection).

bier with the flag carried by his regiment during the Mexican War offering the simple ornamentation. A Boston reporter interviewed a lawyer whose shop was along the procession from Metairie Cemetery. "You asked me what the demonstration means, and my answer to that question is that it is merely a sentimental regard of the people to the memory of the man who was the leading figure in the cause which they believed in, who was the head and

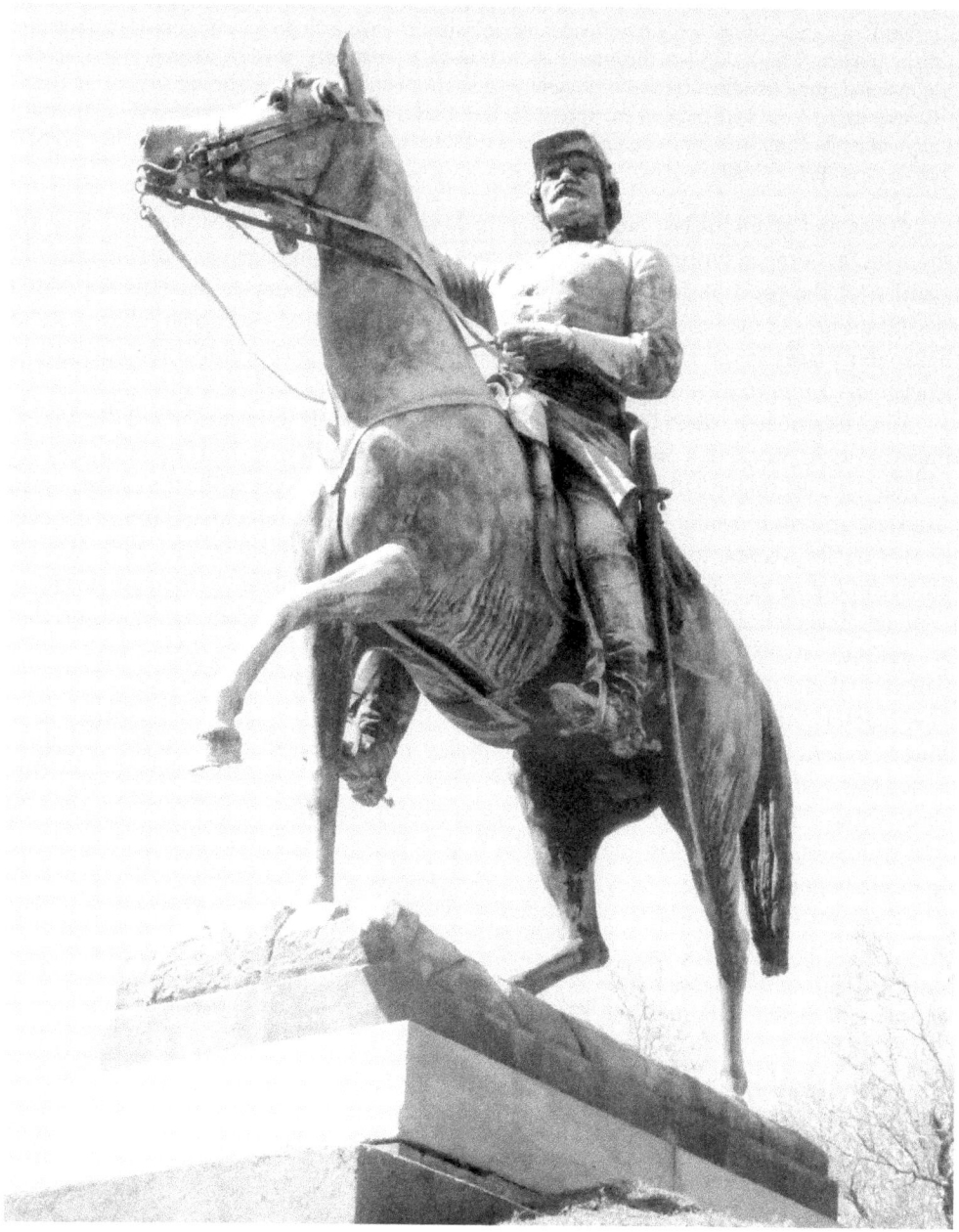

The statue of Albert Sidney Johnson was unveiled in 1887 on the 25th anniversary of the Battle of Shiloh where he had been mortally wounded. Dr. Tebault was chosen to escort his widow to its unveiling. The sculptor, Alexander Doyle, used a horse from the same bloodline as the general's beloved horse, *Fire Eater*. Photograph by author.

front of the movement, and who, in his person, embodied all the ideas which they held to be right and conceived to be just; because you must remember the South and believed they were right in what they did."[111]

Davis's funeral train left Sunday evening, with his body in the first car, which was under guard by Confederate veterans for the 1,200-mile trip to Richmond. The first stop was Beauvoir, Mississippi, Davis's birthplace, followed by Montgomery, Alabama, where his casket was borne from the car to the capitol building where Mr. Davis took the oath of office as President of the Confederacy. Church bells through the city pealed to honor him. Atlanta, Georgia, was the next stop, where his remains were carried to the capitol building for four hours. Other stops were Greeneville, South Carolina, and Raleigh, North Carolina. Finally, the funeral train reached Richmond on the 30th where he was interned. Colonel John B. Gordon, Commander in Chief of the United Confederate Veterans and a U.S. Senator from Georgia, was the chief marshal of the procession. Dr. Tebault, as Surgeon General, was a member of Gordon's staff who accompanied the body during the trip to Richmond. Six southern governors served as pallbearers, and 200,000 people lined the streets with another 100,000 observing the ceremony at the cemetery.

Six years earlier, the equestrian statue of Albert Sidney Johnson had been unveiled in Metairie Cemetery as part of the tumulus of the Army of Tennessee, Louisiana Division. General Johnson had been killed at the battle of Shiloh, and 1887 represented the 25th anniversary of that famous battle. Dr. Tebault was the corresponding secretary and ex-officio chairman of the historical committee of the Benevolent Association of the Army of Tennessee, Louisiana Division and was given the honor of escorting Mrs. Sidney Johnson who had arrived for the event from her home in Los Angeles, California.[112] He took part in the unveiling of the statue, an imposing sculpture of General Johnson astride his spirited horse who was also mortally wounded at the battle. Jefferson Davis had also attended the dedication with his wife and daughter.[113]

5

THE LOST CAUSE

"The preservation of liberty and freedom was the motivating factor in the South's decision to fight the Second American Revolution."
—(The above quote is taken from the website for the Sons of Confederate Veterans.)

Most southerners were devastated economically, emotionally, and psychologically by the loss of the Confederacy in April 1865. And, almost before the smoke cleared from the battlefields, northern and southern literature presented conflicting accounts regarding the responsibility for the war. Former Vice President of the Confederacy, Alexander Stephens, stressed that the war was not over the issue of slavery as those in the North believed, but was instead a conflict brought about by two "opposing principles." Those in the North favored a national and oppressive form of government while those in the South preferred one that incorporated the principles of Federalism and liberty.[1] Following their defeat, many southerners sought consolation by blaming the Union for initiating the hostilities and attributing their loss to factors beyond their control. They also felt the need to justify their actions, including the treatment of Union prisoners at such infamous prisons such as Andersonville and Libby.

Edward Pollard of Virginia penned his famous tome, *The Lost Cause,* in 1867 as a southerner's view of the history of the war.[2] His book is relatively accurate with respect to the actual history of the war. But he attempted politically to redefine the Civil War as a war of northern aggression with the position of the Confederates as defenders of freedom and states' rights. In the first chapter Pollard wrote: "Unfortunately, the world has got most of its opinions of Southern parties and men from the shallow pages of Northern books; and it will take it long to learn the lessons that the system of negro servitude in the South was not '*Slavery*'; that John C. Calhoun was not a '*Disunionist*'; and that the war of 1861, brought on by Northern insurgents against the authority of the Constitution, was not a '*Southern rebellion.*'"[3] (John C. Calhoun was a leading politician from South Carolina known for his outspoken defense of states' rights and the principles of nullification, under which states could nullify any federal laws that they viewed as unconstitutional. He defended the institution of slavery as a "positive good.")

Edward Pollard was a lawyer, a clerk of the Judiciary Committee of the U.S. House of Representatives, and a newspaper editor. He was also a staunch racist and white supremacist. In 1859 he had published his first book, *Black Diamonds Gathered in the Darkey Homes of the South*.[4] The book was a collection of eleven letters describing and justifying slave life as it was practiced in the South. In the book, Pollard felt that abolitionists failed to understand how well off slaves were on southern plantations: "well cared for, and even religiously educated, than his condition in Africa, where he is at the mercy of both men and beasts…."[5] He wrote condescendingly of his "love" for the slaves he knew: "I love the simple and unadulterated slave, with his geniality, his mirth, his swagger, and his nonsense; I love to look upon his continence, shining with content and grease; I love to study his affectionate heart."[6] But Pollard also describes his disgust and anger whenever he saw a "negro gentleman" who "affect[ed] superiority over the poor, needy, and unsophisticated whites."[7] Pollard's books represented terribly biased viewpoints, and his *Lost Cause* and its sequel, *The Lost Cause Regained*, did much to promulgate the concept of white superiority at a time when former Confederates were trying to rationalize and understand their wartime sacrifices and the new South that had been turned upside down by Reconstruction and the 13th, 14th, and 15th Amendments to the U.S. Constitution.[8]

Other notables joined the voices supporting the Lost Cause doctrine, including Lieutenant-General Jubal Early and Jefferson Davis in his two-volume history of the war.[9] Davis used his book to justify and romanticize the antebellum South.

Dr. Tebault used the pulpit of the United Confederate Veterans to further the concept of the Lost Cause. He passionately spoke of three specific issues: (1) The responsibility for the war; (2) the question of slavery; and (3) the medical treatment of prisoners.

There appear to be seven major tenets of the Lost Cause that are consistently presented by its proponents:

1. Secession was justifiable and legal, and a number of northern states, including Massachusetts, had previously threatened secession.

2. The primary cause of the war was the defense of states' rights and not the continuation of slavery; most Confederate soldiers did not own slaves.

3. Confederate generals such as Robert E. Lee and Thomas "Stonewall" Jackson represented the virtues of southern nobility compared to the relatively low moral standards exemplified in such obscene acts as Sherman's march to the sea and Sheridan's destruction of the Shenandoah Valley.

4. Slavery, as practiced in the South, was a benign institution where benevolent masters took care of African slaves, who themselves were illiterate, child-like and incapable of caring for themselves.

5. The industrial North had superior equipment and almost unlimited manpower, which overwhelmed the agrarian South.

6. Certain Confederate generals, such as James Longstreet, were incompetent and showed insubordination to their revered commander, Robert E. Lee; had Longstreet listened to Lee, for example, Gettysburg would have been a Confederate victory.

7. Prisoners in the South were treated to the same food and medicine as Confederate soldiers, but due to the blockade there were shortages—the North had also discontinued exchanges resulting in the large number of Union prisoners for which the Confederacy had to somehow provide.

The psychological trauma resulting from the defeat of the South was enormous. The economy of the South had completely collapsed, including its currency, banks, and insurance companies. Millions of dollars in investments vanished. In 1860 there were approximately four million slaves worth over $3 billion in the southern states; the institution and its investments evaporated.[10] The war had resulted in over a quarter of a million dead; these were a generation of young men who would have contributed significantly to the southern economy. On top of this, approximately 200,000 Confederate soldiers had been wounded during the war, many of whom had lost limbs and the ability to work in a largely agrarian society.

Confederate veterans especially used the Lost Cause to justify their actions and sacrifices. They needed to believe that their efforts were honorable, justified and meaningful; that they were patriots of a just cause and not simply "rebels" or traitors.

Justice Jeremiah Black and Edwin Stanton

At the 1902 reunion of the United Confederate Veterans, Dr. Tebault presented an open letter that had been written by Justice Jeremiah Black to Congressman and future President, James Garfield, in which the Judge lays out the case for the North's responsibility for starting the Civil War. (James Abram Garfield [1831–1881] was strongly opposed to secession and served during the war as a Major General. After the war he continued as a Congressman and supported the Radical Republican movement that pushed for punishing Reconstruction laws. He was elected the 20th President of the United States in 1881 and assassinated 200 days after taking office.)

Jeremiah Sullivan Black (1810–1993) served as U.S. Attorney General (1857–1860) and Secretary of State (1860–1861) under President James Buchanan. Buchanan, Attorney General Black and the Chief Justice of the Supreme Court Roger B. Taney (1777–1864) are considered largely responsible for the 1857 Dred Scott decision, which served as a catalyst for plunging the country into war. To put into context Dr. Tebault's speech at the 1902 Reunion, it is helpful to briefly review that decision as well as some of the personalities involved.

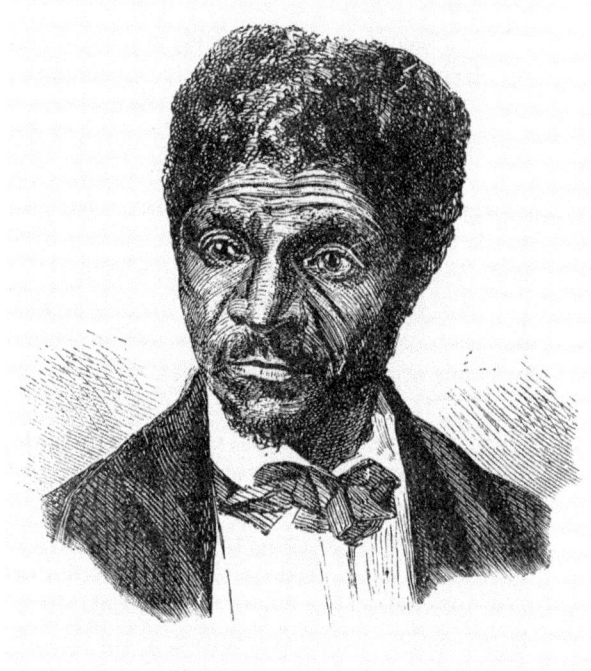

Dred Scott had been a slave owned by Dr. John Emerson, a surgeon in the U.S. Army who frequently brought Scott with him on his travels, which included to states where slavery was illegal. After Dr. Emerson died in 1843, Scott tried to buy the freedom of his wife and his family from Emerson's widow, but she refused. In 1846 he filed suit in St. Louis through the help of a local attorney. He argued that he and his wife had been illegally held in states where slavery was illegal—Illinois and Wisconsin Territory (now Minnesota)—and they should therefore be granted their freedom. The case ultimately made it to the Supreme Court in 1857. President-elect Buchanan pushed to have their decision rendered before his inauguration.

Dred Scott was a slave who accompanied his owner on his frequent travels. Following his owner's death, Scott filed suit arguing for his freedom since he had been held in states where slavery was illegal. The case was heard by the U.S. Supreme Court in 1857, which determined Scott to be a non-citizen with no legal rights. The decision was applauded in the South, although many northern states refused to abide by the verdict, adding to the already smoldering tensions. Library of Congress Brady-Handy Photograph Collection LC-USZ62-5092.

5. The Lost Cause

He believed that a decision recognizing Dred Scott to be a slave, with no rights even in the free states and territories, would suppress the growing discontentment in the South over the North's desire to contain the expansion of slavery.

The court, by a 7–2 decision, found that Scott was a non-citizen with no legal rights; the decision additionally raised the question of whether Congress had authority to restrict the expansion of slavery into federal territories:

> A free negro of the African race, whose ancestors were brought to this country and sold as slaves, is not a "citizen" within the meaning of the Constitution of the United States.
>
> When the Constitution was adopted, they [slaves] were not regarded in any of the States as members of the community which constituted the State, and were not numbered among its "people or citizens." Consequently, the special rights and immunities guaranteed to citizens do not apply to them. And not being "citizens" within the meaning of the Constitution, they are not entitled to sue in that character in a court of the United States, and the Circuit Court has not jurisdiction in such a suit.[11]

Taney quoted from the Declaration of Independence in summarizing the Court's opinion:

> We hold these truths to be self-evident: that all men are created equal; that they are endowed by their Creator with certain unalienable rights; that among them is life, liberty, and the pursuit of happiness; that to secure these rights, Governments are instituted, deriving their just powers from the consent of the governed.
>
> The general words above quoted would seem to embrace the whole human family, and if they were used in a similar instrument at this day would be so understood. But it is too clear for dispute that the enslaved African race were not intended to be included, and formed no part of the people who framed and adopted this declaration, for if the language, as understood in that day, would embrace them, the conduct of the distinguished men who framed the Declaration of Independence would have been utterly and flagrantly inconsistent with the principles they asserted, and instead of the sympathy of mankind to which they so confidently appealed, they would have deserved and received universal rebuke and reprobation.
>
> Yet the men who framed this declaration were great men—high in literary acquirements, high in their sense of honor, and incapable of asserting principles inconsistent with those on which they were acting. They perfectly understood the meaning of the language they used, and how it would be understood by others, and they knew that it would not in any part of the civilized world be supposed to embrace the negro race, which, by common consent, had been excluded from civilized Governments and the family of nations, and doomed to slavery. They spoke and acted according to the then established doctrines and principles, and in the ordinary language of the day, and no one misunderstood them. The unhappy black race were separated from the white by indelible marks, and laws long before established, and were never thought of or spoken of except as property, and when the claims of the owner or the profit of the trader were supposed to need protection.[12]

Since the U.S. Supreme Court had determined that slaves were private property, many southerners believed that Congress did not have the power to regulate slavery in the states and territories. Scott and his family were subsequently returned to the Emersons, who gave them to the Peter Blow family, their original owners who had sold them to the Emersons. Blow had since become an abolitionist and had moved to Missouri where he finally emancipated the Scott family three months after the Supreme Court ruling.[13]

Many in the South felt exonerated by the Dred Scott decision, which in their minds validated their right to own slaves and move them into other territories and states with impunity. On the other hand, many in the North saw the decision as spreading slavery, an institution that they had tolerated as long as it was confined to a few southern states. Northerners and the Republican Party had hoped for the gradual extinction of slavery, believing that labor performed by free men was far superior to that accomplished by forced slave labor. Southerners felt that preventing the expansion of slavery into the West challenged their autonomy and was a slap in their faces. Instead of suppressing the growing discontent within the country, as Buchanan had hoped, the Dred Scott decision fueled further division and suspicions.

The Fugitive Slave Act of 1850 had previously been passed by Congress demanding that any runaway slaves be returned to their owners upon capture, and it specifically mentioned free states and territories, fining any citizens who ignored the law up to $1,000. But, a number of northern states openly defied that federal law. Vermont passed legislation affirming the right of any detained fugitive to a trial by jury. Similar personal liberty laws were passed in Connecticut, Maine, Massachusetts, Michigan, New York, Ohio, Rhode Island and Wisconsin. In 1859 the Supreme Court examined these personal liberty laws (*Ableman v. Booth*), with Chief Justice Taney again weighing in that states could not create legislation that contradicted federal law.[14] But by then, the Fugitive Slave Act and the Dred Scott case had been ignored numerous times in the North, with abolitionists becoming more vocal and violent.

Harriet Beecher Stowe published *Uncle Tom's Cabin* in 1852, expounding the evils of slavery and awakening sentiment in northern citizens who had largely ignored the abolitionists up until that time. A number of runaway slaves were hidden and smuggled into Canada, which had become a major destination for escaped slaves and the Underground Railroad. It was estimated that as many as 5,000 blacks moved across the border into Canada within a few months of the Fugitive Slave Act's passage.[15]

Examples of northern states ignoring federal law were frequently cited by southerners as validating their right to secession; they argued that if states were not required to abide by federal laws, then the Constitution itself was invalid. The state legislature in Virginia described the personal liberty laws being passed in northern states as a "disgusting and revolting exhibition of faithless and unconstitutional legislation." They further claimed the northern resistance to the federal legislation as "palpable frauds upon the South, calculated to excite at once her indignation and her contempt."[16] The famous southern statesman, John C. Calhoun, declared:

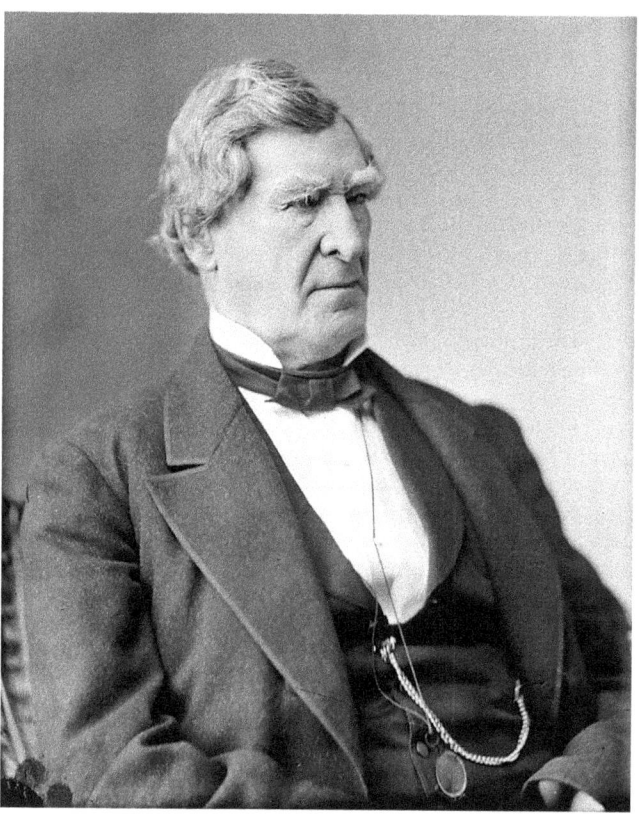

Jeremiah Sullivan Black served as Chief Justice of the Supreme Court of Pennsylvania (1851–1854), and U.S. Attorney General (1857–1860) and Secretary of State (1860–1861) under President Buchanan. After the war Black supported President Johnson's veto of the Reconstruction Act, which was overridden. Credit: Library of Congress Brady-Handy Photograph Collection, LC-BH826-30049.

The citizens of the South, in their attempt to recover their slaves, now meet, instead of aid and co-operation, resistance in every form; resistance from hostile acts of legislation, intended to baffle and defeat their claims by all sorts of devices, and by interposing every description of impediment—resistance from judges and magistrates—and finally, when all these fail, from mobs, composed of whites and blacks, which, by threats or force, rescue the fugitive slave from the possession of his rightful owner. The attempt to recover a slave, in most of the Northern States, cannot now be made without the hazard of insult, heavy pecuniary loss, imprisonment, and even of life itself.... The want of Union and concert in reference to it has brought the South, the Union, and our system of government to their present perilous condition.[17]

To many in the South, secession was a reasonable and legal response as a result of the North's choosing to ignore the Supreme Court's decisions and federal law.

Another personal target of southern frustrations was Edwin M. Stanton. Stanton had become good friends with Jeremiah Black, who at the time was Chief Justice of the Pennsylvania Supreme Court. That friendship would prove fruitful for Stanton as Black was made Attorney General under President Buchanan. Stanton eventually became a frequent advisor to both Buchanan and Black. During this time, he defended Congressman Daniel Sickles (1819–1914) who was later to earn fame as a politically appointed general who famously lost his leg in the Battle of Gettysburg. The 33-year-old Sickles had married 16-year-old Teresa Bagioli Sickles in 1852. Sickles was known to be a notorious womanizer, and his Washington duties along with his various love affairs eventually isolated Teresa, who began an affair of her own with Phillip Barton Key. Key was a U.S. District Attorney whose father, Francis Scott Key, had famously written *The Star-Spangled Banner*. Sickles eventually discovered his wife's infidelity, and, on Sunday, February 27, 1859, he confronted and shot Key to death across the street from the White House. Sickles then retreated to the home of Attorney General Black where he admitted his crime. Stanton subsequently

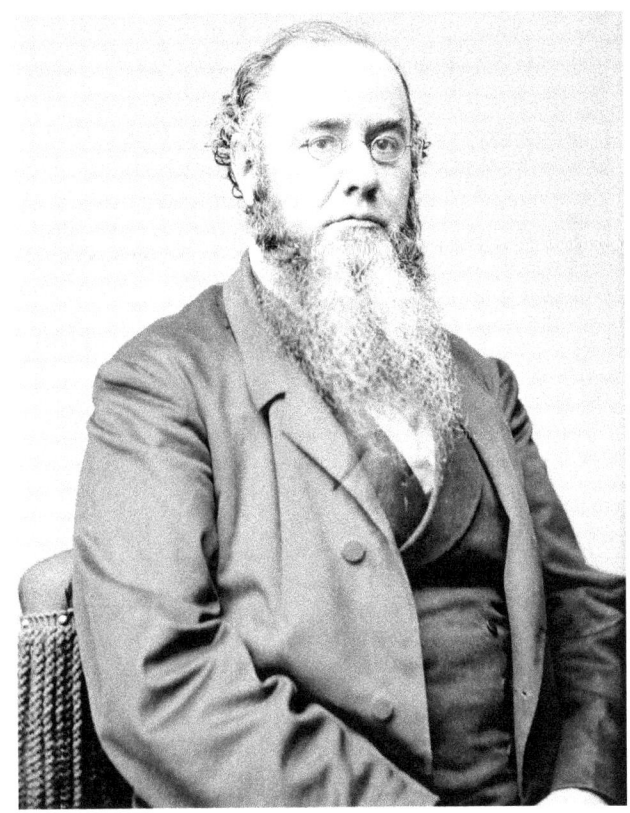

Edwin Stanton served as Attorney General under President Buchanan and Secretary of War under Presidents Lincoln and Johnson. Stanton understood the political arena and was an effective manipulator. He worked to undermine Buchanan's presidency and convinced Massachusetts Senator Charles Sumner that secessionists were plotting to capture Washington and not merely leave the Union. He befriended General George McClellan even while he plotted to diminish McClellan's power. He supported much of the Radical Republican agenda for Reconstruction, and Johnson's attempt to remove him from office was one of the catalysts that led to Johnson's impeachment. Credit: Library of Congress Brady-Handy Photograph Collection CWPBH.00958.

was recruited to become part of Sickles's defense team, and they successfully argued for acquittal based on Sickles being temporarily insane at the time of the crime. This was the first use of the insanity plea.[18]

A little over a year later, Stanton was confirmed as President Buchanan's Attorney General. In a December 26, 1860, letter to a Pittsburgh friend, W.B. Copeland, Stanton mused: "After much hesitation and serious reflection, I resolved to accept the post [of Attorney General] to which in my absence I was called, in the hope of doing something to save this Government. I AM WILLING TO PERISH IF THEREBY THIS UNION MAY BE SAVED. We are in God's hands and His almighty arm alone can save us from greater misery than has ever fallen upon a nation. I devoutly pray for His help; all men should pray for succor in this hour. No effort of mine shall be spared."[19]

The next day, December 27, Stanton and Buchanan's cabinet learned that Major Robert Anderson had abandoned Fort Moultrie and occupied Fort Sumter in Charleston Harbor. Stanton vigorously opposed the measure and expressed his displeasure in one of the more fiery cabinet debates: "Mr. President, it is my duty as your legal adviser to say that you have no right to give up the property of the Government, or abandon its soldiers to its enemies, and the course proposed is treason and, if followed, will involve you and all concerned in it is treason."[20] Stanton strongly opposed secession. He became duplicitous and acted as a spy for the Republicans, with whom he aligned himself.

Stanton met with Senator Benjamin Butler and stated his concerns regarding Buchanan. Butler later recalled:

> I knew Mr. Stanton. He related fully to me the proceedings of the preliminary meeting between the President and the South Carolina commissioners and of the scene in the cabinet consultation, which he had just left. He was full of wrath. He said that I must go to both Black and Buchanan and protest against the fatal course the administration was pursuing. He told me that the so-called ambassadors had actually rented a house in Washington—which I subsequently learned was a fact—expecting to remain permanently as representatives of the South as a foreign nation. He said that he had informed the President that the South Carolina agents were traitors; that the President had no power to negotiate with them, and that I must tell the President that if he should continue negotiating with traitors he would place himself on the same plane with traitors and be liable to impeachment if not something worse.[21]

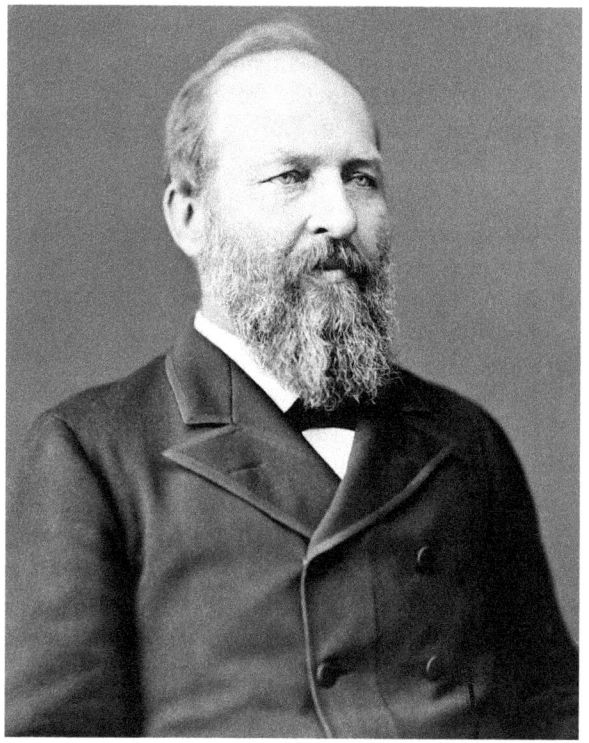

James A. Garfield was a senator from Ohio (1859–1861), elected to Congress in 1862. He served as a Major General in the Union Army during the war, and afterwards sided with the Radical Republicans, supporting black suffrage, the Freedmen's Bureau, and reparations. Garfield was elected President in 1881 and assassinated 200 days later. Library of Congress Brady-Handy Photograph Collection CWPBH.03744.

Stanton continued to transmit tales of President Buchanan's weakness and indecisiveness to the incoming Secretary of State, William Seward. He surreptitiously informed Massachusetts Senator Charles Sumner that the Buchanan administration was rife with corruption. He was able to convince Sumner that secessionists were plotting to capture Washington; that they were not merely intending to leave the Union but in fact to conquer it.[22]

Stanton lost his job as Attorney General after President Lincoln had assembled his Cabinet, but he served as a counsel for the War Department, and during that term he befriended the newly appointed commander of the Army of the Potomac, George McClellan. Based partially on Stanton's enthusiastic endorsement, McClellan replaced the elderly Winfield Scott as commander of the entire U.S. Army. Meanwhile Simon Cameron had become President Lincoln's Secretary of War and frequently used Stanton for legal advice. Cameron was receiving widespread criticism due to his lack of administrative abilities, and Lincoln saw an opportunity to rid himself of him by assigning him as Minister to Russia. Secretary of State Seward suggested to President Lincoln that Stanton assume the role, a recommendation that Lincoln accepted.

As Secretary of War, Stanton aligned himself with the increasingly powerful Radical Republicans who wished to purge the army of disloyal members who resisted their goal of emancipation. McClellan was one of their targets and someone whom Stanton now viewed as a competitor. Stanton undoubtedly helped to poison the waters regarding Lincoln's assessment of General McClellan, and as Stanton praised McClellan to his face, he was secretly leaking information to newspapers to encourage public criticism of the General in the press.[23] Stanton also took control of the telegraph system, effectively enabling him to regulate the news.[24] Now he was not only able to control wire communications between reporters and the press, he also issued press passes with a bias to reporters who supported the administration.[25]

Shortly before Lincoln's assassination, Mr. Stanton had expressed his wish to retire due to his failing health and dwindling finances. President Lincoln convinced him to stay. Senator Henry Wilson (1812–1875), in an *Atlantic Monthly* article, recalled that Lincoln said: "Stanton, you have been a good friend and a faithful public servant; and it is not for you to say when you will no longer be needed here."[26] Stanton, however, remembered the meeting a bit more colorfully after Lincoln's death, claiming that Lincoln had actually said: "Stanton, you cannot go. Reconstruction is more difficult and dangerous than construction or destruction. You have been our main reliance; you must help us through the final act. The bag is filled. It must be tied, and tied securely. Some knots slip; yours do not. You understand the situation better than anyone else, and it is my wish and the country's that you remain."[27] Henry Wilson served as chairman of the Military Affairs Committee of the Senate and oversaw the conscription act passed by Congress and endorsed by Stanton.[28]

Following President Lincoln's assassination, Stanton remained as Secretary of War under President Andrew Johnson. He was accused of disloyalty to President Johnson as he openly criticized Johnson over the President's lenient treatment of former Confederates. While working for President Johnson, Stanton was not only vocal in his criticism of the President, he also continued to leak information damaging to him.[29] In 1867 Congress approved the Tenure of Office Act that sought to shield cabinet members who disagreed with Johnson, specifically Stanton. Johnson summarily ignored the Act and tried to remove Stanton from office, causing Stanton to barricade himself in his office at one point. Much of the Articles of Impeachment of President Johnson were based on Johnson's violation of the Tenure of Office Act and his threats to dismiss Stanton.

Stanton was later blamed by historians for the 1866 New Orleans Riot due to his control of the War Department's official telegraph system. When General Absalom Baird, the acting commander of New Orleans, wrote to President Johnson requesting instructions should violence break out, Stanton withheld the message.

Dred Scott—The Tipping Point

In April 1902 the United Confederate Veterans met in Dallas, Texas. Dr. Tebault, as Surgeon General, presented a lengthy letter written by Justice Jeremiah Black to then Congressman James Garfield in 1876. The letter was in response to a speech of Garfield's, and Justice Black's lengthy response was applauded by southerners as he discusses the history of slavery, the hypocrisy of northern abolitionists and the responsibility for the war.[30] Dr. Tebault's report began:

The history of the War between the States, 1861–1865, would be imperfectly presented without the following history which speaks for itself, and needs no introduction:

To Hon. James A. Garfield, Member of Congress from Ohio:

I have read the speech you sent me. I am astonished and shocked.... You trace back the origin of present parties to the earliest immigrations at Plymouth and Jamestown, and profess to find in the opposing doctrines then planted and afterward constantly cherished in Massachusetts and Virginia, the germs of those ideas which now make Democracy and Abolitionism the deadly foes of each other. The ideas so planted in Massachusetts, were, according to your account, the freedom and equality of all races, and the right and duty of every man to exercise his private judgment in politics as well as religion. On the other hand, you set forth as irreconcilably hostile the doctrine of Virginia, "that capital should own labor, that the negro had no rights of manhood, and that the white man might buy, own and sell him and his offspring forever." Following these assertions with others, and linking the present with the long past, you employ the devices of your rhetoric to glorify the modern Abolitionist and to throw foul scorn, not merely on the Southern people, but on the whole Democracy of the Country....

TOLERANCE IN NEW ENGLAND. The men of Massachusetts, so far from *planting* the right of private judgment, extirpated and utterly *extinguished* it, by means so cruel that no man of common humanity can think of them even now without disgust and indignation.... Did you never hear of the frightful persecutions they carried on systematically against Baptists and Quakers and Catholics? How they fined, imprisoned, lashed, mutilated, enslaved and banished everybody that claimed the right of free thought? How they stripped the most virtuous and inoffensive women, and publicly whipped them on their naked backs, only for expressing their conscientious convictions? Have you never, in all your reading, met with the story of Roger Williams? For merely suggesting to the public authorities of the colony that no person ought to be punished on account of his honest opinions, he was driven into the woods and pursued ever afterwards with a ferocity that put his own life and that of his friends in constant danger. In fact, the cruelty of their laws against the freedom of conscience and the unfeeling rigor with which they were executed, made Massachusetts odious throughout the world.

These great crimes of the Pilgrim Fathers ought not to be cast up to their children; for some of their descendants (I hope a good majority) are high-principled and honest men, sincerely attached to the liberal institutions planted in the more Southern latitudes of the Continent. But if you are right in your assertion that the Abolitionists derive their principles from the ideas entertained and planted at Plymouth, that may account for the course and brutal tyranny with which your party has, in recent times, trampled upon the rights of free thought and free speech.

SLAVERY IN MASSACHUSETTS. Nor are you more accurate in your declaration that the old Yankees planted the doctrine of freedom and equality, or opposed the domination of one race over another.... The Plymouth colony and the province of Massachusetts Bay were pro-slavery to the backbone.... The Plymouth immigrants planted precisely the doctrine which you ascribe to the Jamestown colonists; that is to say, they held that "the negro had no rights of manhood; that the white man might buy, own and sell him, and his offspring forever." ... Whenever it was demonstrated by actual experiment that any people were too weak to defend their homes and families against an invader who visited them with fire and sword, they might lawfully be stripped of their property, and they, themselves, their wives and their children, might justly be held as slaves or sold into perpetual bondage. That was the idea they planted in their own soil, propagated among their contemporaries and transmitted to the Abolition party of the present day....

THE MASSACHUSETTS SLAVE FRAUDS. "They executed this theory to its fullest extent in their own wars with the Indians. Without cause or provocation, and without notice or warning, they fell upon the Pequots, massacred many of them, and made slaves of the survivors, without distinction of age or sex...."

The Indians make bad slaves. They were hard to tame, they escaped to the forest, and had to be hunted down, brought back and branded. They never ceased to be sullen and disobedient. The Africans always, on the contrary, "accepted the situation," were easily domesticated, and bore the yoke without murmuring. For that reason, it became a settled rule of public and private economy in Massachusetts to exchange their worthless Indians for valuable negroes, cheating their West India customers in every trade....

"YANKEE HUMANITY. ... Their precept and example established the slavery of white persons as well as Indians and negroes. As their remorseless tyranny spared no age and no sex, so it made no distinction of color.... One instance is worthy of special attention. Lawrence Southwick and his wife were Quakers, and accused at the same time with many others of attending Quaker meetings, or syding with Quakers, and "absenting themselves from the publick ordinances." The Southwicks had previously suffered so much in their persons and estates from this kind of persecution that they could no longer work or pay any more fines, and, therefore, the general court, by solemn resolution, ordered them to be banished on pain of death. Banishment, you will not fail to notice, was in itself equivalent to a lingering death, if the parties were poor and feeble; for it meant merely driving them into the wilderness to starve with hunger and cold. Southwick and his wife went out and died very soon. But this is not all. This unfortunate pair had two children, a boy and a girl (Daniel and Provided), who, having healthy constitutions, would bring a good price in the slave market. The children were taken from the parents and ordered to be sold in the West Indies. It happened, however, that there was not a shipmaster in any port of the colony who would consent to become the agent of their exportation and sale. The authorities, being thus balked in their views of the main chance, were fain to be satisfied in another way; they ordered the girl to be whipped; she was lashed accordingly, in company with several other Quaker ladies, and then committed to prison, to be further proceeded against. History loses sight of her there. No record shows whether they killed her or not....

As a side note, history has actually not lost sight of the Southwick family. Lawrence and Cassandra Southwick were famously persecuted for being Quakers in Puritan Massachusetts, receiving repeated lashings, fines and imprisonment as a result of their religious beliefs. In 1657 Lawrence, Cassandra and their oldest son were arrested for associating with known Quakers. A son and daughter, Daniel and Provided, were sentenced to be sold into slavery in Barbados for unpaid fines related to their religion. A few months later, Lawrence and Cassandra were sent to Shelter Island off the eastern part of Long Island, New York. There they soon perished due to exposure in 1660. Their children, however, survived the affair.[31]

THE YANKEE SLAVE CODE. The slave code planted in Massachusetts was the earliest in America and the most cruel in all its provisions. It was pertinaciously adhered to for generations, and never repented of, or formally repealed. It was gradually abandoned, not because it was wrong, but solely because it was found, after long experiment, to be unprofitable....

SECESSION A YANKEE PRODUCT. As a part of this conflict of theories, and resulting from it, you describe the South as "insisting that each State had a right, at its own discretion, to break the Union, and constantly threatening secession, where the full rights of slavery were not acknowledged." In fact and in truth secession, like slavery, was first *planted* in New England.... John Quincy Adams in 1839, and Abraham Lincoln in 1847, made elaborate arguments in favor of the *legal right* of a State to go out....

> HOISTED BY HIS OWN PETARD. Speaking of reconstruction, and seeing your broad accusations of treason, I am tempted to ask if you are sure that you, yourself, and your associates did not commit that crime. In March 1867, the then existing Government of the Union was supreme all over the country, and every State had a separate government of its own for the administration of its domestic concerns. That Government was entitled then, if it ever was, to the universal obedience of all citizens, and you, its officers, had taken a special oath of fidelity to it. Nevertheless, you made a deliberate arrangement, not only to withdraw your support from it, but to overthrow it totally in ten of the States; and this you did *by military force*. In all the South you levied war against the nation and against the defenseless States, destroyed the free governments of both, and substituted in their place an untempered and absolute despotism.... I cannot describe to you how unpleasant is the sensation produced by your professions of a desire for peace. Why do you not give us peace if you are willing, we shall have it? You need but to cease hostilities and the general tranquility will be restored. You refuse to do that because peace would endanger your party ascendancy. To maintain your plunderers in power you have uniformly resorted to the bayonet—you have made civil war the chronic condition of the country—wherever you have displaced liberty, fraternity and equality, and given nothing instead but infantry, artillery and cavalry. You are at this moment openly engaged in preparing your battalions for armed intervention in the struggle of the people with the carpet-baggers.
>
> What makes this worse is your closing declaration that you will take no step backward. There is to be no repentance, no change of policy, and consequently no peaceful or honest government. "Onward," you say, is the word. Onward—to what? To more war, more plunder, more oppression, more universal bankruptcy, heavier taxes and still worse frauds on the public treasury?[32]

Dr. Tebault's presentation of Black's open letter supported the Lost Cause thesis that slavery originated in the New England states; that it was abolished in those states, not because it was unjust, but because it was uneconomical in the industrial North; and that slavery was cruel and vicious as practiced in the North compared to the more benign institution that was practiced in the South.

Dr. Tebault next concluded his report by presenting another letter written by Black to Charles Francis Adam regarding a speech of Adams extoling the virtues and character of William Seward. Charles Francis Adams (1807–1886) was the son of President John Quincy Adams. He served two terms in the Massachusetts State Senate and served under President Lincoln as the U.S. Minister to Great Britain.[33] Dr. Tebault writes:

> In conclusion, I have the pleasure of presenting the following extract from the same author, and most pertinent in this connection. I take it from his reply to Charles Francis Adams' speech on the Character of William Seward.
>
> ... Mr. Seward, as soon as he came into office, concocted a scheme for the surrender of Fort Sumter into the hands of the Secessionists; that he drew General Scott into it, and tried to get the President's assent also; that the President having declined to surrender, and determined to re-enforce the place, a confidential friend and protégé of Mr. Seward notified his confederates in the South of the movement about to be made; that the whole plan and arrangement of the Administration for the relief of the fort was brought to nothing by a series of secret, deceptive, and underhand maneuvers which Mr. Seward carried on without the knowledge of the War or Navy Department; and that, while he was thus betraying his associates, he wrote to Secessionists that his faith pledged to them would be fully kept. These accusations seem to be proved by overwhelming evidence....
>
> When the troubles were at their worst, certain Southern gentlemen, through Judge Campbell, of the Supreme Court (of the U.S.), requested me to meet Mr. Seward and see if he would not give them SOME GROUND ON WHICH THEY COULD STAND WITH SAFETY INSIDE OF THE UNION. I consented, and we met at the State Department.... I told him what I felt perfectly sure would stop all controversy at once and forever. I PROPOSED THAT HE SHOULD SIMPLY PLEDGE HIMSELF AND THE INCOMING ADMINISTRATION TO GOVERN ACCORDING TO THE CONSTITUTION. AND UPON EVERY DISPUTED POINT OF CONSTITUTIONAL LAW TO ACCEPT THAT EXPOSITION OF IT WHICH HAD BEEN OR MIGHT BE GIVEN BY THE JUDICIAL AUTHORITIES. HE STARTED AT THIS, BECAME EXCITED, AND VIOLENTLY DECLARED HE WOULD

DO NO SUCH THING. "THAT," SAID HE, "IS TREASON THAT WOULD MAKE ME AGREE TO THE DRED SCOTT CASE."

In vain I told him that he was not required to admit the correctness of any particular case, BUT MERELY TO SUBMIT TO IT AS THE DECISION OF THE HIGHEST TRIBUNAL, FROM WHICH THERE COULD BE NO APPEAL EXCEPT TO THE SWORD.

You will see that if such a pledge as this had been given and kept, THE WAR COULD NOT HAVE TAKEN PLACE; IT WOULD HAVE LEFT NOTHING TO FIGHT ABOUT; and the decent men of the Anti-Slavery party would have lost nothing by it which they pretended to want, for even the Dred Scott case had enured to their practical benefit.... I HAD NEVER BEFORE HEARD THAT TREASON WAS OBEDIENCE TO THE CONSTITUTION AS CONSTRUED BY THE COURTS.

Dr. Tebault had chosen carefully the words written by Justice Black. They were well received at the Reunion. Southern sympathizers had praised Black's letter. William Browne wrote Black after reading the letter thanking Black for his "recent scathing exposure of Yankee intolerance, cruelty, lawlessness, hypocrisy, and dishonesty ... it was one of the ablest defenses of the Constitution I have read during the last fifteen years."[34] (William Montague Browne [1827–1883] was a well-known Confederate politician and had served as a General during the war as well as Secretary of State to President Jefferson Davis. He was a lawyer and taught Constitutional Law at the University of Georgia after the war.)

Dr. Tebault also spoke of slavery as having its seeds in New England during a 1901 speech:

> The slave code planted in Massachusetts was the earliest and the most cruel in all its provisions. It was pertinaciously adhered to for generations, and never repented of, or formally repealed. It was gradually abandoned, not because it was wrong, but solely because it was found, after long experiment, to be unprofitable.... The African slavery, like the slavery under the Roman dominion, originated in the law of nations, or in the common practice

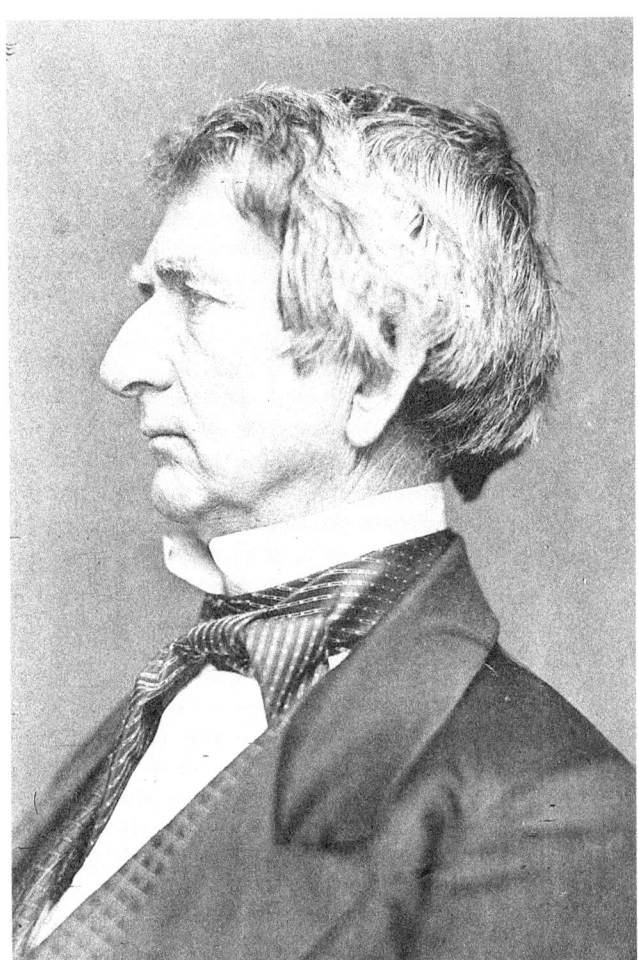

William H. Seward became President Lincoln's Secretary of State and remained in that position under Johnson's administration. In an attempt to avoid secession of the southern states, Seward proposed a constitutional amendment that would protect slavery, a proposal that angered the Radical Republicans in Congress. When Fort Sumter was being held by Union forces, he also argued against resupplying the garrison as doing so would be viewed as a provocative move by many in the South, including the crucial border states. Library of Congress, Alfred Whital Stern Collection of Lincolniana.

of European States in dealing in negroes as ordinary merchandise, with no rights to be respected, as it was thought, an inferior order of beings, is in fact of history so indubitable, that only egregious ignorance or a blinding fanaticism can deny it. As an inferior order of beings, having no human rights, negroes were brought as property, called slavery, into all the colonial settlements of America. They were property on the shores of Africa, were received as property into slave-ships, were held as property on the ocean, and were sold as property to the white inhabitants of the American colonies.... All the wealth of New England, and all her institutions, have their roots in the nefarious traffic of men and women torn from their African homes, and subjected to the sufferings and cruelties of a prison-ship, to be sold into perpetual slavery to a different people.[35]

Responsibility for the War

Dr. Tebault, along with many Lost Cause proponents, felt that history supported the legal right of states to secede, and this became a common theme to many of his reunion presentations. In his report given during the 11th Annual Reunion of the United Confederate Veterans in 1901, he outlined the position: "It was the right of Southern States to *withdraw* from the Union as they did withdraw. It is now almost unanimously agreed that it is best for all of us to be united as we are at present, in a stronger Union of States, but this might have been accomplished by just and peaceful and constitutional methods, without all the past expenditures of human life and treasure, and the still more terrible reconstruction period, for all of which the North alone must stand responsible before the bar of conscience and of history."[36]

He again reminded reunion attendees that some northern states had previously threatened to secede: "John Quincy Adams in 1839, and Abraham Lincoln in 1847, made elaborate arguments in favor of the *legal right* of a State to go out of the Union.... In fact and truth, session, like slavery, was first planted in New England. There it grew and flourished and spread its branches far over the land, long before it was thought of in the South, and long before the full rights of slavery were called in question by anybody."[37]

Quoting Leon Prince, Tebault added[38]:

But the capital instance of the exercise of imperial powers by the United States government and its sanction by a majority of the people is the American civil war. Now, as a question of purely abstract right, the seceding States were undoubtedly correct in their position. [Leon Prince graduated from Dickinson College in 1898 and taught history and economics there for 30 years. He served as a Pennsylvania state senator between 1928 and 1936. Dr. Tebault quoted from Prince's article, "The Passing of the Declaration," his contention that the United States was an imperial nation and that the principles of the Declaration of Independence were frequently discarded in favor of political need, which Prince thought was actually necessary and moral in order to move the country forward and achieve peace.]

The Constitution was originally a compact between thirteen independent sovereignties whereby certain rights were surrendered by them to the Federal government and certain others were retained. Among the latter the rights of secession was expressly reserved by the States of New York and Virginia, and Rhode Island and South Carolina refused to enter the Union until that right had been put beyond the shadow of reasonable doubt. The right of secession was subsequently affirmed and reaffirmed by different States on different occasions; notably in the Virginia and Kentucky resolutions of 1798–99, three times by the Legislature of Massachusetts (in 1802, 1844, and 1845), and by all the New England States during the war of 1812.... But there was another philosophical reason to support the principle of secession. It is to be found in the fact that, since the parties to the contract were sovereign States, there was no superior tribunal to which the question of State rights could be referred. The Federal courts were not competent to pass upon it, because they were the creatures of the Union and the Union was in turn the creature of the States.... Manifestly the seceding States had the right to go. They had the right under the Constitution and they had the further right of revolution, expressly affirmed by the

Declaration of Independence as being inherent in all communities and upon which each of the thirteen States had justified its secession from the mother country in 1776. But when the seceding States attempted to enforce that right, what did the government of the United States do? It invaded their territory with all the military force at its command, terrorized their inhabitants, destroyed their homes, violated their constitutionally guaranteed right of property by an executive act of unparalleled usurpation, and put to death on the fields of battle as many as possible of those inhabitants who dared openly to resist. And when at last the United States government, by virtue of its superior resources and greater strength, had reduced the seceding States to subjection, it deprived them of their Statehood, overturned their home rule; nullified their statutes, displaced their civil by military jurisdiction, and forced upon them the alternative of either accepting the thirteenth, fourteenth, and fifteenth amendments to the Constitution or remaining forever in the status of subjugated territory.... No reasonable man believes to-day that the result should have been in any wise different from what the stern arbitrament of war decreed. For while, logically and in principle secession was right, yet it was most fortunate for the South and for the country at large that it did not succeed.... But the point I make is that the entire action of the United States government toward the South, from 1860 until the last seceding State was 'reconstructed,' was imperialistic and usurpative in the extreme and there is no possible constitutional or legal aspect that can make it anything else.[39]

While Dr. Tebault rightly felt that Prince had made a strong and intelligent argument regarding the states' right to secession, Prince also felt that the usurpation of such individual states' rights was necessary to achieve peace for the nation.

The bombardment of Fort Sumter was viewed in the South as an unlawful seizure of state property by the Federal Government. Dr. Tebault noted that Lincoln's cabinet "voted six to one *in favor of surrendering* Fort Sumter.... The President, if he did not yield to the majority, must have wavered a considerable time; the Secretary of State was so sure of him, that he caused the South Carolina authorities to be informed that the *fort would be given up*."[40] Alexander Stephens who had served as Vice President of the Confederacy, also described a similar view of the responsibility for the war in his book, *A Constitutional View of the War Between the States*:

I maintain that it [the war] was inaugurated and begin, though no blow had been struck, when the hostile fleet, styled the "Relief Squadron," with eleven ships, carrying two hundred and eighty-five guns and two thousand four hundred men, was sent from New York and Norfolk, with orders from the authorities at Washington, to reinforce Fort Sumter peacefully, if permitted—"but forcibly, if they must." The war was then and there inaugurated and begin by the authorities at Washington. General Beauregard did not open fire upon Fort Sumter until the fleet was, to his knowledge, very near the harbor of Charleston, and until he had inquired of major Anderson, in command of the Fort, whether he would engage to take no part in the expected blow, then coming down upon him from the approaching fleet.[41]

The position of Dr. Tebault and many southerners was that it was the Federals who tossed aside negotiation and compromise and forced the hand of the South to take action, an act that they also believed the U.S. Constitution supported. "It was felt by all who could forecast coming events, that the question was now presented in the political issue, whether the Constitution and Union were to be one and inseparable in the future, as they had been in the past, or the Union preserved and the Constitution disregarded."[42]

Dr. Tebault further quoted from Lincoln's inaugural address, noting that Lincoln had made it clear that he would disregard the ruling by the Supreme Court on the Dred Scott case. The part of Lincoln's first inaugural address that Dr. Tebault quoted is as follows:

I do not forget the position assumed by some that constitutional questions are to be decided by the Supreme Court, nor do I deny that such decisions must be binding in any case upon the parties to a suit as to the object of that suit, while they are also entitled to very high respect and consideration in all parallel cases by all other departments of the Government. And while it is obviously possible that such decision may be erroneous in any given case, still the evil effect following it, being limited to that particular case, with the chance that it may be overruled and never become a precedent for other cases, can better be borne than could the evils of a different practice. *At the same time, the candid citizen must confess that if the policy of the Government upon vital questions affecting the whole people is to be irrevocably fixed by decisions of the Supreme Court, the instant they are made in ordinary litigation between parties in personal actions the people will have ceased to be their own rulers, having to that extent practically resigned their Government into the hands of that eminent tribunal.*

Dr. Tebault put into italics the last sentence, which in his opinion substitutes the whims of a political party to make changes to law over that of the Constitution. "The lines which I have put in italics proclaim the most pernicious political heresy ever uttered in the politics of our country."[43] He then went on to state: "Every publicist knows that it is not the party which fires the first shot that is responsible for the war but the party which makes war necessary.... For there is no question but a just fear of an imminent danger, though there be no blow given, is a lawful cause of war."[44] (A publicist is an expert in public or international law.)

The Treatment of Prisoners

In 1861 both sides felt that the armed conflict would soon be over, and therefore there was no need to plan for prisons to hold large numbers of captured enemy combatants. Military convention at the time held that prisoners were subject to immediate exchange or parole with the promise from the parolee not to fight or aid the enemy in any way. This philosophy avoided the burden of moving, sheltering, feeding and caring for large numbers of prisoners.[45] The anticipated short conflict became a drawn-out war, however, and paroled prisoners returned to their regiments to again join in the fight, thus making this rather noble idea unfeasible and burdening both sides with a sudden influx of hordes of captured and wounded enemy.

The war would create thousands of prisoners on both sides, and the high death rates recorded in makeshift prisons became a controversy that both sides would debate long after the war's end. Four hundred and ten thousand men would become imprisoned, and 56,000 prisoners would die, accounting for almost 10 percent of all deaths during the war. Much of the suffering was the result of a lack of preparation as well as generally unresponsive bureaucracies. In the South, plans for the construction of prison facilities occurred only out of desperation, as Richmond prisons overflowed. The Andersonville stockade was rushed to completion. Located near Andersonville, Georgia, the prison experienced a high mortality rate, largely as a result of the Confederacy's failure to prepare and a general lack of bureaucratic vision. In the summer of 1861, Brigadier-General John Winder was placed in charge of the Confederate prisons. Winder possessed no particular experience that qualified him to address the myriad details associated with the management of prisons. He was known to be short-tempered and aloof.[46] Winder was soon overwhelmed. "He was expected to return deserters, enforce martial law in all of its ramifications, guard Federal prisoners, oversee the camps of instruction, and discharge disables or ill soldiers."[47] Winder died suddenly in February 1865 from what appears to have been a massive heart attack. Had he survived the war, he may have been tried and executed for war crimes, as was his subordinate Henry Wirz.

In a letter to the *Richmond Times* that was published in 1915 after his death, Dr. Tebault noted that the Confederate policy towards the treatment of prisoners had been established by law shortly after the commencement of the war: "prisoners of war should have the same rations in quantity and quality as Confederate soldiers in the field. By an act afterward passed, all hospitals for sick and wounded prisoners were put upon the same footing with hospitals for sick and wounded Confederates. This policy was never changed. There was no discrimination in either particular between Federal prisoners and Confederate soldiers."⁴⁸ While noble, these policies were certainly not enforced uniformly through southern prisons.

The Union prison bureaucracy was better organized and produced more complete records than that of the Confederacy, but they were not more efficient. Colonel William Hoffman was appointed as Commissary General of Prisons in April 1862, a time when scattered makeshift prisons already overflowed with captured Confederate soldiers. Hoffman issued a circular on July 7, 1862, that called for the humane treatment of prisoners, including medical care under the charge of the senior surgeon, requisitions of clothing, a general fund to be established for the benefit of prisoners, the distribution of articles contributed by friends and families of prisoners, sutlers who would offer items at "reasonable prices," letter writing, and the maintenance of detailed prison records.⁴⁹ While the circular describes what one would consider to be quite reasonable conditions for prisoners, the treatment of prisoners in the North was at least as dreadful as that of southern prisons, with a lack of food, clothing, shelter and medical attention as common complaints. Prisons such as Camp Douglas in Chicago, like Andersonville, had its share of cruel guards and daily atrocities.⁵⁰ In 1864 Hoffman wrote to Secretary of War Edwin Stanton, with the suggestion that rations be reduced "considerably." Stanton forwarded the suggestion to Major-General Halleck, who replied, "Why not dispense with tea, coffee, and sugar and reduce the rations to that issued by the rebel Government to their own troops?"⁵¹ When Surgeon General Barnes heard of

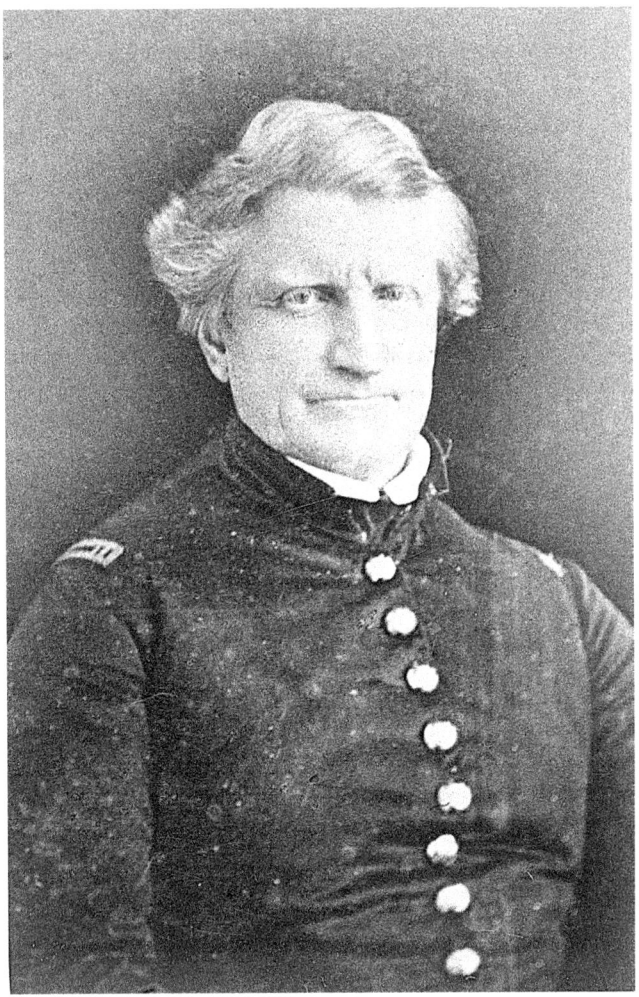

General Winder (1800–1865) served in the U.S. Army during the Mexican War when this photograph was taken. A lack of food, poor sanitation, and overcrowding led to high mortality rates at Andersonville Prison during his tenure. He died suddenly from a heart attack in February 1865. Civil War Photographs, 1861–1865, Library of Congress, Prints and Photographs Division, LC-B812-8967.

the change, he wrote Major General Halleck: "The reduction proposed by Major-General Halleck could be carried out with the exception of the ration for the sick and wounded."[52] Halleck quickly agreed that the sick and wounded would be allowed to have tea, coffee, and sugar in their rations.

Hoffman completed the construction in February 1862 of a new prison on Johnson's Island that was designed to hold 1,280 men just as Grant captured 15,000 prisoners at Fort Donelson.[53] Both sides struggled to care for the multitude of prisoners they never expected nor planned for.

There would be a total of more than 150 prisons created by both sides to house the hordes of prisoners. The conditions within these prisons varied from open stockades such as Andersonville to much more reasonable accommodations such as Fort Warren in Boston Harbor and Raleigh Prison (barracks) in North Carolina. The principle prisons in the North and South are shown in Tables 7 and 8 compiled from the records that were kept following Hoffman's July 1862 circular. This is an incomplete record as no information is available prior to July 1862, and even after the issuance of the circular, there were prisoners held in the custody of provost-marshals, in civil prisons, and in hospitals for whom there is no record. Additionally, monthly records were not always completed. While four New York prisons are listed, there were a total of 13 different prisons in that state.[54]

Table 7: Major Federal Prisons

Union Prisons[55]	Year Opened	Max. Held	Died
Allegheny City Penitentiary, Pennsylvania	1863	118	0
Alton, Illinois	1862	1,891	1,508
Camp Butler, Illinois	1862	2,186	866
Camp Chase, Ohio	1862	9,423	2,260
Camp Douglas, Illinois	1862	12,082	4,454
Camp Morton, Indiana	1862	5,000	1,763
Elmira, New York	1864	9,441	2,993
Fort Delaware, Delaware	1862	12,600	2,460
Fort Lafayette, New York	1862	163	2
Fort McHenry, Maryland	1862	6,957	33
Fort Mifflin, Pennsylvania	1863	215	3
Fort Pickens, Florida	1862	146	2
Fort Warren, Massachusetts	1862	394	12
Fort Wood, New York	1863	108	3
Gratiot Street, Missouri	1862	1,800	1,140
Hart's Island, New York	1865	3,446	235
Johnson's Island, Ohio	1862	3,256	235
Little Rock, Arkansas	1864	718	217
Louisville, Kentucky	1863	6,737	343
McLean Barracks, Ohio	1863	179	4
Morris Island, South Carolina	1864	558	3

Union Prisons[55]	Year Opened	Max. Held	Died
Nashville, Tennessee	1863	7,460	359
New Orleans, Louisiana	1863	1,856	213
Newport News, Virginia	1865	3,490	168
Ohio Penitentiary, Ohio	1864	68	0
Old Capital, District of Columbia	1862	2,763	457
Point Lookout, Maryland	1863	22,000	3,584
Rock Island, Illinois	1863	8,607	1,960
Ship Island, Mississippi	1864	4,430	103
Wheeling, West Virginia	1863	497	2

Table 8: Major Confederate Prisons

Confederate Prisons	Year Opened	Max. Held	Died
Andersonville, Georgia	1864	32,899	12,919
Belle Isle, Virginia	1862	10,000	300+
Boerne, Texas	1862	350	0
Cahaba, Alabama	1863	3,000	225
Camp Ford, Texas	1863	4,900	232+
Camp Groce, Texas	1863	500±	20
Castle Pinckney, South Carolina	1861	300	0
Castle Thunder, Virginia	1862	3,000	?
Charleston, South Carolina	1861	1,100	?
Charlotte, North Carolina	1865	1,200	?
Columbia, Tennessee	1864	2,000	?
Danville, Virginia	1863	4,000	1,297
Libby Warehouse, Virginia	1862	4,221	20+?
Ligon's Warehouse, Virginia	1861	600	?
Macon, Georgia	1861	1,900	?
Meridian, Mississippi	1863	700	?
Millen, Georgia	1864	10,299	488+
Raleigh, North Carolina	1861	500	?
Richmond, Virginia	1861	13,500	200+
Roper Hospital, South Carolina	1864	200±	?
Salisbury, North Carolina	1861	10,321	3,700
Savannah, Georgia	1864	6,000	2+?

On Wednesday, August 23, 1865, the trial of Henry Wirz began in Washington.[56] Wirz had been the commander of the infamous Andersonville Prison, and the trial and his subsequent execution brought much negative attention to the treatment of Union prisoners held in the South. Most southerners perceived Wirz as a scapegoat and his execution an appeasement to those in the North who sought revenge. Jefferson Davis wrote about Wirz's trial in his two-volume history of the war and provided a detailed account:

> Meanwhile certain persons of influence and public position at that time, either aware of the fabricated character of this testimony or convinced of its insufficiency to secure my conviction on a trial, sought to find ample material to supply this deficiency in the great mortality of the soldiers we had captured during the war and imprisoned at Andersonville. Orders were therefore issued by the authority of the United States government to arrest the subaltern officer Capt. Henry Wirz, a foreigner by birth, poor, friendless, and wounded, and held a prisoner of war. He had been included in the surrender of Gen. J.E. Johnston. On May 7, he was placed in the "old capital" prison at Washington. The poor man was doomed before he was heard, and the permission to be heard according to law was denied him. The first charge alleged against him was that of conspiring with myself, Secretary Seddon, Gen. Howell Cobb, Gen. Winder, and others, to cause the death of thousands of the prisoners through cruelty, etc. The second charge was alleged against himself for murder and violation of the law and customs of war. The military commission before which he was tried was convened by an order of President Johnson, of August 29, directing the officers detailed for the purpose to meet as a special military commission on August 20, for the trial of such prisoners as might be brought before it.... The so-called trial afterwards came on, and lasted for three months, but no evidence whatsoever was produced showing the existence of such a conspiracy as had been charged. Wirz, however, was pronounced guilty, and, in accordance with the sentence of the commission he was executed on November 10, 1865.
>
> On April 4, 1867, Mr. Louis Schade, of Washington, and the attorney of Wirz on the trial, in compliance with the request of Wirz to do so as soon as the times should be propitious, published a vindication of his character. The following is an extract from this publication: "On the night previous to the execution of the prisoner, some parties came to the confessor of Wirz (Boyle, Rev. Father) and also to me. One of them informed me that a high cabinet officer wished to assure Wirz that if he would implicate Jefferson Davis with the atrocities committed at Andersonville, his sentence should be commuted. He (the messenger, whoever he was) requested me to inform Wirz of this. In the presence of Father Boyle, I told him next morning what had happened. The captain simply and quietly replied: 'Mr. Schade, you know that I have always told you that I do not know anything about Jefferson Davis. He had no connection with me as to what was done at Andersonville. If I knew anything of him, I would not become a traitor against him or anybody else to save my life.'"[57]

Former Confederate Vice President Alexander H. Stephens published a two-volume history after the war. In a chapter devoted to "Prisoners of War," Stephens writes: "Neither Libby nor Belle Island nor Salisbury nor Andersonville would have had a groaning prisoner of war but for the refusal of the Federal authorities to comply with the earnest desire of the Richmond government for an immediate exchange upon the most liberal and humane principles. Had Mr. Davis's repeated offers been accepted, no prisoner on either side would have been retained in confinement a day."[58]

The process of exchanges came to a halt after Jefferson Davis's proclamation on Christmas Eve, 1862. Davis's General Orders, No. 111 mostly dealt with pronouncing Union General Benjamin F. Butler a criminal deserving of death as a result of Butler's iron fist in ruling over New Orleans. Davis then turned to the subject of how they should treat black troops in his General Orders: "all negro slaves captured in arms be at once delivered over to the executive authorities of the respective States to which they belong to be dealt with according to the laws of said States ... like orders be executed in all cases with respect to all commissioned officers of the United States when found serving in company with armed slaves in insurrection against the authorities of the different States of this Confederacy."[59] Since his proclamation equated black soldiers in the Union Army to slaves in revolt, the States could treat blacks in Federal uniform as rebellious slaves in any way they saw fit, including exe-

5. The Lost Cause 131

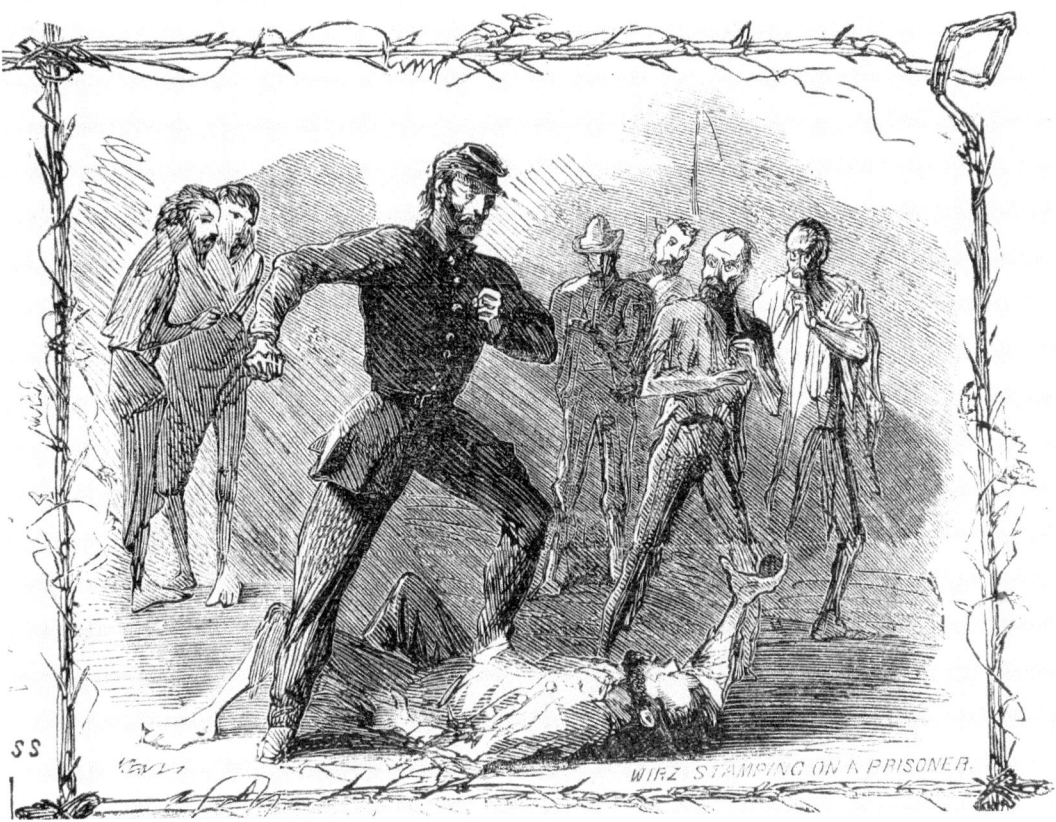

This illustration was published in *Harper's Weekly* just before the much-publicized trial of Henry Wirz commenced and was meant to show the brutality of Andersonville's commander. Wirz was found guilty and subsequently executed on November 10, 1865. *Harper's Weekly*, September 16, 1865, 585.

cution on the battlefield. This is the same manner in which slave revolts were handled in the antebellum South. The clear implication was that rebellious slaves would be executed, and white abettors to slave revolts (officers) would likewise be executed. In denying black Union soldiers the customary protections accorded enemy troops, it made their military service riskier than for soldiers in white regiments and gave the North an excuse for halting all prisoner exchanges.

The North became rather obsessed with reports of the poor treatment of Union prisoners in the South. Prisoners who either escaped or who were exchanged wrote books and articles in newspapers describing their ordeals, with undoubtedly some exaggeration. In the preface of one such book, the author states that "The evidence all goes to show that instead of trying to save the lives or alleviate the sufferings of those whom the fortunes of war had thrown into their hands, they [Confederates] practiced a systematic course of starvation and cruelty, that, in this nineteenth century, seems scarcely believable."[60] In another book, its author voices a similar opinion: "We are even led to conclude, by the usage which we have received at the hands of our captors and brutal prison keepers, that it was their deliberate intention to maim, and thereby render us completely unfit for future service."[61] And still another started his description of imprisonment and escape with the following: "In presenting the following narrative of suffering while a prisoner of the so-called Southern Con-

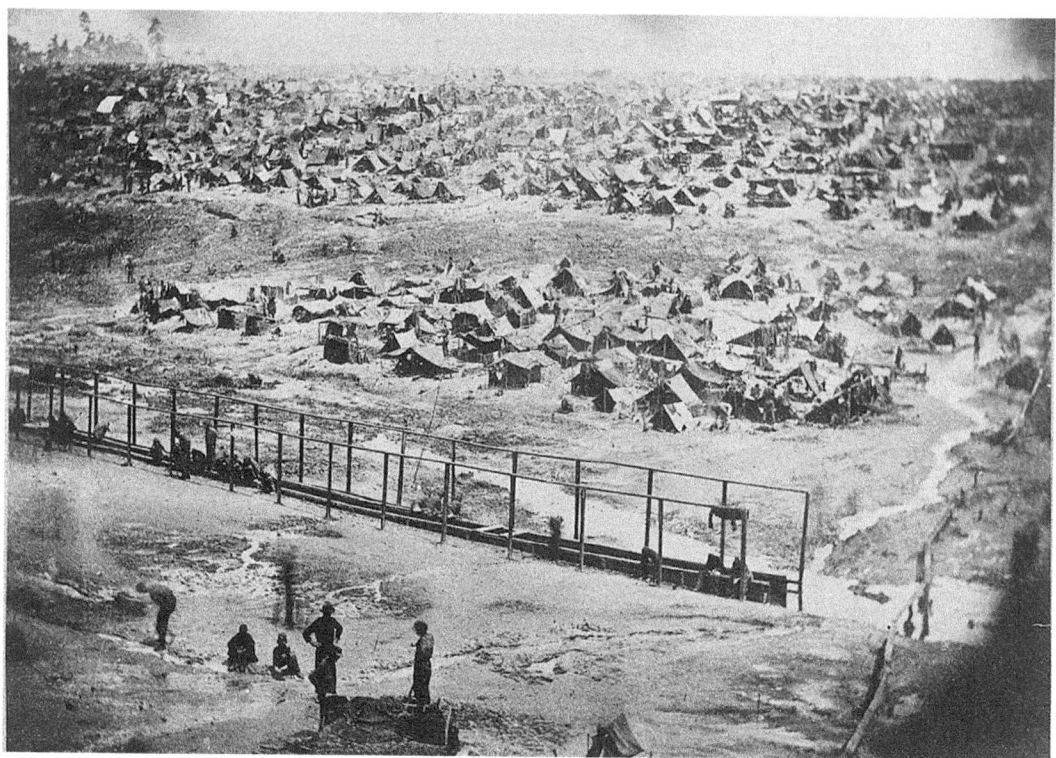

This photograph shows the conditions of Andersonville, with men living in improvised shelters and tents. Stockade Creek can be seen running from the lower left to the bottom; men in the foreground are obtaining water from the creek's runoff, while the wooden structure just above them is the prison's latrine, which ran along the creek. Disease ran rampant. Library of Congress, Prints & Photographs Division, Civil War Photographs, LC-DIG-ppmsca-33769.

federacy, the principal object had in view by the author, is to place before those into whose hands this volume may come, a plain, straightforward, unvarnished account of facts."[62]

While these written accounts shocked northerners, no prison in the South or North had a higher death rate than Camp Douglas in Chicago until the stockyard at Andersonville was built in 1864.[63] On February 18, 1862, two well-known civilian physicians, Thomas Hun and Mason Cogswell, inspected Camp Douglas at the request of the Sanitary Commission and described it as an "extermination camp." "In our experience we have never witnessed so painful a spectacle as that presented by their wretched inmates; without change of clothing, covered with vermin, they lie in cots without mattresses or with mattresses furnished by private charity, without sheets or bedding of any kind except blankets often in rags, in wards reeking with filth and foul air."[64]

Much of the criticism from the South regarding northern prison abuse came in the period after the war when southerners were pushing the Lost Cause and defending their civility from northern accusations. Dr. Tebault used his position as Surgeon General to defend the Confederate treatment of prisoners, especially regarding their medical management.[65] A major part of his argument was based on the fact that the North stopped prisoner exchanges later in the war due to the fact that the same prisoners, once exchanged, would return to the fight. Dr. Tebault quoted General Grant from Grant's telegram to Major General Butler in 1864:

5. The Lost Cause

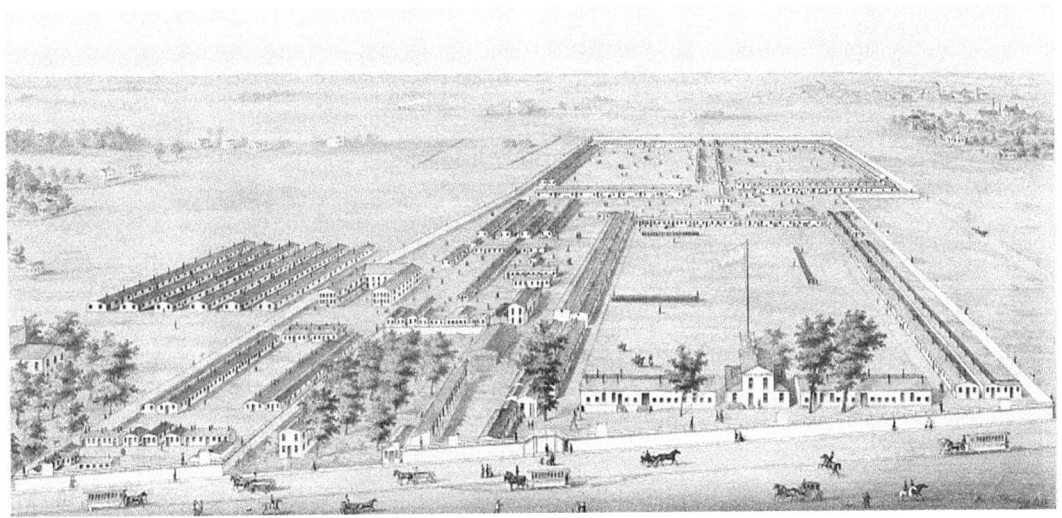

The conditions at Camp Douglas were certainly better than those of the Andersonville stockade, although prisoners were at times deliberately underfed, and diseases such as typhus and dysentery were common. Prisoners also had to contend with the harsh winter weather of Chicago. Library of Congress, Prints & Photographs Division, Civil War Photographs, CPH 3a17854.

CITY POINT, VA., August 18, 1864.

Major-General Butler,
 ...It is hard on our men held in Southern prisons not to exchange them, but it is humanity to those left in the ranks to fight our battles. Every man we hold, when released on parole or otherwise, becomes an active soldier against us at once either directly or indirectly. If we commence a system of exchange which liberates all prisoners taken, we will have to fight on until the whole South is exterminated. If we hold those caught they amount to no more than dead men. At this particular time to release all rebel prisoners North would insure Sherman's defeat and would compromise our safety here.
U.S. Grant, Lieutenant-General[66]

The South had proposed the use of Federal surgeons to treat their own men who were being held in southern prisons. On January 24, 1863, Colonel (Judge) Robert Ould, Confederate Agent for Prisoner Exchange, wrote his counterpart in Washington, General Ethan A. Hitchcock:

In view of the present difficulties attending to the exchange and release of prisoners, I propose that all such on each side shall be attended by a proper number of their own surgeons, who, under rules to be established, shall be permitted to take charge of their health and comfort. I also propose that these surgeons shall act as commissaries, with power to receive and distribute such contributions of money, food, and clothing and medicines as may be forwarded for the relief of the prisoners. I further propose that these surgeons shall be selected by their own Government, and that they shall have full liberty at any and all times through the agents of exchange to make reports not only of their own acts, but of any matters relating to the welfare of prisoners.[67]

While Ould's proposal was a logical one, he never received any reply from Hitchcock.[68]

In a letter written to Dr. Tebault, Dr. V.G. Hitt of Atlanta recalled Judge Ould's proposition to aid Union prisoners in southern prisons.[69] Ould had refused to meet with General Benjamin Butler, who at the time was the Federal agent for exchanges, as President Jefferson Davis had proclaimed "Beast" Butler to be an outlaw based on his treatment of women in New Orleans. Ould instead met with Major John Elmer Mulford, who became the Federal

Exchange Agent. Their meetings were quite civil, according to Hitt, and Mulford would often bring Ould "luxuries" not obtainable in the South such as coffee and French sardines. In his letter, Hitt described Ould's proposal:

> He [Ould] prefaced by stating to Major Mulford that we had no medicine or scarcely anything pertaining to the proper equipment of the surgeon in field or hospital—the same being contraband and shut off from us by reason of the blockade—that if the United States Government would send these medical equipments, they would be devoted exclusively to the Federal prisoners—and he added, furthermore, that if they sent their doctors they would be allowed to treat all the Federal sick without question as to their methods.... Major Mulford expressed himself as being delighted with this proposition, and dwelt on the satisfaction the entire northern people would hail this really humane feature.

Mulford left to confer with northern authorities while the Confederates waited a reply. Mulford came back with the statement: "Not only [is the proposal] not accepted, but the exchange of sick will no longer continue."[70]

In his report given at the 1896 reunion, Dr. Tebault mentioned the difficulties of providing medical care to prisoners of war:

> During the first two years of the war whenever the Confederate surgeon was made a prisoner while at his post of duty, his instruments, for professional work, were taken from him, and during the entire period of the war all medicines were made contraband of war, though thousands of Federal prisoners were held by the Confederacy because the Federal authorities refused to exchange them. The record will show that prior to the immediate surrender of the Confederate armies, the number of Federal prisoners captured much exceeded the captures made on the side of our then enemies, and in spite of this important fact, and though medicines were contraband of war, the casualties, by death, of prisoners held by the Southern Confederacy, were far less, than the death rate of Confederate prisoners held by the United States government, with unlimited means at its command.[71]

At the next year's reunion, Dr. Tebault provided statistics regarding northern and southern prisoners:

> In the first report, presented at the Richmond reunion, I showed that the medical roster for the Army of Tennessee has been preserved in duplicate. I shall offer in a more detailed report data to prove indisputably important facts relating to the prisoners of war upon both sides, with the purpose of establishing the death-rate responsibility in the premises. It will suffice to mention here that the report of Mr. Stanton, as Secretary of War, on the 19th of July, 1866, exhibits the fact that of the Federal prisoners in Confederate hands during the war only 22,570 died; while of the Confederate prisoners in Federal hands 26,436 died. This report does not set forth the exact number of prisoners held by each side respectively. These facts were given more in detail in a subsequent report by Surgeon-General Barnes, of the United States Army. That the whole number of Federal prisoners captured by the Confederates and held in Southern prisons from first to last during the war was in round numbers 270,000, while the whole number of Confederates captured and held in prisons by the Federals was in like round number only 220,000. From these two reports it appears that with 50,000 more prisoners in Southern stockades or other modes of confinement, the deaths were nearly 4,000 less. According to these figures the percentum of Federal deaths in Southern prisons was under nine; while the percentum of Confederate deaths in Northern prisons was over twelve. These mortuary statistics are of no small weight in determining on which side there was the most neglect, cruelty and inhumanity, proclaiming as they do a loss by death of more than 3 per cent, of Confederates over Federals in prisons, while the Federals had an unstinted command of everything.[72]

The controversy over the treatment of prisoners would not go away. Both sides argued bitterly during Reconstruction. In 1879 the future president of the United States, James Garfield, gave an impassioned speech to the survivors of Andersonville. "From Jeff Davis down it was a part of their policy to make you idiots and skeletons.... We can forgive and forget all other things before we can forgive and forget this."[73]

The Spanish-American War of 1898 would finally do much to put to rest the bitterness between the former rivals as they united in a spirit of reconciliation. Thereafter, monuments would be built on such hallowed ground as the site of Andersonville prison, and former soldiers from both sides would make pilgrimages to battlefields and prison sites in nostalgic reminiscences, paying homage to the heroic sacrifice and bravery on both sides of the conflict.

6

THE UNITED CONFEDERATE VETERANS

"to do justice to our common country, care for our needy and disabled comrades in their declining years, and assist the needy widows and orphans of our comrades."[1]

One year after the end of the war, the Grand Army of the Republic (GAR) was formed as a fraternal group of northern veterans offering camaraderie and support. It eventually became a strong political force in supporting Republican candidates and legislation that benefited veterans, including pensions, medical care, and the creation of old age homes to house indigent veterans. As the veterans grew old, a splinter group was formed for the sons of the veterans. The Sons of Union Veterans of the Civil War (SUVCW) was thus created, which continues today to honor and remember Union soldiers.

There were no such organized groups in the South until 1889 when Colonel J.F. Shipp and Leon Jastremski organized the United Confederate Veterans (UCV) in New Orleans, modeled after the GAR in the North. Before that time, some states had formed loose associations of veterans ("camps") based on the different state regiments who served. In 1889, however, there was a need to provide assistance to aging veterans, a need that was becoming more compelling with each passing year. Frederick Stith Washington (1840–1893) served as the first president of the UCV. He had served in the war as a private in the 7th Louisiana Infantry. Washington was related to President George Washington, and his father was an editor of the *Daily Picayune*, one of the more influential Democratic newspapers published in New Orleans.

A circular announcing the formation and convention of the UCV was sent from New Orleans to be published in southern newspapers.

> *To the Veteran ex–Soldiers and Sailors of the Confederate States*: COMRADES: In view of the ideas which permeate our minds that we, of the South, should, in a spirit of amity and friendship, in the interest and for the benefit of our whole Republic, form a federation of associations, and that all ex–Confederate soldiers and sailors now surviving, who were in good standing, be invited to join with us for that purpose, we beg to suggest:
>
> The formation of an association for such benevolent, historical and social purposes, as will enable us to do justice to our common country, care for our needy and disabled comrades in their declining years, and assist the needy widows and orphans of our comrades, in a spirit of mutual friendship, fraternity and good will….[2]

The purpose of the UCV had been described by Dr. Joseph Jones as encompassing two noble objectives:

1st. The preservation of the story of our heroic struggle, with its victories, defeats, privations and sufferings.

2nd. The relief of the sufferings, diseases and wounds of veterans of the Confederate army and navy.[3]

Interestingly, included in the constitution was Article 14 that banned political or religious discussions: "The discussion of political or religious subjects, nor any political action shall be permitted within the organization of the United Confederate Veterans, and any camp, bivouac or association that will have acted in violation of this article, shall be declared to have forfeited its membership in this association."[4]

The New Orleans chapter of the UCV came into being on June 10, 1889. The UCV selected as its first commander-in-chief the former United States senator and then governor of Georgia, ex–Major General John B. Gordon. Gordon exemplified the New South politician who capitalized upon his fame with the Confederacy to obtain political and financial rewards. Gordon served the UCV well until his death in 1904. He had survived the war after receiving numerous severe wounds.[5] Joseph Jones (1833–1896) became the Surgeon General of the UCV. He had served in the Confederacy as a surgeon and was known for his scientific inquiries into the diseases and injuries in Confederate hospitals. Originally from Georgia, he held a teaching position at the University of Louisiana in New Orleans.[6]

While the organization originated in New Orleans, the first reunion of the UCV was held in Chattanooga, Tennessee, in July 1890. During that first reunion, Surgeon General Jones leveraged his personal interests in medical research and identified two important objectives for his new role in the UCV: "First. The collection and preservation of the records of the Medical Corps of the Confederate Army and Navy; Second. The determination by actual investigation and inquiry the numbers and condition of the surviving Confederate soldiers who have been disabled by wounds and diseases, received in their heroic defense of the rights and liberties of the Southern States."[7]

The fires in Richmond, Virginia, on April 3, 1865, had destroyed most of the Confederate medical records. Because of his interest in research and statistics, Jones recognized the need to compile as many medical records from as many of the surviving medical corps as possible to create a medical legacy. To help accomplish his objective, Jones issued the following circular before the reunion in the hope of collecting important medical data:

To the Survivors' of the Medical Corps of the Confederate States Army and Navy: COMRADES—The surrender of the Army of Northern Virginia on this day, twenty-five years ago, practically ended the struggle for independence of the Southern States, and during this quarter of a century death has thinned our ranks, and our corps can now oppose but a broken line in the great struggle against human suffering, disease and death. S.P. Moore, Surgeon-General of the Confederate Army is dead; Chas. Bell Gibson, Surgeon-General of Virginia; Surgeons L. Guild, A.J. Ford, J.A.A. Berrian, J.T. Darby, W.A. Carrington, S.A. Ramsay, Samuel Choppin, Robert J. Breckenridge, E.N. Covey, E.S. Galliard, Paul F. Eve, O.F. Manson, Louis D. Foard, S.E. Habersham, James Bolton, Robert Gibbes, and a host of medical officers of the Confederate States Army are dead. The Association of the United Confederate Veterans was formed in New Orleans June 10, 1889, the objects of which are historical, social and benevolent. Our illustrious commander, General John B. Gordon, of Georgia, has ordered the United Confederate Veterans to assemble at Chattanooga, Tennessee, on July 3, 1890. It is earnestly hoped that every surviving member of the Medical Corps of the Confederate Army and Navy will meet upon this important occasion, and promote by his presence and his counsels the sacred interests of the United Confederate Veterans. It is of the greatest importance to the future historian, and also to the honor and welfare of the medical profession of the South, that careful records should be furnished to the Surgeon-General of the United Confederate Veterans, embracing the following data:

1st. Name, nativity, date of commission in the Confederate States Army and Navy, nature and length of service of every member of the Medical Corps of the Confederate States Army and Navy.

2. Obituary notices and records of all deceased members of the Medical Corps of the Confederate Army and Navy.

3d. The titles and copies of all field and hospital reports of the Medical Corps of the Confederate Army and Navy.

4th. Titles and copies of all published and unpublished reports relating to military surgery, and to diseases of armies, camps, hospitals and prisons.

The object proposed to be accomplished by the Surgeon-General of the United Confederate Veterans, is the collection, classification, preservation, and final publication of all the documents and facts bearing upon the history and labors of the Medical Corps of the Confederate States Army and Navy, during the civil war, 1861–65. Everything which relates to the critical period of our national history, which shall illustrate the patriotic, self-sacrificing, and scientific labors of the Medical Corps of the Confederate States Army and Navy, and which shall vindicate the truth of history, shall be industriously collected, filed and finally published. It is believed that invaluable documents are scattered over the whole land, in the hands of survivors of the civil war of 1861–1865, which will form material for the correct delineation of the medical history of the corps which played so important a part in the great historic drama. Death is daily thinning our ranks, while time is laying its heavy hands upon the heads of those whose hair is already whitening with the advance of years and the burden of cares. No delay, fellow comrades, should be suffered in the collection and preservation of these precious documents.

To this task of collecting all documents, cases, statistics and facts relating to the medical history of the Confederate Army and Navy, the Surgeon-General of the United Confederate Veterans invites the immediate attention and cooperation of his honored comrades and compatriots throughout the South.[8]

Dr. Jones served as Surgeon General for the UCV until his death in 1896. Even though his health had been slowly failing, he continued to work on his research and teach Chemistry and Medical Jurisprudence at the newly renamed Tulane University. His death came rather suddenly on February 17, 1896.[9] Following Dr. Jones's death, Dr. Tebault was appointed to replace him as Surgeon General of the UCV. The two men had known each other well, not only from their New Orleans connections, but also during their war experiences. While Dr. Tebault was not the scientific researcher that Jones had been, his passion for the cause of aiding veterans certainly helped him in transitioning into the position left vacant by his predecessor.

In his first address to the UCV, Dr. Tebault acknowledged Dr. Jones's legacy: "Let me express my own heartfelt sorrow, in common with all true Confederates, at the losses by death our Association had sustained during the past year, and among others that of the lamented Surgeon General Joseph Jones, my predecessor, who passed away ripe in honors, beloved by all who knew him, and as true and devoted a Confederate as our heroic and immortal and constitutionally sustained cause possessed."[10] Even in his eulogy to Jones, Tebault felt the need to remark about the "constitutionally sustained" secession.

The UCV provided much-needed assistance for aging and destitute veterans. The New Orleans camps offered veterans employment assistance and collected money to support veterans' homes and pension assistance.[11] UCV memorial associations were also created, which raised donations to create memorials honoring Confederate generals and soldiers, a point of contention in today's political climate as they also promoted the Lost Cause doctrine.

Reunions were probably the most important aspect of the UCV, with parades, drinking, enthusiastic and adulatory speeches, and the attention of young admirers, especially the young girls selected to be "sponsors" each year. Being together with old comrades and like-minded people supported the notion that theirs had been an honorable fight and that all their sacrifices were worthwhile. Many of the speeches were in support of the Lost Cause, citing legal and emotional reasons that the war was unjustly started by those in the North. It

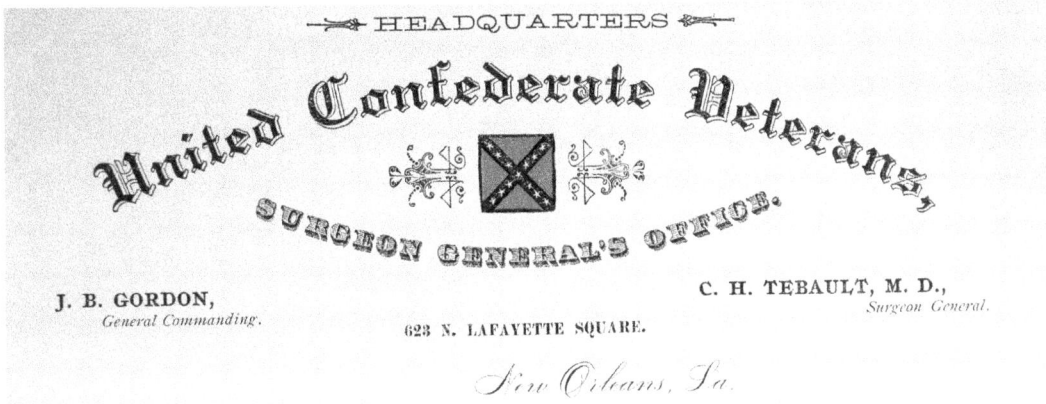

Dr. Tebault listed his home address (623 N. Lafayette Square) as his headquarters while serving as Surgeon General of the UCV. Photograph by author (letter owned by author).

also gave veterans a voice where they could proudly recall, with some embellishments, their service and the heroism of fellow soldiers. Reunions were expensive affairs, but southern cities vied for the publicity and economic income from the gatherings, especially during the early years when the numbers of veterans attending were great; as the years went on, the dwindling number of veterans still brought much attention to the host city, although the economic benefits of hosting veterans and their families were diminished.

Remarkably, the participation of black veterans was not uncommon. A black man who fought in the 12th Louisiana Regiment attended the 1903 reunion in New Orleans.[12] For the white veterans, the participation of blacks in their reunions may have validated their relationships with former slaves, one of their Lost Cause arguments.

Like the GAR, a splinter group, the Sons of Confederate Veterans (SCV) was formed in 1896 at the first annual meeting of the UCV.[13] The SCV is still active today, with the goal of serving "as a historical, patriotic, and non-political organization dedicated to ensuring that a true history of the 1861–1865 period is preserved."[14] The SCV website also includes references to Lost Cause tenets. "The preservation of liberty and freedom was the motivating factor in the South's decision to fight the Second American Revolution."[15] It also includes a quote from Stephen Dill Lee, Commander of the UCV, from a speech he gave during the 1906 reunion: "To you, Sons of Confederate Veterans, we will commit the vindication of the cause for which we fought. To your strength will be given the defense of the Confederate soldier's good name, the guardianship of his history, the emulation of his virtues, the perpetuation of those principles which he loved and which you love also, and those ideals which made him glorious and which you also cherish." The SCV is committed to preserving and honoring Confederate gravesites and memorials.

Afterword

> *"Though men deserve, they may not win, success;*
> *The brave will honor the brave, vanquished none the less."*
> —(The above couplet served as the tagline for the
> *Confederate Veteran* magazine, published between
> 1893 and 1932.)

In many ways, Christopher Hamilton Tebault typified the southern patriot. He was quick to volunteer to fight for his state and a cause he considered to be just. He was a creative physician who, during the war, served his fellow soldiers well and earned their respect. After the war he decided to devote his medical career to helping children, a noble focus that may have been the result of all the bloodshed he faced during the war. Dr. Tebault left many positive contributions to the city of New Orleans. He participated as a delegate to the Constitutional Convention of 1898, helped to create boards of health throughout the state, and produced much-needed benefits and relief for aging Confederate veterans. He founded the Real Estate and Direct Taxpayers' Union as a means of fighting the onerous taxes levied on New Orleans by Reconstruction policies. He fought the corrupt Louisiana Lottery Company. His persistence paid off: taxes were reduced, and the Louisiana Lottery was eventually closed, although corruption at the state and local levels continued to pervade Louisiana politics for decades to come.

In 1899 the *Times-Picayune* published a rather stirring tribute to Dr. Tebault and his daughter Corrine Tebault who was actively involved in the Daughters of the American Revolution, the United Daughters of the Confederacy and other organizations. The paper's tribute noted a lineage of patriotism and public service:

> He shouldered a musket in defense of the people's rights on the celebrated Fourteenth of September, which emancipated Louisiana. He was one of the professors at the Charity Hospital Medical College, health officer of the city, and has served the state and city in a number of other capacities, among them as chairman of the committee on health, quarantine and state medicine, and was also a member of the veterans' committee, which secured pensions to the old veterans in the constitutional convention of 1898, of which he was a member for the parish of Orleans. He was also one of the very earliest, most active and prominent members of Confederate Camp No. 2, Army of Tennessee, U.C.V. Dr. Tebault s distinguished record as surgeon in the confederate states army is fully mentioned in the *Life of General Beauregard* written by Judge Roman.[1]
>
> Miss Tebault's paternal ancestor, Baron Tebault, who left valuable memoirs, was general-in-chief of the French army just before Napoleon's time. Her paternal great-grandfather, Christopher Hall, of Norfolk, Va. was in the Revolutionary war and was a warm friend of General Lafayette. When Lafayette visited America, he was entertained by Hon. Christopher Hall who was then in the Virginia legislature. The next year Hon. Christopher Hall made a tour of Europe, when he was entertained by General Lafayette at his favorite chateau, *La Grange* in France, and Lafayette presented him when he left France with four views of *La Grange*. Miss Tebault's father now has in his possession one of the views. Colo-

nel Hall was also an officer in the celebrated Indian wars. Miss Tebault's paternal grandfather, Major E.J. Tebault, was a banker and planter, being cashier of the famous Bank of Louisiana just prior to the war. Miss Tebault's maternal revolutionary ancestor was Governor Win. Bradford, the first governor of Massachusetts. Her maternal great-grandfather, Hon. Seaton Grantland, represented Georgia in the legislature and in congress; he founded the first newspaper in middle Georgia, the *Southern Recorder*, and was also one of the founders of the Whig party in Georgia, and was one of the wealthiest men in Georgia. Her maternal grandfather, Hon. J. Bailey [David Jackson Bailey], of Griffin, Ga. was colonel of the thirtieth Georgia Regiment in the army of Tennessee, and he also served during the Indian war during the entire time the country was engaged in battling with the Seminoles and Creeks, and was promoted to a captaincy. Colonel Bailey served the state of Georgia as speaker of the House of Representatives, and as president of the Senate, and for several terms in the United States Congress. At the time of his death he was the oldest congressman in Georgia, and here occurred a remarkable incident in the history of the country. Colonel Bailey and his father-in-law, Hon. Seaton Grantland, both in Congress at the same time, from the same state, one a Whig and the other a Democrat. Miss Tebault, on her father's side and through her Huguenot ancestry, is related to the Manderville and Rutledge families of South Carolina. [John Rutledge (1739–1800) was one of the signers of the Declaration of Independence and was a member of a large family living near Charleston.] Miss Tebault, as well as her mother, are both Daughters of the American Revolution and Colonial Dames; Miss. Tebault is also a member of the United Daughters of the Confederacy, Louisiana division, and was appointed a delegate to represent them at the Charleston convention. Miss Tebault also had one great uncle killed under General Jackson in the Battle of New Orleans.[2]

Dr. Tebault died on May 24, 1914, after a long illness. Numerous obituaries and tributes were published honoring his service and contributions, but perhaps the most thorough tribute was made in the May 25, 1914, issue of the *Times-Picayune*:

DEATH TAKES OLD SOLDIER; DOCTOR TEBAULT PASSES.

Well Known Figure in New Orleans Yields at Last to Long Illness.

Dr. Christopher Hamilton Tebault, scion of a distinguished family of stock from which sprang ex–President Theodore Roosevelt, died late Sunday evening at his residence, 623 North Street. He had been ill many months.

Dr. Tebault's passing removes an interesting figure. A distinguished Confederate veteran, for twenty-five years or more he served as Surgeon General of the United Confederate Veterans. He was also a member of the Confederate Cavalry Camp and the Army of Tennessee. He was one of the city's best known and oldest physicians.

Attended by his son, Grantland L. Tebault, his figure was a well known one in the vicinity of Lafayette Square, facing which he made his home for many years. He was accustomed to taking long walks on the arm of his son. He won laurels in the army through his introduction of modified inoculation in smallpox cases.

Returning to New Orleans after peace had been declared, Dr. Tebault published

The above photograph was published in the 1914 *Confederate Veteran* as part of Dr. Tebault's obituary.

in the first issue of the *Medical and Surgical Journal* his war experiences with modified inoculations and its advantages over vaccination. For the first two years succeeding the war he taught anatomy in the medical college where he had graduated and was elected to the Board of Health to the important position of Health Officer of the Second District.

He has been visiting physician of the Charity Hospital at different times, and filled the chair as professor of the diseases of children, and was associated in the chair of obstetrics and diseases of women with Professor Warren Brickell, Professors Samuel Choppin, J. Dickinson Bruns, Schuppert, Loeba, Warren Stone Jr., Schruggs, Ford and Schmidt.

He organized in New Orleans the Real Estate and Property Holder's Union and was made its President. In fact of what had been termed a "hopeless dream" by many legislators, Dr. Tebault in the Constitutional Convention reduced the municipal taxation of New Orleans from thirty to ten mills, and the State taxation from twenty-one and a half mills to six mills.

He is survived by his widow, two sons, Grantland L. and Dr. C.H. Tebault, Jr., and a married daughter, Mrs. Howard V. Harper.

Dr. Tebault was a prominent member of the Constitutional Convention of 1898. Much of his work in the war is detailed in the *Photographic History of the Civil War*[3] and in the *Confederate Military History*.[4] Though a lad hardly out of his teens, Dr. Tebault was designated "one of the four distinguished physicians of the Civil War."

The *Confederate Military History* summarized Dr. Tebault's war record and life:

After the retreat from Corinth to Tupelo, Tebault was promoted to surgeon as assigned to the 10th SC, with which he served during the KY campaign and until the battle of Murfreesboro, when he was detailed for service in a hospital in Cleveland, TN. He remained on duty there until the post was evacuated and afterward served in the hospitals at Calhoun, Griffin, Albany and Macon, GA of the Army of TN. His performance of duty was so faithful and devoted, and marked by such professionalism, as to win him the love and admiration of many soldiers. He became an eminent surgeon in New Orleans, also holding the position of health officer of the city, demonstrator of anatomy at the college, professor of diseases of children and associate professor of gynecology at the Charity Hospital of New Orleans. Though not taking an active part in politics, his influence was such as to cause his election to the state constitutional convention of 1898, in which he served on several prominent committees, among them the Confederate committee and as chairman of the committee of Health, Quarantine and State Medicine. These reports of the surgeon are also the storehouses of facts testifying to the humanity of the South in caring for Northern prisoners, a fact which, thanks to General Tebault, and other patriotic Southerners, has been placed in a position of unassailable historic verity.[5]

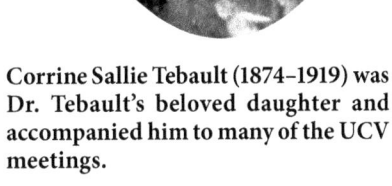

Corrine Sallie Tebault (1874–1919) was Dr. Tebault's beloved daughter and accompanied him to many of the UCV meetings.

On May 26, two days after his death, the *Times-Picayune* published the final funeral arrangements that included a remarkable list of distinguished pallbearers, which included past and present Louisiana Governors, United States Senators, City Mayors, Chief Justices, ministers, physicians and prominent businessmen:

Afterword

The funeral of Dr. C.H. Tebault, prominent physician and Confederate army surgeon, will be held at the family home, 623 North Street, at 3:30 o'clock Tuesday afternoon. The Rev. A. Gordon Bakewell, Confederate chaplain and the Rev. Dr. Robert S. Coupland, rector of Trinity Church, will officiate. Interment will be in the tomb of the Army of Tennessee in Metairie Cemetery. The active pallbearers will be Dr. Ernest E. Lewis, Dr. Y.R. LeMonnier [City Physician and Coroner], Pearl Wight [owner of a ship chandlery and supply business in New Orleans], James D. Hill [Confederate veteran and prominent sugar planter in Louisiana], J.A. Harral [Confederate veteran actively involved in the UCV], and W.O. Hart [prominent New Orleans lawyer and author of a number of books and articles on New Orleans].

Honorary pallbearers will be: Former Governor Newton C. Blanchard [United States Senator who became the 33rd Governor of Louisiana, 1904–1908], Martin Bohrman, John Fitzpatrick [Mayor of New Orleans, 1892–1896], Dr. J. Dickson Bruns [Confederate surgeon and chair of physiology at Tulane; he was one of the main speakers at the mass meeting in front of the Clay statue that led to the Battle of Liberty Place in September 1874], Dr. Paul Rees, Dr. Edward Jones, Dr. J.D. Bloom [House Surgeon at Charity Hospital], Hon. Luther E. Hall [State Senator and District Judge who was elected the 35th Governor of Louisiana, 1912–1916], Robert Ewing [Publisher of the *Morning Chronicle*; he served along with Dr. Tebault as a Democratic delegate to the 1898 Constitutional Convention], Thomas G. Raspier, C. Taylor Gauche, Lee Marrero, Charles A. Larendon [husband of P.G.T. Beauregard's daughter, Laure Beauregard], Judge Breaux [Confederate veteran and Chief Justice of the Louisiana State Supreme Court], Judge Monroe [Confederate veteran actively involved in the UCV; in 1914 he became Chief Justice], Judge Claiborne, Judge St. Paul, Judge Godehaux, Henry Denis, Sol Wexler [President of the Whitney-Central National Bank of New Orleans], Lewis Guion [Confederate veteran and attorney who was a staunch fighter against Reconstruction; his obituary noted he was considered "an authority on Southern history and was instrumental in correcting many of the historical errors found in books used in public schools of the South"], Walter Guion [district judge who later became a United States Senator from Louisiana in 1918], H.A. Morine, A.J. Peters, John J. Gannon [Vice President of the New Orleans Railway & Light Company], W.R. Irby [managed the W.R. Irby Tobacco Company, a branch of the American Tobacco Company], George W. Nott [Postmaster of New Orleans], John Wait, Wm. Winans Wall, John Tobin, George W. Flynn [Secretary of the Democratic State Committee under Governor Nicholls], Judge Provosly, Fred Schmidt, A.G. Ricks, W.B. Thompson [President of the W.B. Thompson & Company cotton manufacturing company and President of the New Orleans Cotton Exchange], E.E. Lafaye, Gen. W.J. Behan [Washington Artillery of New Orleans, twice elected as Major-General of the Louisiana Division UCV, participated along with Dr. Tebault in the Battle of Liberty Place in 1874, and elected Mayor of New Orleans in 1882], Harold W. Newman [President of the New Orleans Stock Exchange], Judge Sommerville [Associate Justice of the Supreme Court of Louisiana], A.H. Annan, Robert Marr, the Rev. John Caldwell, the Rev. I.L. Leucht, the Rev. Max Heller, the Most Rev. Archbishop Blank, Judge Skinner, Hugues de la Vergne, Gen. Albert Estopinal [sugar cane planter who served as a Democrat in both houses of the Louisiana State Legislature between 1876 and 1900 and in the United States House of Representatives from 1908 until his death in 1919], Bishop Davis Sessume, the Rev. S.H. Weriein, Dr. Hermann B. Gessner, Dr. W.F. McKee, Carlton Hunt, Dr. Brickell, the Rev. Dr. George H. Cornelson, Jr., Col. George Soule [Confederate veteran who founded Soule College in New Orleans just before the war in 1856; the college closed in 1983], Victor Mauberret, Capt. T.J. Woodward, and Alden McLellan.[6]

The impressive list of pallbearers underscores the influence and esteem Dr. Tebault held in New Orleans society. Dr. Stanford E. Chaillé paid his old friend Dr. Tebault a moving tribute, a portion of which was published as the final paragraph in Dr. Tebault's obituary that appeared in the August 1914 issue of *Confederate Veteran*. Dr. Chaillé was addressing the Association of the Medical Officers of the Confederate Army and Navy at the 1903 UCV reunion in New Orleans:

> But, while your armed comrades were dying for the south, where were the noncombatant medical officers of the Confederacy? Close by their sides, whether sick, wounded or dying; whether on the bare ground, in tent, in hospital, or on the battle field. How close you clung to your suffering comrades, let this small fraction of the woeful truth testify. The war-record of only a small portion of the gradu-

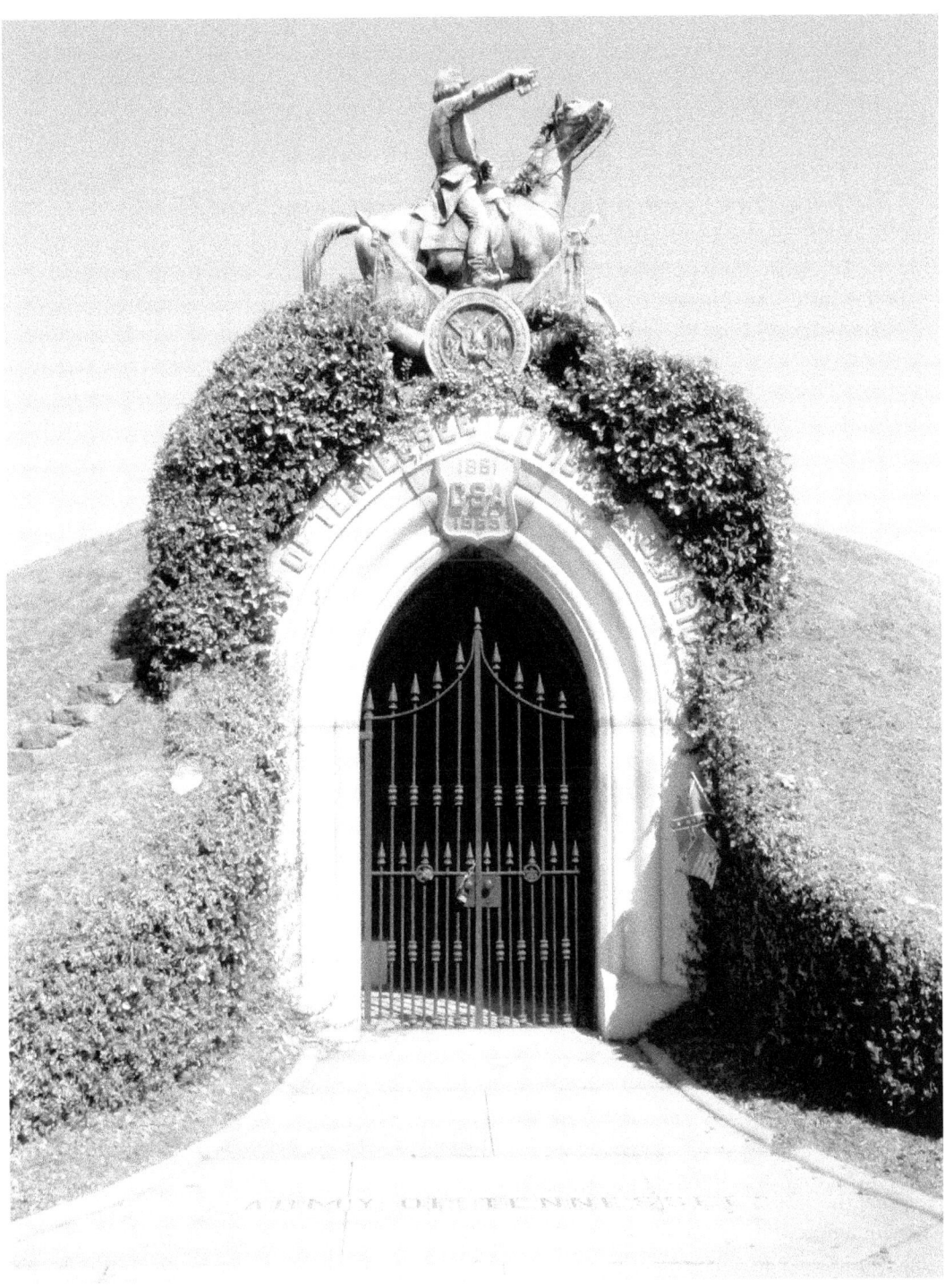

The Army of Tennessee Tumulus in Metairie Cemetery is a 30-foot-high earthen mound topped with a statue of Alfred Sidney Johnson riding his horse, *Fire Eater*. The tumulus contains 48 crypts. General P.G.T. Beauregard was entombed there after his death in 1893. Dr. Tebault's body was originally placed in the tumulus but later removed to a nearby family tomb (author's collection).

ates of the Medical Department of Tulane University has been traced. Yet, of this fraction of this one medical college, twenty-four died or were permanently disabled by wounds received and thirteen were killed in battle. Medical officers still living incurred like risks and, of these, not one was more unselfish, efficient and faithful than the present Surgeon General of Confederate Veterans, Dr. C.H. Tebault.[7]

The Failure of Reconstruction and the Rise of the Lost Cause

Dr. Tebault was an esteemed physician and publicly minded patriot. But how can we today justify his support of the Lost Cause and his fight against Reconstruction, whose main purposes were to readmit the Confederate states into the Union, to help rebuild the southern states, and to secure equality for black citizens—all admirable goals? It is easy to judge the past using today's social values. We may feel intellectually superior when reading Dr. Tebault's writings regarding his defense of secession and the North's responsibility for the war. We may feel morally superior when reflecting on his support of the Crescent City White League and his participation in the Battle of Liberty Place. Today numerous protesters crusade to remove from town squares and buildings Confederate monuments and the names of Confederate heroes as they believe such markers wrongly celebrate the southern rebellion, its support of slavery, and the subsequent years of oppression of black Americans. There are even those who advocate for the purging of Thomas Jefferson's and Andrew Jackson's names from buildings and currency because Jefferson owned slaves and Jackson waged genocide against Native Americans. But assuming such moral high ground ignores the social, political, and economic reasons behind viewpoints that we might today feel to be odious and offensive. Without understanding and listening to the voices from the past, how can we improve ourselves and our country? Isn't this lack of understanding why many of the Lost Cause tenets are still commonly espoused in southern states today?

While not a member of the White League, Dr. Tebault actively joined with them in the Battle of Liberty Place. From a southern viewpoint, the event heroically drove the carpetbaggers from the state and restored democracy after the punishing period of Reconstruction; a period where native white citizens saw their government being run by outsiders and scalawags. Additionally, there had been efforts by the Radical Republicans in Congress to disenfranchise ex–Confederates from voting; anyone who had voted for secession or had openly advocated for it, including newspaper editors and ministers, were considered unqualified to vote. To be exempted from such disqualification, one had to take an oath favoring Radical Reconstruction.[8] In the 1868 Louisiana election returns calling a constitutional convention, almost twice as many blacks as whites had registered to vote—45,218 whites versus 84,436 blacks.[9] Whites in Louisiana were outraged. Today we view the September 14 event as whites and battle-hardened ex-Confederates joining a paramilitary group to overturn the state government and repress Republicans and black citizens; essentially, that was what the Battle of Liberty Place signified. But it is also understandable how and why it came about given the circumstances existing at the time.

As the Surgeon General of the UCV, Dr. Tebault left a written legacy that promoted the doctrines of the Lost Cause; his focus was largely on the legal aspects of secession, the responsibility for the war, and the treatment of prisoners. The end of the Civil War put to rest the debate regarding whether states had the right to secede from the Federal union, but at the time this was not an illogical position. In 1814 delegates representing Massachusetts, Connecticut and Rhode Island had discussed secession during the Hartford Convention;

New Englanders were angered by the continuing war with England and the recent Louisiana Purchase, which they viewed as diluting their political influences.[10] While the Hartford Convention did not seriously contemplate secession, the fact that they had considered it to be a legal option was not inconsequential. The Declaration of Independence can also be construed as giving states the legal right to secede:

> We hold these truths to be self-evident, that all men are created equal, that they are endowed by their Creator with certain unalienable Rights, that among these are Life, Liberty and the pursuit of Happiness.—That to secure these rights, Governments are instituted among Men, deriving their just powers from the consent of the governed,—<u>That whenever any Form of Government becomes destructive of these ends, it is the Right of the People to alter or to abolish it, and to institute new Government</u>, laying its foundation on such principles and organizing its powers in such form, as to them shall seem most likely to effect their Safety and Happiness.[11]

The underlined text supported the view that secession was legal.

Many northern states had been actively ignoring the Supreme Court's Dred Scott decision and the Fugitive Slave Law of 1850 and had passed so-called "personal liberty laws" as a result. While today we view the Dred Scott case as morally, constitutionally, and legally wrong, southerners at the time saw it as a vindication of slavery in the face of the increasingly violent protests from northern abolitionists. If some northern states could ignore Federal law then perhaps the Constitution itself was invalid, so they thought. Dr. Tebault's arguments at the time were rational and, of course, warmly embraced by southerners seeking to justify their sacrifices.

Dr. Tebault's second focus regarding the Lost Cause was on the responsibility for the Civil War. He quoted from the letters of Justice Jeremiah Black of Pennsylvania who had opposed Congress's plan for Reconstruction. Black had met with Lincoln's Secretary of State, William Seward, and suggested that the southern states would stay with the Union if Seward would pledge himself to accept the decisions of the Supreme Court as the final word on any legal dispute. Seward replied that he would not do so, and he added that he considered it to be "treason" to try to trick him in that manner to agree with the Dred Scott case. Black believed that had such a pledge been made, the war would not have taken place as all sides would be satisfied.[12]

Dr. Tebault argued that the attack on Fort Sumter was also a legal act. "The Fort was within the jurisdiction of South Carolina. It was built especially for her protection, and belonged to her."[13] He pointed out that Lincoln's cabinet "voted six to one in favor of surrendering Fort Sumter...."[14] Dr. Tebault quoted from Alexander Stephens, the former Vice President of the Confederacy: "I maintain that it [the war] was inaugurated and began, though no blow had been struck, when the hostile fleet, styled the 'Relief Squadron,' with eleven ships, carrying two hundred and eighty-five guns and two thousand four hundred men, was sent from New York and Norfolk, with orders from the authorities at Washington, to reinforce Fort Sumter peacefully, if permitted—'but forcibly, if they must.'"[15]

President Lincoln certainly did not want to alienate the border states, most being against secession. He, however, underestimated the impassioned reactions in the South when he called for 75,000 troops to quash the "rebellion." Many southerners may have not liked the idea of secession, but they hated coercion more and now felt that they were about to be invaded by hostile troops.

Dr. Tebault's third focus was the treatment of prisoners during the war. His opinions regarding such treatment are also not entirely incorrect, even by modern historical views. While the conditions at Andersonville Prison were incredibly difficult, a number of northern prisons were no better. Camp Douglas in Chicago was described at the time by respected northern physicians, Drs. Hun and Cogswell, as an "extermination camp." The memoirs published during and immediately after the war by northern soldiers described sadistic prison guards and deplorable conditions at southern prisons and did much to fan northern anger and calls for retributions towards the South. The stories of Camp Douglas and other Union prisons, however, went largely unreported by northern newspapers. Southerners felt unjustly criticized, and Dr. Tebault's rather lengthy statistical reports comparing prison mortality on both sides offer an interesting perspective.

The commander of Andersonville Prison, Henry Wirz, was tried and executed immediately after the war. Today, the appropriateness of his execution is still debated. Northerners were demanding retribution, and Wirz represented the perfect scapegoat.[16] In his defense, Wirz never received the money or the materials necessary to build an acceptable prison. Food, building materials, medical care, inspectors and religious leaders were entirely out of his reach. The lines of responsibility were also confusing at best; Wirz oversaw the prison's daily operations, but others had responsibility for the Confederate post, of which the prison was part. Prison guards, the hospital, and the quartermaster departments also reported to different lines of command.[17] Wirz acknowledged in a newspaper interview before his execution, however, that he used threats as a tool to maintain control of the prison population. These included withholding food and physical punishments.[18] Thus, he was certainly not without blame.

But, as Dr. Tebault described, Wirz was viewed by most southerners as a martyr. In 1909 the United Daughters of the Confederacy erected a monument to Wirz about one mile from the site of Andersonville prison. On the base of the monument are four plaques, one of which clearly portrays Wirz as a victim: "Discharging his duty with such humanity as the harsh circumstances of the times, and the policy of the foe permitted, Captain Wirz became at last the victim of a misdirected popular clamor. He was arrested in time of peace while under the protection of a parole, tried by a military commission of a service to which he did not belong and condemned to ignominious death on charges of excessive cruelty to federal prisoners. He indignantly spurned a pardon proffered on condition that he would incriminate President Davis and thus exonerate himself from charges of which both were innocent." His monument is also a shrine to the Lost Cause.

The Lost Cause Continues

Through its efforts to vindicate and rationalize the southern cause, the Lost Cause denied the issue of slavery as the principle cause of the Civil War and deprived African Americans of their rightful place as participants and victims in one of the country's defining events. Denying the crucial role they played in the Civil War further placed black Americans in an inferior position during and after the Reconstruction period of the South. By not giving African Americans their true history and contributions to building America, the Lost Cause effectively buried the truth.

Edward Pollard, the author of *The Lost Cause*, was one of the architects of the doctrine. A 2019 article entitled "White Liar" depicts Pollard's *The Lost Cause* as "an atrocious cornucopia of the crackpot idea modern historians call 'the Lost Cause mythology….' Pollard's preposterous portrait of genteel aristocrats, mindlessly happy slaves, and evil carpetbaggers was a balm for Southerners depressed by defeat."[19] This rather frank sentiment dramatizes today's view of the Lost Cause, but to label it as "crackpot ideas" and "mythology" ignores its true genesis.

Pollard was by all measures a racist, white supremacist and propagandist rather than a historian. He wrote in *The Lost Cause*:

> The war has not swallowed up everything. There are great interests which stand out of the pale of the contest, which it is for the South still to cultivate and maintain. She must submit fairly and truthfully to *what the war has properly decided*. But the war properly decided only what was put in issue: the restoration of the Union and the excision of slavery; and to these two conditions the South submits. But the war did not decide negro equality; it did not decide negro suffrage; it did not decide State Rights, although it might have exploded their abuse; it did not decide the orthodoxy of the Democratic party; it did not decide the right of a people to show dignity in misfortune, and to maintain self-respect in the face of adversity. And these things which the war did not decide, the Southern people will still cling to, still claim, and still assert in them their rights and views. This is not the language of insolence and faction. It is the stark letter of right, and the plain syllogism of common sense. It is not untimely or unreasonable to tell the South to cultivate her superiority as a people; to maintain her old schools of literature and scholarship; to assert, in the forms of her thought, and in the style of her manners, her peculiar civilization, and to convince the North that, instead of subjugating an inferior country, she has obtained the alliance of a noble and cultivated people, and secured a bond of association with those she may be proud to call brethren![20]

His sentiments would permeate the South and complicate reconciliation efforts during Reconstruction and thereafter.

The doctrines of the Lost Cause continue to distort our views of history and civil rights, but it is understandable how white southerners after the war embraced such dogma as a way to maintain their honor and rationalize the results of their defeat—the staggering losses of human life, the ruined southern economy, and the new world order where former slaves were now in positions of power. The punishing Reconstruction period that followed further exasperated white southerners and made martyrs of those who fought and died in fighting back, the Battle of Liberty Place and the New Orleans Riots being two examples. White supremacy groups such as the White Leagues and the Ku Klux Klan had foundations based on racial fears. Newspapers at the time suggested that former slaves, now encouraged by Reconstruction policies and protected by Federal military rule, were hell-bent on taking vengeance against their former owners and white society. Such reports often included threats of white women being raped by former slaves, a topic that was sure to stoke panic in the white population. One cannot justify in any way the disenfranchisement of black voters and the persecution of black Americans for the next one hundred years, but one can understand how it began.

The recent controversies over Confederate monuments can also be traced back to the Lost Cause doctrine. While memorials commemorate and honor Robert E. Lee, Jefferson Davis, and other Confederate heroes, many were erected around the war's 25th anniversary (1886–1890), which also coincided with the era of the oppressive Jim Crow laws. In many cases, the monuments served as strong, unspoken statements to black citizens. Many people, both black and white, protested their construction at the time they were erected.

One can see Civil War monuments in almost every northern and southern community, with many placed prominently in city squares and parks. Many of these memorials list the names of the local men who fought and died in the war. The monuments were often later expanded in tribute to local men who lost their lives in later wars, such as World Wars I and II. Many additional memorials were built on the sites of battlefields, commemorating both the northern and southern men who fought and lost their lives there. On the Gettysburg battlefield there are over 1,300 such monuments, markers and memorials, of which about half are dedicated to Confederate units. As soldiers' bodies were retrieved from their temporary graves and reinterned in local cemeteries, more monuments were constructed in remembrance. Such tributes can remind us of our history and honor those who served and paid the ultimate sacrifice for our communities, states and nation. But when does a monument distort or serve as a veiled affront to history? This is an important question as there are those who wish to remove all traces of Confederate monuments, even those in cemeteries and on battlefields.[21]

Many proponents of removing Confederate memorials argue that no monuments were erected in Germany honoring the Nazi party; in fact, all traces of Hitler, the swastika and the Nazi party were effectively removed from public and private property, libraries and schools.[22] Top Nazi leaders were also put on public trial, with many of them subsequently imprisoned or executed. So why do we still see such memorials to the leaders of the Confederacy? Why weren't the leaders of the Confederacy tried in court for their traitorous actions? Why has the "War of the Rebellion" now become known as the "War between the States"? To address these questions, it is helpful to consider the differences between the aftermath of World Wars I and II.

Germany signed the armistice ending World War I on November 11, 1918. Earlier that year President Wilson had offered "Fourteen Points" for creating a stable, long-lasting peace. His proposals called for relatively benign peace terms that would result in a "peace without victory." President Wilson fell gravely ill during the Paris Peace Conference, however, and French Prime Minister Clemenceau was then able to institute much more vindictive policies. Notably, Article 231 of the Treaty of Versailles, which became known as the "War Guilt Clause," demanded reparations from Germany: "The Allied and Associated Governments affirm and Germany accepts the responsibility of Germany and her allies for causing all the loss and damage to which the Allied and Associated Governments and their nationals have been subjected as a consequence of the war imposed upon them by the aggression of Germany and her allies."

The Treaty required Germany to pay some $63 billion in reparations, later reduced to $33 billion to the Allied nations.[23] Most Germans did not believe that they had been the cause of the war, however; a majority believed that they were forced into the war when Russia mobilized its army.[24] Blaming Germany for the war made no sense to the average German, and forcing them to pay reparations was incendiary. The Weimar Republic was further destabilized by European inflation following the war, leading to hyperinflation and the rise of National Socialists and other radical political parties that promised to overturn the harsh penalties and economic suffering.

By contrast, the European Recovery Program, better known as the Marshall Plan, helped restore a defeated Germany after World War II by offering economic assistance to rebuild the country, remove trade barriers, and modernize its industry. Secretary of State George Marshall justified his plan for U.S. aid:

> The modern system of the division of labor upon which the exchange of products is based is in danger of breaking down. Aside from the demoralizing effect on the world at large and the possibilities of disturbances arising as a result of the desperation of the people concerned, the consequences to the economy of the United States should be apparent to all. It is logical that the United States should do whatever it is able to do to assist in the return of normal economic health to the world, without which there can be no political stability and no assured peace. Our policy is not directed against any country, but against hunger, poverty, desperation and chaos. Any government that is willing to assist in

recovery will find full co-operation on the part of the United States. Its purpose should be the revival of a working economy in the world so as to permit the emergence of political and social conditions in which free institutions can exist.[25]

The reparations and restrictions on Germany following World War I led to great poverty during the Weimar Republic. The German people felt they were being unfairly punished by the Western powers. The National Socialists subsequently rose to power with promises to restore normalcy and pride. The Marshall Plan following World War II prevented such radical economic conditions from developing and helped reconstruct the war-torn cities.

Similarly, white southerners felt they were being unfairly blamed for the cause and cost of the American Civil War. Like French Prime Minister Clemenceau, the Radical Republicans in Congress sought retributions, with some wanting to try and execute Confederate leaders as traitors. President Lincoln had advocated for a relatively benign reunion of the southern states, but his untimely death left the Radical Republicans in charge.

The above is a rather simplified accounting and comparison; a version of the Marshall Plan was untenable politically following World War I. But the similarities in the political and economic conditions in Germany following World War I and in the South after the American Civil War are interesting to compare. In both cases, citizens felt falsely accused and punished.

Following World War I, many monuments were erected in Germany honoring their "Lost Cause." Most were destroyed during World War II bombardments, and those that survived were removed by Allied forces as part of the deliberate destruction of any symbols of German patriotism.

Battlefield monuments, such as the ones erected at Gettysburg and Antietam, memorialize the sacrifices and bravery of soldiers and their leaders as they fought across the field. Their construction by the survivors of the respective regiments was largely apolitical. Veterans from both sides of the conflict frequently journeyed back to those hallowed fields and woods in annual reunions. Likewise, the Confederate and Union memorials that are commonly seen in almost every town square across the country are primarily unbiased tributes to the soldiers from those towns who fought and died during the conflict. But other Confederate monuments were meant to support the doctrines of the Lost Cause. Instead of simply memorializing, these monuments glorified the old South, its leaders, and their principled sacrifices. The monument to the Battle of Liberty Place was an example of a symbol erected to honor the whites who died in trying to overthrow the Republican government in Louisiana and who fought against a largely black Metropolitan Police force. When that monument was erected, it failed to mention any black men who died during the "battle." Nowhere does one even see in the South a monument to the slaves, who were certainly an important part of American and Civil War history. Likewise, many of the monuments to Confederate leaders serve to continue the concept of the nobility of the Lost Cause.

A recently published article in *Smithsonian Magazine* discusses the impact today of these Confederate monuments and sites such as Beauvoir, Jefferson Davis's home. The authors note that "a century and a half after the Civil War, American taxpayers are still helping to sustain the defeated Rebels' racist doctrine, The Lost Cause.... It maintains that the Confederacy was based on a noble ideal, the Civil War was not about slavery, and slavery was benign."[26]

The Lost Cause is still with us; while we should repudiate its use as a premise for white supremacy, disenfranchisement, and violence, it is important to understand how and why it

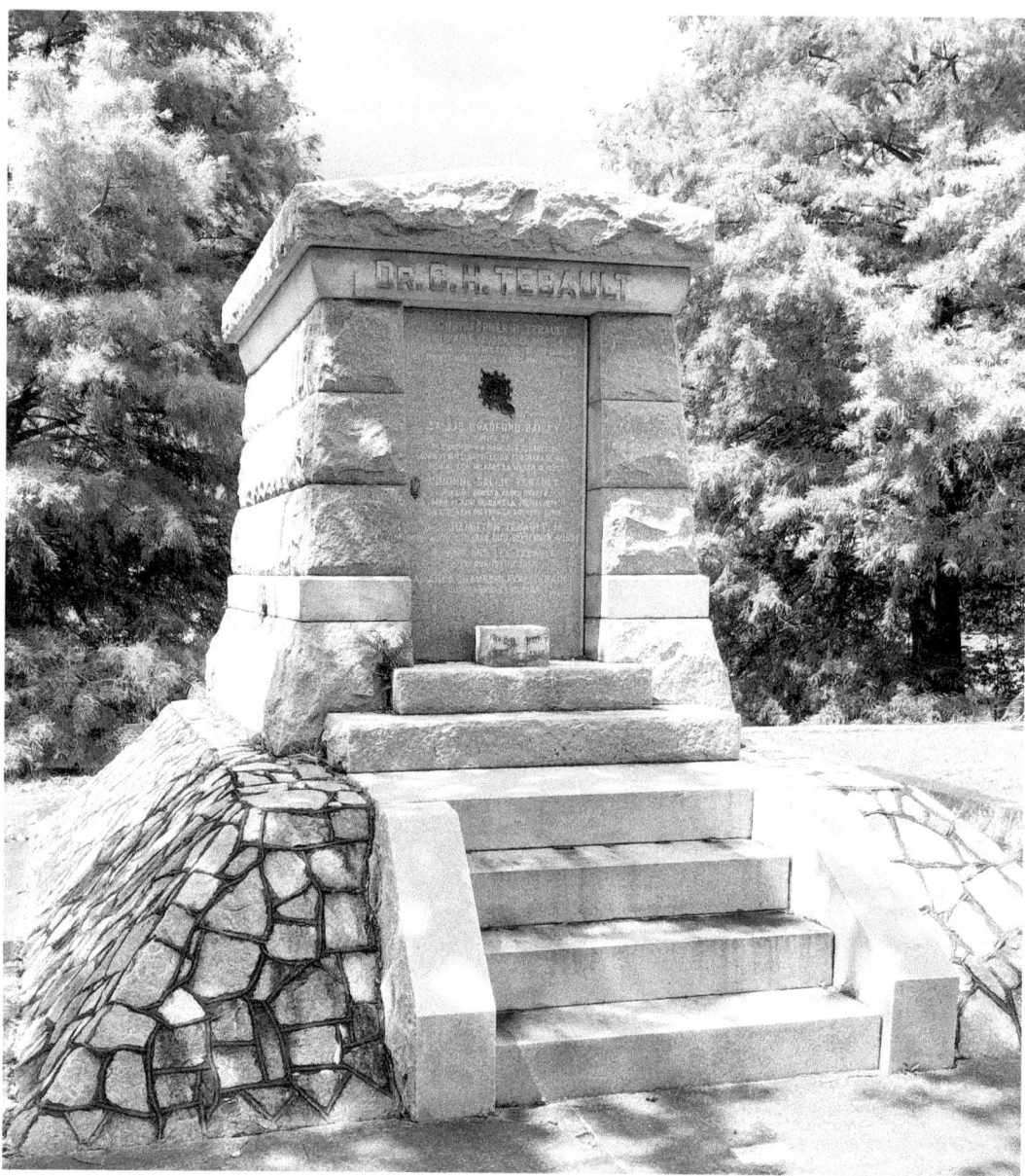

Dr. Christopher H. Tebault is buried in Metairie Cemetery alongside his wife, Sallie, and his children, Corrine Tebault Harper, C. Hamilton Tebault, Jr., Grantland Lee Tebault, and Amanda Tebault, who died shortly after birth. The bronze circular marker on the tomb identifies Sallie and Corrine as members of the Daughters of the American Revolution. Photograph by author.

came about if we are to finally eliminate its dissemination and comprehend the true history of the war and its ramifications.

While many southerners consider Confederate memorials to be an important part of their heritage, many of these memorials were erected during the days of oppression and disenfranchisement of blacks. The Lost Cause doctrine needs to be acknowledged as a distortion of the reasons behind the war and its devastating results. We can certainly understand and even empathize with the reasons why the Lost Cause was so important immediately after the war to rationalize the sacrifices of brave Confederate soldiers, as southerners felt they were being unfairly prosecuted and censured by the North. But the monuments to the Lost Cause need to be re-examined; after 150 years, we still are unnecessarily "fighting" the war.

The challenge is to ensure the we are not covering up or further distorting history in such re-examinations. Hiding monuments, statues, writings, and views we may deem to be offensive is much less effective than exploring and understanding their history. We should remove icons that represent the notion of white supremacy. The monument to the Battle of Liberty Place has now been removed. With today's polarized politics and media, however, it is at times difficult to grasp the truth. But the better we understand our true history, the better we will be prepared to move forward and make a difference for today and tomorrow.

Let me end with a quote attributed to Robert E. Lee:

"A nation which does not remember what it was yesterday does not know where it is today."

Dr. Tebault's Writings— A Selection

As Surgeon General for the United Confederate Veterans, Dr. Tebault submitted official annual reports for each reunion beginning with the 6th Annual Meeting and Reunion in Richmond, Virginia (1896), when he took over the position from Joseph Jones who had passed away. After the 14th reunion, instead of UCV reports he started making presentations to the Association of the Medical Officers of the Army and Navy of the Confederacy, whose meetings ran concurrently with the UCV reunions. In 1909 and 1910, he submitted general reports for the 19th and 20th UCV reunions. His last report was published in 1915, a year following his death.

The following is a selection of four of his most important writings, as they add to our knowledge of Confederate medicine. Included are the following articles:

1. Modified Inoculation (1866);
2. The Drainage System Peculiar to New Orleans (1889);
3. Confederate Resources (1902);
4. Hospitals of the Confederacy (1902).

Modified Inoculation (1866)

New Orleans Medical and Surgical Journal 19 (July 1866): 36–42.
Art. IV—MODIFIED INOCULATION:
By C.H. Tebault, M.D., Visiting Physician Charity Hospital, New Orleans, Louisiana.

In offering the present paper for publication, I am influenced by no other motive than a desire to bring into somewhat more prominent, and I trust, too, more favorable notice, a subject hitherto attracting but a fugitive interest in the profession. I allude to modified inoculation. My attention was first directed to this subject by the accompanying note from George B. Wood, M. D., *Treatise on the Practice of Medicine*, fifth edition, page 406:

> It was an easy inference from the modifying influence of the system of the cow on the variolous contagion, that a similar effect might be produced by the milk of the cow on small-pox matter; and M. Thiele, of Kassan, and M. Robert, of Marseilles, proposed the use of such a mixture in vaccination. M. Bracket, of Lyons, in the year 1832, made some experiments with satisfactory results; and these have been recently repeated on a much larger scale at La Charité, in Lyons, by M. Bouchocourt. Equal parts of cow milk and variolous matter taken from the pock in the vesicular stage were mixed, and then children inoculated with the matter.
>
> Others were inoculated from matter proceeding from the vesicles thus produced, and others again

from these secondary cases. Of twenty-one cases, eighteen presented solitary vesicles, confined to the place of puncture, having all the character of genuine vaccine disease; others, but a few additional pocks. The inoculation thus performed proved protective." (See *London Medical Times and Gazette*, April 1854, p. 412.)

From the month of October 1864, until the surrender of General Johnston, I was connected with the Ocmulgee Hospital at the Confederate Post of Macon, Georgia, and together with other duties, was appointed superintendent of vaccination. It was imperative at this date, by orders, so requiring, that every soldier, before receiving his discharge from the military hospitals, should be closely scrutinized with reference to the probable degree of immunity he enjoyed against variolous contagion; if he were adjudged sufficiently fortified against the disease, a certificate, so stating, was furnished him by the surgeon in charge, which he deposited with his ranking medical officer on returning to the army. If, per contra, he was not deemed properly secured, vaccination, or revaccination, was required to be performed, as the case might be; and a certificate, giving date of operation, statement of result, etc., supplied him, to be likewise surrendered on rejoining his regiment or company.

The numerous vaccinations and revaccinations which such orders imposed, proved, were long, too exhausting for the supply of reliable virus on hand. It hence occurred, that many of our soldiers were vaccinated from scabs, procured indiscriminately from each other; and it was precisely from just this quality of material that nearly all (excepting, probably, a fractional few which may have taken on erysipelas or gangrene), those distressing cases originated, jeopardizing at times life itself, as well as limb.

These anomalous cases were by no means of rare occurrence, nor were they confined within the pale of the army. Liberal details of medical men were sent throughout the country to vaccinate all the healthy children, so that an ample supply of the purest vaccinia should be ever at hand for the use of the medical staff. (Author's note: children were considered to be ideal donors of vaccination matter as they would not have syphilis, a disease thought to be transmitted via vaccinations when using the crusts covering the vaccination sites of other inoculated men.)

This admirably designed arrangement was destined to defeat itself. At first, moved by the double motive of patriotism and a desire to protect their offspring from the contagion of small-pox, at this time widely diffused through every State of the Confederacy, mothers unhesitatingly yielded the arms of their infants and older children to the charmed lancet of the surgeon. And thus for a while this most necessary work went successfully on without hindrance. But can it be wondered at that this spirit, but lately all aglow, on the part of mothers, should wane and dim into well-nigh extinction, when spurious matter, by some accident or other, was used on their nurselings, developing, in lien of simple vaccine disease, ugly, phagedenic sores, spreading into unmanageable and destructive ulcers, ending occasionally in the forfeiture of life, or else seriously compromising the future usefulness of the limb?

[Author's note: "Spurious vaccination" was generally used to describe infections at the vaccination site. Deep ulcers, swelling and soreness would often result from the use of non-sterile lances and questionable vaccination matter. Many physicians at the time believed such infections were caused by syphilis contracted from using the vaccination crusts of infected men. While some "spurious" cases could have been attributed to syphilis, most undoubtedly resulted from a variety of infections in immunodeficient men compromised by poor diets, exposure and fatigue.]

In this last view of the matter, it cannot be a subject of surprise that our legitimate virus could no longer sustain the ceaseless drain upon it. It was at this epoch in the history of the army, that I decided on testing the value of the note above quoted, being unprovided with reliable matter, and quite unwilling to compel soldiers to submit to the introduction of a virus, of which I could procure no history.

Accordingly, with every possible caution under the circumstances, and strictly conforming to the recommendations contained in the note adverted to, I engrafted one soldier after another with the modified lymph, until thirty-odd had swelled the list of my experiments. Of thirty-five persons thus successfully inoculated, three only exhibited a few additional pocks, in no case more than six, in addition to the seat of puncture.

No perceptible difference could be detected, whether in the course of the pock, or in its effects on the system at large, when contrasted with the phenomena attendant on simple, uncomplicated vaccine. None of these cases had been previously vaccinated. The wards of the Ocmulgee Hospital, at the time of these experiments, were more than usually crowded—the result of an order transferring the greater number of the hospitals in this department to the Carolinas. It was thus rendered impossible to prevent the inoculated patients from freely intermingling with the rest of the inmates of the hospital, many of whom even at this late day had never been vaccinated; still, in the face of these facts, not even a single case of varioloid occurred within its walls, during or after the suspension of this practice. Previously, from time to time, an occasional case had offered.

The accidental information of which I became possessed, at this juncture, at the hands of a friend in the profession, to-wit: that the laws of the State of Georgia were especially severe concerning any other procedure than vaccination, as a security against small-pox, influenced me to discontinue the practice, which I had so far kept to myself. A further inducement to avoid all possible conflict with the State laws, consisted in the fact of my now being in possession of a moderate supply of good material, secured from healthy children, whom I had recently vaccinated.

My observations on the subject, however, did not close here. A large small-pox encampment had been established on the outskirts of Vineville, about three miles distant from Macon. I use the term "encampment" purposely, for the patients were all treated in tents. It was under the direction of Assistant Surgeon L. Carter, at that time in the service of the Confederacy, and was an appendage to the Floyd House Hospital, Surgeon Dabney Herndon in charge.

I omitted to state a very important fact when recording the results of my own cases, which define in this history, I shall correct at once. I had neglected to mention that those soldiers whose arms had perfectly cicatrized, permitted me, with some persuasion, to test, by a second inoculation, the degree of immunity so conferred, and this time with pure unmodified small-pox lymph. The material used on them, I intentionally secured from a case of confluent variola, and introduced the same in great abundance into numerous incisions. All that remains to be added is, that the second inoculation with confluent variola lymph, had no effect in the three cases thus experimented on.

At the encampment above mentioned, this modified inoculation was in general use, vaccination being entirely ignored. It was practiced, I believe, previous to the date of my own experiments, though unknown to me at the time. To this station all cases of variola or varioloid occurring at any of the Post Hospitals, were immediately sent for treatment.

As the result of too much precaution, it frequently happened that soldiers were sent out to this place, because their symptoms were suspicious, and associated with the fact that they had never been vaccinated, or had never taken, when, in truth, they were not laboring under the supposed disease. Such cases, after a systematic exposure of the kind, were constrained to remain here, till they were armed against the disease by measures looking to immunity, or had successfully passed through its several stages and sufficiently recovered therefrom.

The immunity never failed to follow successfully modified inoculation, as far as could be ascertained. In no instance, after the pock had attained to maturity, have I ever seen varioloid ensue. I cannot speak so favorably of vaccination, for I have seen small-pox itself occur again and again under exactly such circumstances, and, in spite of the unquestionable purity of the virus used. Hundreds of cases at this encampment were subjected to this modified inoculation, yet not a case found it necessary to take to bed.

Their identity in every sense with vaccinia, was as noticeable and as thorough as could be. The people of the neighborhood and their children, on applying to be vaccinated, were likewise inoculated, and the same favorable results were obtained. They visited and intermixed with each other without any restrictions on their freedom; yet, in this locality variola and varioloid were scarcely known. The few cases that did occur, were distinctly traceable to exposure to small-pox itself.

It would seem that this immense focus of contagion, here centralized, would have invited numerous attacks of variola or varioloid among the dwellers of this immediate vicinage; but the converse was the case, whilst in Macon, these diseases were alarmingly prevalent. As far as could be determined by investigation, the few seized by either of the affections were confined exclusively among the nonvaccinated and the vaccinated—not a case occurring among such as had been protected by modified inoculation. The scabs derived from such inoculation in healthy children, were used with like happy results.

It is to be hoped that Dr. Carter will find an early occasion to make known his very extended experience in the premises.

Dr. C.B. Gamble, of Florida, our estimable and respected Surgeon of the Post, on my apprising him of such procedure, in contravention of the State laws on the subject, was about to take instant means for its suppression. I entreated of him a little delay that he might inquire into its results, at the same time expressing how favorably I viewed its workings. I saw Dr. Gamble some two weeks later, and, in lieu of discountenancing and frowning down its further practice, he had become one of its advocates, in so far as to send scabs procured as above stated from healthy children, to his friends and acquaintances writing for vaccinia. These, he afterwards informed me, had behaved admirably in every case.

In the *Revue Medico-Chirurgiale*, No. 13, published by Dr. A. Martin Lauzer, for 1865, may be found on p. 543, the following, which I translate into English:

"Inoculation of variola-virus, diluted by admixture with cream."—M. Lanfranchi, Sanitary Officer at Guitera (Canton of Licavo District of Ajaccio), and physician to the Canton, had to contend in 1854 with an epidemic of confluent variola, which carried off more than four hundred victims from the nine parishes of the canton, among whom children were to be found wearing manifest traces of previous vaccination. The variolous inoculation attempted in some of the parishes did not lessen the intensity of the malady. M. Lanfranchi conceived the idea of testing on his son a mixture of variolous matter and cream from cow milk, after the ensuing method: Having made a small incision about the middle of the anterior aspect of the fore-arm, he deposited virus, just secured from a small-pox vesicle, into the same; and then taking a small quantity of cream from cow-milk, on the point of the same instrument, he introduced it into the same incision, spreading it to mix it with the virus; then covering up the slight wound with a light coating of the same cream, which he required to dry before permitting the readjustment of the child's dress.

The result of this operation was not long waited on; a slight irritation followed soon after the inoculation of the modified variolous virus. It formed a small scab which fell off or became indolent on the third or fourth day; when on the sixteenth or seventeenth day a well pronounced inflammation manifested itself at the incision; fever was kindled, and variolous pimples exhibited themselves in diverse places on the body, to the number of seven or eight.

The fever was mild in character, and the child recovered without having evinced the least restlessness. Six other children of the parish, not yet seized by the epidemic, were subjected to the same mode of inoculation, and like the son of M. Lanfranchi had a benign type of varioloid. Last summer a fresh epidemic of variola occurred in one parish, and successively invaded the entire canton. As in 1854, this epidemic seized on the vaccinated alike, as on the unvaccinated children. The small-pox was confluent, claiming many victims, and disfiguring those who did not succumb under its violent usage. Now, in this instance, M. Lanfranchi practiced, as he practices still at this moment, his inoculation of variola-cream, and the children whom he has thus protected enumerate above a hundred. With all, the effects were so exceedingly mild, that a large number did not take to bed, and in no case did such inoculation present more than twenty pocks. It is difficult in families to put to the test the preservative virtue of such inoculation, by afterwards inoculating with the pure variola lymph; but what M. Lanfranchi could not prove on the children of his clients, he verified on his own son, at the suggestion of M. Cauro. With virus taken from a variolous vesicle, without admixture with cream, he inoculated his child ten years after the modified inoculation of 1854, and the result was void. The subject was perfectly refractory against the second inoculation (*Journal de Médecine Pratique*).

M. Lanfranchi's method is somewhat different from that pursued at Macon. His cases were something severer, and may be due to the difference in his plan of inoculating. In his severest cases, however, twenty pocks were the largest number that ever occurred in his practice. There are few persons, it occurs to me, who would not accept immunity from the disease at this cost. He found this procedure infinitely superior to vaccination.

Let us briefly, in conclusion, draw what may be considered fair inferences from the foregoing facts:

1st. We hope to have demonstrated that its operation is equally benign with vaccination—in fact that their action is identical, and resting this statement on an experience of fully five hundred cases.

2nd. That the disease so ingrafted, like vaccinia, is not communicable by contact.

3rd. That the immunity it confers would seem to be more lasting, and otherwise superior to that responding to vaccination.

4th. That simultaneously with the occurrence of small-pox, we are supplied with a seemingly all-potent means for its arrestation.

The Drainage System Peculiar to New Orleans (1889)

Its Demonstrated Possibilities and Its Bearing When Properly Enforced Upon the General Health of the City, Under a Most Crucial Test.

By C.H. Tebault, M.D.

Gaillard's Medical Journal 49 (October 1889): 325–338.

From the "Report on Drainage to the City Council of New Orleans, by Maj. B.M. Harrod, City Surveyor, November 22, 1888," I am indebted for the following:

> The removal of the entire surface drainage of a city by pumping is very exceptional, there being no other instance in this country in which it is necessary. Hence, but few observations on this subject have been made or recorded. The importance of a careful study in this case is, therefore, apparent. The following table is submitted, for the time, based on the assumption that rainfalls of six inches are of sufficient frequency to make it necessary to provide for the removal, within twenty-four hours of such part as is not retained by cisterns, absorbed by the soil, or consumed by vegetation.

Table 9: Proportion of Six Inches of Rainfall to be Pumped from Each Drainage District in Twenty-Four Hours

Drainage Districts	Total Area, Acres	Total Volume of 6-inch Rainfall, Cubic Feet	Area of Improved Lands, Acres	Areas of Unimproved Lands, Acres	Proportion of Drainage from Improved Lands, %	Proportion of Drainage from Unimproved Lands, %	Volume of Drainage from Improved Lands, Cubic Feet	Volume of Drainage from Unimproved Lands, Cubic Feet	Total Volume of Drainage, Cubic Feet
First District, between New and Old Canals	2,213	48,308,040	1,530	688	.75	.30	24,992,550	4,495,392	29,487,942
Second District, above New Canal	8,650	188,397,000	4,630	4,020	.50	.25	50,420,700	21,888,900	72,309,600
Third District, from Old Canal to Lafayette Avenue	4,612	100,449,360	1,820	2,792	.60	.30	23,783,760	18,242,928	42,026,688
Fourth District, below Lafayette Avenue	3,724	81,108,720	1,247	2,477	.50	.25	13,579,830	13,487,265	27,067,095
Entire City	19,204	418,263,120	9,227	9,977	.56	.27	112,776,840	58,114,485	170,891,325

Assuming the mean or average lift from the interior canals to the level of the lake as three feet, there would be required for the removal of this volume of storm drainage an aggregate of six hundred and seventy-four horse power. This would be divided between the different districts as follows: 1st District, 1418,16 horse power; 2d District, 285 horse power; 3d District, 166 horse power; 4th District, 107 horsepower. This power could be concentrated to advantage in one pumping station for each district, except the second, where, owing to the large volume and area, it would be advantageously divided.

It is of vital importance to the inhabitants of Southern cities to weigh well all the facts relating to the origin, causes, and means of prevention of yellow fever. Only through the accumulation of a large number of well observed and undoubted facts can we reach a correct knowledge of the laws which govern yellow fever and all other diseases. Those who are instrumental in the discovery and establishment of the laws which concern the origin and spread of so great a scourge as yellow fever should certainly be considered as honored and useful instruments in the hands of Providence.

The author of the observations immediately to follow is well remembered for his devoted and untiring efforts in the cause of sanitary science, and his recognized ability gives a high character to his testimony upon this or any other subject of hygienic experience, and is, therefore, in every way entitled to the confidence and respectful consideration of the medical profession.

The personal inquiries of Dr. Elisha Harris, with respect to the hygienic history of New Orleans during the late war between the States, were made during the month of July 1865, while pursuing certain investigations relating to the hygienic experience of the military forces. We shall limit the present review to a bare statement in the language of the author, of those facts which are of the greatest interest in their bearing upon the sanitary regulations carried out in New Orleans, and the results growing out of their rigid enforcement. Before proceeding to quote from this valuable contribution, let me add that shortly after the occupation of New Orleans by the United States' forces, the most stringent sanitary requirements were promulgated, and an efficient sanitary police established.

Following is from Dr. Elisha Harris's report:

Throughout the entire period, upwards of two years, the Provost-Marshal, the Military Governor, the Mayor (an appointee of the provisional government), together with the Medical Director of the post, and certain subordinate health officers, have vigilantly administered the regulations relating to municipal hygiene and cleanliness in New Orleans and its vicinity. During all that period the accustomed scourgings of yellow fever have been suspended in that city, while the dire forebodings and prophecies of the inevitable pestilence that would quickly destroy the Northern soldiery on reaching the Gulf coast, remain unrealized. The conditions under which the Crescent City has obtained this remarkable immunity from a doom which her own bitter experience seemed to fasten upon her, are now as well under stood as were the apparently inexorable causes of her former insalubrity.

Such immunity from her accustomed scourgings of yellow fever had not been enjoyed by New Orleans the last half century. Even her wisest hygienists had been generally discredited and often derided when they publicly taught, as Fenner, Barton, Simonds, and Bennett Dowler had most faithfully, that the active and localizing causes of yellow fever and the high death-rate in that city were preventable. There was a truthfulness worthy of the medical profession in the words of Dr. Barton, who, as President of the New Orleans Sanitary Commission, sitting in grave and scientific consultation upon the terrible visitations of yellow fever, unhesitatingly declared the causes of that pestilence and the city's excessive insalubrity "entirely susceptible of cure." But how few persons appreciated the truth of Dr. Barton's words of prophecy when he said that "upon the broad foundation of sanitary measures we can erect a monument of public health, and that if a beacon light be erected on its top, and kept alive by proper attention, this city will be second to none in this first of earthly blessings."

It is the design of the following notes to show what have constituted the chief causes of insalubrity in New Orleans, and by what means the redemption from its fearful doom has been achieved. In doing this it will be shown that for two successive years the threatening pestilence was localized in a fleet of gunboats, moored so close to the city's levees that they menaced the streets with death. It will likewise appear that by the exercise of absolute and relentless military authority, an impregnable system of quarantine was maintained, restraining all the exotic causes of yellow fever, and controlling such causes at a distance of nearly seventy miles from the city; and yet that this dreaded scourge originated spontaneously in more than twenty of the gunboats that were moored in the river, opposite the city; also that those naval vessels were uniformly filthy, ill-ventilated, and over crowded; that of the more active, cleanly, and less crowded steam boats (120 in number) employed in quartermaster's service, no yellow fever occurred; that in all the city not more than three or four cases of yellow fever occurred each year, and that the cause of such immunity from the pestilence of former years was as certainly the direct result of *civic cleanliness* and the hygienic care of the poor, as its accustomed visitations were the result of neglect of these public duties.

Three classes of facts, concerning which neither doubt nor uncertainty can be alleged, have conspired to give precise relations and definite value to the series of events we are about to consider:

First.—The relentless rigor and precision of a military government precluded the ordinary violations of quarantine regulations, while it gave peculiar certainty to the execution of sanitary regulations in the city.

Second.—The official usages and the armed discipline of the naval fleet in the harbor of New Orleans and upon the river, enabled the medical officers to trace to its source every case of yellow fever that occurred in the gunboats.

Third.—That the climate of the city and of the river districts, during the past three years was not perceptibly different from the climate of previous years and the periods of yellow fever epidemics; the same evils from imperfect culture and drainage, imperfect levees, and extensive crevasses, flooding and subsequent evaporation from vast areas of overflowed land, continued to recur in the latter as in the former years. In short, all the physical conditions that are supposed to promote the prevalence of yellow fever—excepting only such as are immediately controllable by sanitary police—prevailed continually and abundantly in the delta of the Mississippi during this period of immunity from that dread disease.

The Sanitary History of New Orleans before the War.—Constantly recurring epidemics of pestilential diseases had, for two generations seemed to pronounce the doom of the "Crescent City," and notwithstanding the vast interests of commerce, there have been dismal forebodings of inevitable decadence of wealth and commerce.

Between the years 1829 and 1852 inclusive, there were not less than *twelve* great epidemics of yellow fever, or one every second year. Those twelve epidemics killed 22,884 inhabitants, or an average of 1,907 in each epidemic, which gives an average of 888 persons killed by that fever, year by year. As the fever prevailed to some extent almost every year, the actual average each year reached about 1,000 persons.

During the epidemic years the average death-rate, from all causes, was nearly 75 deaths to the 1,000 inhabitants. The average annual death-rate during all that period, and up to the year 1861, was about *six and a-half per cent*. There were years when the death-rate exceeded *ten percent*.

Fresh immigration of Northern or foreign born persons was always accredited as the chief source of any excessive mortality; and to become *creolized* (naturalized to the climate) was esteemed almost equivalent to a limited life assurance policy. But we have now seen that during the period of military occupation by the national troops, a hundred thousand Northern men, uncreolized and unacclimated, have annually arrived in or passed through that city without a single individual being smitten with yellow fever, except in a few instances in which soldiers detailed to assist at the boats on the levee in receiving and conveying yellow fever patients to the Naval Hospital on New Levee and Erato streets.

The Summers of 1862, 1863, 1864, and 1865 have now passed without any sign of epidemic disease, except from paludal malaria being manifested at New Orleans, save only the outbreak of small pox last Winter. That epidemic was at once controlled by a house-to-house visitation by a corps of medical inspectors, armed with vaccine virus.

Malarial fever and the ordinary diseases of the climate, not dependent upon a medical police, continued to prevail, but the diarrhoeal and infantile maladies were less fatal than in former years. The following statistics of mortality for the six weeks that are usually the most unhealthful of the year show how the "hygienic barometer" stood during the Summers of 1863 and 1865—the periods when the largest numbers of Northern men and unacclimatized persons were in that city. For the Summer of 1863 the records stand thus:

Table 10: Mortality During the Summers of 1863 and 1865

		No. of Deaths
During the week ending	August 2	169
" " " "	" 9	176
" " " "	" 16	166
" " " "	" 23	139
" " " "	" 30	161
" " " "	September 6	145
" " " "	" 13	203
During the seven weeks of the past summer (1865), of which we have received official returns, the records read as follows*:		
During the week ending	July 2	155
" " " "	" 9	154
" " " "	" 16	154
" " " "	" 22	165

		No. of Deaths
During the week ending	July 30	174
" " " "	August 6	144
" " " "	" 13	168
" " " "	" 22	170
" " " "	" 27	141
" " " "	September 5	149
" " " "	" 10	116

*The total population, including the permanent or the transient military forces, was little less than 200,000.

New York cannot boast a lower death-rate for the same period. The total number of deaths in July was 793, and in August, just past, the number was but 623. Compare this with the mortality in that city in August, 1853, when 6,201 of the inhabitants died. Or compare with the average mortality of the three years, 1853, 1854 and 1855, which gave more than 1,000 deaths per month, though the population was far less than during the past Summer. It cannot be claimed that there were any favoring circumstances in the seasons, the dryness or the humidity,—that can account for such hygienic changes. During the past three years the levees have been cut and crevassed, and the country overflowed as at no former period; and then, in August last, for example, the swampy surfaces surrounding the city were desiccated, less than a single inch of rain having fallen that month; while in the early part of the present month (September), as in the months of Spring and Summer, floods have descended. Now, from the sanitary officers of the city, we learn that diseases and mortality have been chiefly diminished in connection with the abatement of those local conditions that are recognized as the localizing causes. These causes, in the language of Dr. E.H. Barton, consisted mainly in—

1. Bad air.
2. Offensive privies, cemeteries, various manufactories, stables, slaughter-houses, filthy streets, etc.
3. Bad water, stagnant water, bad drainage.

These were the causes of disease first noticed and officially controlled by the military government under the national forces.

The Appliances and Means of Sanitary Reform.—1. The streets, the courts, the market-places, and all the private and public premises of the city, have been cleansed and kept in a state of unusual cleanliness by an absolute authority.

2. The drainage of the city was a matter of constant official concern, and the steam-drainage works kept in great activity night and day. (As all the drainage is superficial, by gutters, ditches and canals, the mechanical appliances for drainage located at the junctions of canals and bayous leading towards Pontchartrain maintain an important relation to civic purity and the public health. *Some of the water-lifting machines exhaust from the canals and basins at the rate of more than 100,000 cubic feet per minute, raising the sewage from the lowest levels of the town, and sending it forward toward Lake Pontchartrain by way of the bayous.*) During the frequent rain-falls, when the water floods the gutters and covers whole streets, cleaners are seen at work with hoes and stiff brooms, adding the effectiveness of their arms to the process of cleaning by water-flushing.

3. The water supply, which is wholly from the river, was, from the beginning of the military government, a matter of first-rate importance. Though the river surface is higher than the plane of the city, the supply depends mainly upon steam-pumps and reservoirs. The pumps were ordered to be kept in the highest activity, and the water company was held accountable for any failure in its works.

4. Street cleaning was literally a cleansing. The faithful broom was immediately and all night long, as constantly as night returned, succeeded by a flushing stream of water from the hydrants, filling and flushing gutters and the pavement joints, and, aided by the sleepless sweepers, thus rendering the Augean work complete. *So clean a city had never before been seen upon the continent.*

5. Scavenging and domiciliary hygiene were enforced by order of the Provost-Marshal. Privies and garbage, stables and butcheries, damp and unventilated quarters, and the haunts of vice and debauchery, were all brought under police control. The privies in populous streets, and those connected with

places of public resort, were some times cleaned as frequently as twice each week. All animals for the markets were impounded at the outskirts of the city, and the cattle boats were there scrubbed and cleansed before proceeding down to the commercial levees. And as an illustration of the salutary exercise of authority over improper habitations, the writer would mention that he saw all the tenements upon the first floor of an entire block vacated by peremptory orders in a single day.

6. The destitute were supplied with wholesome food at the expense of the city.

Such were the leading features of the sanitary government of the Crescent City under military rule. The errors of that government, and the criticisms it may have provoked, were neither the cause nor consequence of the protection it gave to life and health. *All the acts that related directly to the public health can be repeated in any city, and by any enlightened civil government.*

Quarantine.—Perhaps there has never been a more enlightened and faithful exercise of regulations in the nature of quarantine than has been witnessed at New Orleans the past four years. Yellow fever and small-pox were the only infections feared or guarded against. All the exotic and transportable causes or fomites of these maladies were detained at the quarantine anchorage, sixty-five miles down the river, near Fort Philip.

Shall we be told that it was by this very application of a judicious and inviolable quarantine that the city escaped the epidemic visitations of disease? We have seen that small-pox appeared as a wide spread epidemic, and that it was checked by a house-to-house visitation of a medical police armed with vaccine virus.

Yellow Fever.—This disease did not become epidemic in the city. Nearly three and a-half years have passed without so many as a score of sporadic cases occurring in the streets, where that enemy and pest of the city had been wont to destroy its thousand victims every year, and sometimes to kill no less than *five thousand* in a single month!

As the writer's views concerning the *transportability* and the infectious nature of yellow fever are already well known to the Academy, the following statement regarding yellow fever and quarantine at New Orleans, will not require explanation as respects the standpoint from which he has examined the facts. With the peculiar and abundant experience of yellow fever in the ports of the North fresh in mind, the history of this malady at New Orleans and in our naval fleet on the Mississippi, was investigated with all the predilections which such experience could justly impart in favor of the theory of the exotic and imported origin of the disease.

Well-marked and fatal cases of yellow fever occurred in New Orleans in the Autumn of 1863, and in the Autumn of 1864. In the former year the Charity Hospital received two cases, both of which proved fatal. Both were boat hands from the steamer *J.H. Hancock*, a river tug. In 1864 there were five undoubted and fatal cases of yellow fever, terminating in black vomit. The writer conversed with the physicians who attended the patients, viz.: Professor Crawcour, Dr. Bennett Dowler, and Dr. Smythe; and Dr. Huard has furnished notes of a case that occurred in the parish prison. These five cases occurred in persons who resided or daily visited in the vicinity of Erato, Tchoupitoulas, and New Levee streets. They were exposed to known causes of the fever. Other cases may have occurred; if so, they have eluded all search.

We have referred to the two cases from a tug in the river in the Autumn of 1863. *Nearly 100 other cases of the fever occurred in the river fleet and in the Naval Hospital that season.* The history of all these cases, in detail, shows that they were not of imported origin. They nearly all occurred in crowded, filthy, and unventilated gun boats that were at anchor in the river at New Orleans. Owing to the inaccessibility of medical officers who had charge of some of the patients, the tabulated history of these cases gives way, in this place, to the more complete records of yellow fever in the Autumn of 1864.

We have mentioned the five cases of black vomit that occurred near New Levee street in 1864. The Naval Hospital occupies a large pile of old buildings on that street, with yards and accessory buildings towards Erato and Tchoupitoulas streets. One block of buildings—store houses—intervenes between the hospital and the river levee and landings. The accompanying record of yellow fever in that hospital and in the idle gunboats in the stream, sufficiently accounts for the concentration of infection in the particular locality in which the five cases occurred outside of the hospital premises. Other cases occurred, but they were directly dependent on intercourse with the infected vessels, and the bedding brought from those vessels.

The fact, then, is indisputable, that yellow fever visited twenty five vessels in the fleet that was anchored in the river in front of New Orleans during the summer of 1864, and that the disease appeared first, viz.: as early as September 12th in vessels that had been for a long time at anchor there. The brief notes here appended supply the best commentary we could wish. Filthiness, crowding, excessive heat and moisture, lack of ventilation, and the stagnation incident to anchorage in a tideless stream, constitute the leading facts relating to the infected vessels.

To test the merit of this view of the spontaneous origin of the fever, the writer has obtained the written history of every case of which any note was made at the Naval Hospital and elsewhere. He also obtained from the quartermaster in charge of water transportation a record of the 120 steamers and sailing vessels that were under his control. *Of these active vessels only one had yellow fever onboard.* That these ordinary mercantile and transport vessels under control of the quarter master were open, ventilated and moving briskly about from place to place, yet infinitely more exposed to all sources of exotic infection, is the only comment this point in our record requires. Our records show that not less than 191 cases of yellow fever occurred onboard the twenty-five vessels we have mentioned in the fleet at New Orleans in the year 1864; and that of these fifty-seven proved fatal. Also, that in addition to these there were twelve cases and three deaths among employees and guard at the Naval Hospital and landing on Erato Street. *Five other cases of black vomit* occurred in citizens exposed to the same cause in the vicinity of the landing.

The total number of cases was 208, and the total deaths 65. At the quarantine station no other cases or vessels than those mentioned in our record were seen in 1864; and from July 4, 1863, to September 10, 1865, only twenty-three deaths from yellow fever occurred, and only one vessel, besides those we have here designated, brought cases of the fever to the quarantine station—that, a Spanish war ship, in 1863.

The hygienic lessons taught by the events to which these notes refer, abundantly vindicate the principles and the methods of sanitary improvement which are advocated by the medical profession. These lessons may be entitled as follows:

1. The insalubrious circumstances that produce a constantly high death-rate, and the localizing causes of disease generally, are the most important and the most preventable causes of the epidemics that afflict cities.

2. *That the climate and the topographical disadvantages which have hitherto been popularly supposed to be the essential causes of the insalubrity of New Orleans, are but unimportant factors of insalubrity,* which sink into insignificance when the preventable causes of disease in the city are controlled, and that "vanquished Nature yields its empire to man who creates a climate for himself."

3. That yellow fever, the most dreaded scourge of New Orleans, *was unequivocally generated in a large number of filthy and unventilated gunboats and other naval vessels lying idly at anchor within a mile from the densest portions of the city.*

4. That by fomites, or some other material agency, the infection of yellow fever was communicated to the guard, and to certain other persons who were exposed in a narrow district, at the Naval Hospital landing in Erato Street, and near New Levee and Tchoupitoulas streets.

5. That the infected vessels were remarkably close in their exterior construction; that they discharged no cargoes; were under an armed surveillance and discipline; and were seemingly incapable, from the circumstances, of diffusing their own infection, except by the clothing and "dunnage" of the sick when taken ashore.

6. That vessels and river-boats of ordinary construction and in active service, escaped yellow fever almost without exception.

7. That no vessel infected with yellow fever, arriving by way of the Gulf of Mexico, was allowed to pass above the quarantine station 65 miles from the city.

8. That the utility of a rational quarantine system against the fomites of yellow fever was not disproved, but the contrary, rather, by the records studied by the writer at New Orleans.

9. That an epidemic of small-pox was promptly arrested by house-to-house vaccination.

10. That with the prevention of epidemics, and unquestionably by the same agencies of prevention generally, the death-rate from zymotic diseases as a class has been very greatly diminished.

The length of this article is greater than I could have wished, and I trust it will not prove burdensome to either your pages or to your intelligent subscribers. The subject discussed is of vast and growing importance. It should be stated that this sanitary work under the military occupation of this city was not performed by the large forces on duty here—it was done by non-military employees of the city government and paid for out of the city treasury. It is proper, however, to say that the city government was conducted through military appointments, control or direction. The most rigid sanitary regulations during the four years of military control began and ended in the simple and strict enforcement of the privy and drainage systems of our city. Nothing new was practiced or even suggested—not an addition was deemed necessary to be added thereto. Our two peculiar systems just above mentioned were found capable of meeting the most exacting requirements and the very highest duty in the interest of, possibly, the most scrupulous and inflexible sanitary discipline that was ever invoked on the top of the earth, and the constant spur of apprehended danger never relaxed, thus evidencing results never before attained, much less equaled, in any known large community. Indeed it is well averred, "so clean a city had never before been seen upon the continent."

The following represents the total amounts expended under the military occupation of this city during the late war between the States in thoroughly carrying out her drainage system, in thoroughly draining and cleaning her streets, and in the performance of all other works relating to the most exacting and absolute sanitation:

Table 11: Expenditures Used in Draining and Cleaning Streets in New Orleans During the Military Occupation, 1862–1865

	Drainage	*Paving*	*Streets*
1862	$93,185.00	$43,405.96	$270,567.11
1863	33,871.84	none	352,599.75
1864	39,247.33	none	334,971.21
1865	65,481.03	none	396,550.77

Had this system not fulfilled all the vital necessities of the then most urgent and pressing military requirements of an invading army completely unacclimated, it would have been improved, where improvement were possible, under this absolute authority, or in some manner modified. The occupation of this city was a matter of crucial importance, and the very fact that no fault was ever found with its sanitary system, its drainage, etc., pleads eloquently from this source in the splendid and continuous good health of this large army of invasion for the maintenance of our unsurpassed system if rightly administered, and its careful and intelligent perfection to keep pace with our enlarging and growing requirements.

Our open ditches and open canals flushed with our exceedingly pure (from an analytical standpoint) Mississippi River water, and exposed as they are to the constant influence of one or the other of Nature's three greatest and perfect disinfectants, to wit: the general atmosphere, the sunshine, and our heavy rainfalls, it is impossible for noxious and poisonous gases from this source to attack our people, as is too often the case in sewered cities. The ensuing from a high authority is pertinent: "The exaltations from the lungs and skin of a single human body vitiate or spoil for breathing ten cubic feet of air per minute, or about 90,000 gallons per day. This foul air, together with that formed from innumerable other sources of contamination, is perfectly removed by diffusion (an unfailing chemical law) and the atmosphere is thus preserved respirable and pure."

The drainage canals were in a bad condition when the city was occupied by the military, hence the larger expenditure in 1862. In a future contribution, if this meets with a favorable reception, we may have more to say on this subject. We might, with pardonable pride, close with the inquiry, where may we look to find a system equal to our own?

Confederate Resources (1901)

CONFEDERATE RESOURCES.*
BY C.H. TEBAULT, M.D., NEW ORLEANS, LA.,
Surgeon-General United Confederate Veterans.
*Paper prepared for the Memphis meeting of the Association of Medical Officers of the Army and Navy of the Confederacy, May 28–80, inclusive, 1901.
Southern Practitioner 24 (January 1902): 44–50.
Mr. President and Fellow-Comrades:

In the pages following, I beg to contribute for the coming historian a number of interesting facts derived from various sources, in evidence of some of the many grave difficulties encountered by the South during the war between the States, and how undauntedly we met them.

Almost immediately after the Confederate Government was organized at Montgomery it was confronted by strong facts and large figures as to required supplies by the different departments. Agents were sent at once to Europe, most of whom were in London, where they established a weekly newspaper, with local correspondents in nearly every Southern town from Virginia to Texas. Instructions were given, that as there was only two sources of supply, capture and blockade-running, importance was given to securing, first, arms and ammunition; second, clothing, including boots, shoes and hats; third, drugs and chemicals, such as were most pressingly needed, as quinine, chloroform, ether, opium, morphine, rhubarb, etc.

These agents were instructed to see that all blockade-runners or any transport ships, barks or brigantines, that were clearing for Southern ports for cargoes of cotton, were loaded with the above enumerated articles; the cargoes to be consigned to individuals, firms, or agents of the Government at any port for which they cleared.

At the outset, the question of drugs and medicines was thus considered third in importance, and the druggists of the South had either to manufacture what they could from native barks and leaves, herbs and roots, or purchase at Southern ports such supplies as the blockade-runners brought, not intended for the Government. In most cases, these cargoes were offered at auction; this was a custom at New Orleans, Galveston, Mobile, Charleston, Savannah, Pensacola and Wilmington. The gulf cities received large supplies from Cuba, while in Texas there was almost a continuous train of contrabanders or smugglers bringing goods across the Rio Grande from Mexico, but not much of this was medicine. The wagon trains of the enemy, captured from time to time, furnished us some supplies of medicines and surgical appliances, but these were insufficient to meet the most distressing needs in the army; so it may be seen, that home manufacture and blockade-running were the only sources of supply during nearly four years, for between six and seven millions of people.

The interior towns suffered most, such as Jackson, Meridian, Columbus and Aberdeen, in Mississippi; Selma, Montgomery, Eufaula and Huntsville in Alabama; Albany, Columbus, Macon, Augusta, Athens, Rome and Atlanta in Georgia; Spartanburg, Greenville and Columbia in South Carolina; Fayetteville, Goldsboro, Raleigh, Statesville and Charlotte in North Carolina; Danville, Lynchburg, Petersburg and Richmond in Virginia. In nearly all of these towns one or more druggists manufactured from stock on hand of roots, herbs and barks, or from home supply of such medicinal plants, etc., as he could secure, tinctures and like preparations.

> The supply of whiskey was not so short as that of medicine; the so-called "moonshiners" of the mountains of North Carolina, Tennessee, Alabama and Georgia, kept their stills (often made of gum logs), running night and day, and found a ready sale for all they produced. So far as known, no tax was placed on whiskey.
>
> I have in my possession a copy of the following work: *Resources of the Southern Fields and Forests, Medical, Economical and Agricultural, being also a Medical Botany of the Southern States, with practical information on the useful properties of the trees, plants and shrubs*, by Francis Peyre Porcher, M.D., formerly Surgeon in charge of city hospitals, Charleston, and Lecturer on Materia Medica and Therapeutics; Corresponding Member of the Medical and Surgical and the Obstetric Societies, and the Lyceum of Natural History, of New York, and of the Academy of Natural Sciences, of Philadelphia.
>
> The first edition of this volume (to use the language of Dr. Porcher) was prepared during the late war by direction of the Surgeon General of the Confederate States, that the Medical officers, as well the public, might be supplied with information, which, at the time, was greatly needed. I was released, temporarily, for this purpose, from service in the field and hospital. My connection with the last mentioned institution, as physician and surgeon, has extended almost uninterruptedly over a period of twelve years, so that my opportunities for experimental investigations in therapeutics and practical medicine, have been ample.

The edition I now have is the "New Edition—Revised and Largely Augmented," published at Charleston, in 1869. This new edition comprises some 700 pages. I will proceed to quote from his "Preliminary":

> It will, therefore, be observed how important it is for us to understand the flora, as well as the soil of a country, and, as one, at least, of our staple commodities, has suffered, we must seek to diversify our industries, and by a more intelligent observation, we may discover new products adapted to our wants and capable of being produced here. It will be observed that most of our useful plants are not indigenous, many now in the woods may, by careful cultivation, become greatly improved in quality and ten-fold more productive, as has already been done with our wild grapes, apples, cauliflowers, strawberries, etc. Central botanical gardens should be established in place of parks, which may be made useful to the industry of man and are as important to a State as geological surveys. I have introduced a notice of upwards of five hundred substance, possessing every variety of useful quality. Some will be rejected as useless; others will be found, on closer examination, to be still more valuable. The most precious of all textile fibres, grains, silks, fruits, oils, gums, caoutchouc, resins, dyes, fecula, albumen, sugar, starch, vegetable acids and alkalies, liquors, spirits, burning fluid, material for making paper and cordage, grasses and forage plants, barks, medicines, wood for tanning, and the productions of chemical agencies, for timber, ship-building, engraving, furniture, implements and utensils of every description, all abound in the greatest munificence, and need but the arm of the authorities, or the energy and enterprise of the private citizen to be made sources of utility, profit or beauty .

I have but imperfectly hinted at the valuable labor performed by Surgeon Porcher, under his appointment as stated, and later on hope to make future contributions from this immense storehouse, in proof of the inexhaustible and but little dreamed of variety of our as yet slumbering, though teeming, Southern resources. I append a list of substitutes that were used by druggists and physicians during the war, in large quantities, in most instances, being the only medicines of the kind to be had.

Imported articles in italics, substitute following each in Roman type:—

Columbo Quassia.—Yellow root.
Spanish Flies.—Potato bugs, powdered leaves of butter-nuts.
Jalap.—Wild jalap, wild potato vine, fever root.

Aloes.—Wild jalap, mulberry bark, dock, wild potato vine, American Columbo.
Digitalis.—Blood root, wild cherry, pipsisewa, bugle weed, jasamine.
Quinine and Peruvian Bark.—Tulip tree bark, dogwood, cotton seed tea, chestnut root and bark, chinquapin root and bark, thoroughwort, Spanish oak bark, knob grass, willow bark.
Conium.—American hemlock.
Opium.—Motherwort, American hemlock.
Sarsaparilla.—Wild sarsaparilla, soapwort, yellow parilla, China briar, queen's delight.
Chamomile.—Dogwood.
Flaxseed.—Watermelon seed.
Gum Arabic.—Low mallows, apple, pear and quince gum, balm, watermelon seed.
Ergot—Cottonroot.
Guaiacum.—Boxwood, poke, prickly ash.
Ipecac.—Wild jalap, Carolina hipps.
Mezereon.—Prickly ash.
Kino and Catechu.—Cranesbill.
Senna.—Wild senna.
Colocynth.—Alum-root.
Tannin.—Smooth sumac.
Olive oil.—Peanut oil, beechnut oil, cottonseed oil.
Laudanum.—Hops, motherwort.
Acroia.—Slippery elm bark, sassafras pith.
Bougies.—Slippery elm bark.
Corks.—Black gum roots, tupelo wood, corn cobs.
Allspice.—Spice bush.
Pink root.—Cardinal flower.
Assafoetida.—Wild chamomile.
Calomel.—Dandelion, pleurisy root, butterfly weed.
Belladonna and Hyoscyamus.—Jamestown weed.
Valerian.—Lady's slipper.
Colchicum.—Indian poke.

Wood anemone was employed as a vesicatory in removing corns from the feet. Powdered may-apple, mixed with resin, was used as a caustic in treating bones, the farriers using it for escharotic purposes. On the farms, the juice of the pulp of the maypop seeds was made into a summer drink, in place of lemonade. Powdered blood-root snuffed up the nose made a powerful sternutatory and was applied as an escharotic to fungous flesh. Pond-lily poultice was extensively applied to ulcers, button snake root, or globe dower, was used largely as an expectorant and diuretic. Toothache bark (aralia spinosa) was used to allay pain caused by carious teeth, and in South Carolina the negroes relied on it almost exclusively for rattle-snake bite. Side-saddle or flycatcher was used in the various forms of dyspepsia. Ink was made from the rind of the pomegranate fruit and poke berries. During convalescence, or as an astringent tonic, dogwood supplied the need. Thism, with blackberry and gentian and pipsissewa, as tonics and diuretics, and sweet gum and sassafras for mucilaginous and aromatic properties, and with jalap as a cathartic, supplied the surgeon in camp with easily procured medicinal plants, which proved sufficient in times of need.

Palmetto leaves, split into shreds with fork and hackle, boiled and dried in the sun, for a few days, made a light, clean, healthy and durable mattress. Palmetto pillows were light and comfortable, and used by our soldiers on the coast. The negroes were employed making palmetto hats for the army. A bed made from the downy swamp plant, which was called "cat's tail," took a premium at an agricultural fair in South Carolina.

Phytolacca decandra, or poke root plant, was largely used in diseases affecting the scalp, and in ulcers, eruptions, itch and hemorrhoids. Knot grass was considered a powerful astringent in diarrhea, and in uterine hemorrhage. Mountain laurel was employed with claimed success in rheumatism, gout, and glandular enlargements. Black alder was used as a wash in cutaneous troubles. Pinckneya pubens, Georgia bark was said to be useful in intermittent fevers—it is said to contain a considerable amount of cinchonine. Woodbine was given in asthma, and a decoction of the flowers administered to calm the pains following child-birth . A decoction made by pouring boiling water over the leaves, dowers and berries of the elder bush, was used as a wash for wounds, to prevent injuries from flies.

As a substitute for hemp the following were used: the sundower stalk, asclepias syriaca, urtica dioecia, and yucca filamentosa, or bear grass. The juice of the skin of the blue fig made a red ink. Fig twigs were used for pipe stems. Rope was made of wahoo (ulmus alata), and used in baling cotton.

Wax myrtle (myrica cerifera) was employed in making candles, and as a basis for fine soap. The soap was obtained from the berries by boiling and skimming. Four pounds of the wax made forty pounds of the soap, with the other ingredients counted. Candles made by the addition of grease are of a green color.

The following is from the *Charleston Courier,* of 1861: "The low-bush myrtle, indigenous to our coast from Virginia *ad libitum* South, the berries of which are now mature, will afford a supply of wax that, with the addition of one-third tallow, will furnish candles sufficient to light every house in the Confederacy for the next year. So also, on every plantation, nay, in almost every kitchen, the monthly waste of ashes and grease, with the addition of a little lime and salt, and the labor of one person for one day, will make soap enough for our purposes." Candles were made of resin. A model, economical candle, sixty yards long, was recommended for the camp and for plantation purposes. It was said to burn six hours a night for six months, and all at a cost of only a few cents. One pound of beeswax was added to three-fourths pound of rosin and melted together; four threads of slack twisted cotton was used for a wick, and drawn through the melted wax and rosin three or four times, and wound into a ball, which on pulling the end up and lighting, furnished a good candle. I conclude this paper with the following: W. Gilmore Sims wrote a friend that "the persimmon beer made in Orangeburg District, South Carolina, by Hon. J.M. Felder, equaled the best sparkling Jersey champagne, or carbonated cider." The old Southern song ran, "Christmas comes but once a year, eggnog and 'simmon beer.'" It was customary to mash the fruit, strain through a coarse sieve, knead with wheat bran and bake in an oven; the bread could be put away for winter use in making beer when wanted.

The foregoing are some of the instructive facts connected with the old days in the Southern Confederacy. On another occasion I hope to make further contributions on this most interesting subject, but what I have here recorded establishes some at least, of the many difficulties of our situation, the straits to which we were forced, and the unflagging energy with which we met them in our fight for the preservation of the pure Constitutional Government of our fathers.

Hospitals of the Confederacy (1902)

HOSPITALS OF THE CONFEDERACY*
BY C.H. TEBAULT, M.D., SURGEON-GENERAL, U.C.V.,
of New Orleans, La.
* Paper Submitted at Dallas Reunion for Publication in the Official Organ
Southern Practitioner 24 (1902): 499–509

Mr. President and Comrades of the Association of Medical Officers of the Army and Navy of the Confederacy:

It is a great pleasure independently of meeting each other to find ourselves at the home of our dear old Octogenarian Comrade, the venerable S.H. Stout, M.D., Surgeon and Medical Director of the Hospitals of the Confederate Army and Department of Tennessee, who administered so successfully and brilliantly this great medical arm of the military service, so fortunately committed to him. Confusion very largely prevailed at first. The ablest surgeons and assistant surgeons, the most experienced, were in the field, while the hospital service was chiefly under the management and direction of the little experienced contract physicians, not immediately connected with the service. The required examinations that shortly followed as the service became better organized, weeded many of these out, and placed in charge of established medical posts, and in immediate charge of the Confederate hospitals, our very ablest surgeons and assistant surgeons.

Out of the chaos above described, soon order and perfect organization ensued, and the splendid hospital system which continued from this date uninterruptedly to the termination of the war, and for which result the chief credit is justly due to the superb administrative ability and tireless energy of our distinguished comrade and always friend, Medical Director of the Hospitals, S.H. Stout, M.D. Vastly more could and should be said respecting the official work of our beloved director of this great department, but time forbids, and I must pass on to the consideration of other points.

On the moment of an expected battle a telegram would be sent by the Medical Director of Hospitals to the hospital post surgeons within easy and rapid communication with the expected battle-field, to forward to the more distant hospital posts all the sick and wounded who could bear transportation, and immediately to telegraph for available supplies for the impending emergency. The able Medical Director in the field was always in instant official communication with the Medical Director of Hospitals. Thus there obtained no loss of time or confusion in knowing where to send the sick and wounded on such instant and momentous occasions, and hospital posts were thus always in readiness to receive and care for our wounded and desperately sick comrades whenever a battle was joined between the contending armies; and our unequalled women, God bless them all, likewise duly notified, were also prepared with the needed delicacies possible to provide with their own dainty and loving hands that our straightened circumstances permitted.

When the wounded and sick were received, all who could stand a bath were given one, and those who could not were carefully sponged off, and all were dressed in clean cotton material for the bed and placed upon neat and comfortable bunks. The surgeons and assistant surgeons, the nurses and our superb womanhood were all now actively and zealously employed under a systematic and well organized authority.

Our corps of nurses were detailed from the hospital sick and wounded who were convalescent, and were at once most faithful and efficient in the discharge of their duties under the close, vigilant and devoted eyes of our surgeons and assistant surgeons, who were unwearying in the performance of their tremendous and highly taxing duties. The prescriptions, written in a book kept for that purpose, were put up by soldiers detailed for that express purpose, but always under the direction and supervision of the ever-watchful medical officers of the hospitals. In all this important service the writer cannot recall a single instance in which an accident of any moment occurred, so careful and exacting was the supervision.

Again, on the eve of expected battle the nearby hospital posts would send on special cars a delegation from their medical staff accompanied by nurses, all of our nurses being men, and all needed appliances within our means and a supply of such delicacies as our precious and always ready women could prepare with their own hands for their loved ones in peril of death.

Thus we stood prepared for our responsible duties on the edge of the battlefield, ready to use our best skill there and then in caring for the wounded as they were being conducted to the nearest hospital posts.

Every hospital had its officer of the day, who was in authority on that day. Each hospital surgeon and assistant surgeon discharged in turn this important office, and concluded his day's inspection with a written report which was strictly examined by the surgeon in charge of the hospital, and then transmitted by him to the surgeon of the hospital post.

The surgeon in charge of the hospital had highly responsible duties; he received and disbursed all money under proper vouchers, looked after and cared for all hospital belongings, drugs, instruments, etc., bought all provisions and made regular monthly reports to the surgeon of the post.

The surgeon of the post supervised the entire hospitals at the post, received and gave all post orders and transmitted the hospital reports to our vigilant Medical Director of Hospitals. The assistant surgeons were the real active workers among the hospital sick and wounded, they were in immediate charge of the most commanding obligations and responsible duties, and excepting the associated duty of officer of the day, were restricted to these two duties of unsurpassed gravity and importance, and which together with being members of the examining boards claimed their well nigh ceaseless occupation. Chickens, eggs, butter, vegetables, etc., were foraged for by convalescent soldiers detailed for this purpose who frequently were out for a week at a time. Towards the last it was necessary to trade off certain articles valued by the country people, which were supplied us at these posts, as our money became valueless.

In the Confederate Hospitals it was the daily custom when the weather permitted to remove all bedding from the building and expose it to the sun and air. Those too ill to leave their beds were carried out in their bunks and placed in the shade of the hospital, or in the sun if desired, or under the shade of trees. Thus the hospitals were frequently cleaned and scrubbed and thoroughly ventilated and kept neat and sweet.

Hospitals frequently conducted vegetable farms by renting land in near reach which was worked by the convalescents; and fresh vegetables thus secured for the sick and wounded. Every day committees of Southern ladies would visit the hospitals, bringing the delicacies wrought by their ever busy hands, and as they passed from bunk to bunk speaking kind, cheering and comforting words to the occupants, and so ministering as loving and Christian and especially only Southern womanhood could.

All this was done with the utmost harmony and under the advice and directing eye and in hearty concurrence with the medical officers in charge. Lady matrons were connected with every hospital and discharged their assigned and invaluable duties with the utmost efficiency and devoted faithfulness. In many instances they were of the very best families of the South driven from their desolated homes, refugees in consequence.

The strict professional courtesy and co-operation between the members of the medical staff whether in hospital or field service, was a matter of wondering animadversion. The medical men of that day were men of the highest honor and standing at home. Their social rank was among the first; their unvarying unity of purpose; their social intercourse; their official relationship; their strict attention to every duty; their strict obedience to recognized necessary authority; their unbroken friendship and respect one for the other whenever they met; the complete and perfect harmony with which they worked together in the discharge of every duty assigned them was the marvel and always favorable comment of all other departments of our military service. Their great-hearted, broad-minded humanity needs no better epitaph than this:

With 50,000 more prisoners of war to care for, prisoners of war whom the Federal Government refused to exchange for Confederate prisoners held in Federal prisons, and knowing the very scant and limited resources of the Confederate Government to properly provide for them, still in the face of this never to be forgotten fact, the Confederate medical staff lost 4,006 less of Federal prisoners than the Federals lost in prison of Confederate prisoners whose exchange they persistently refused.

Smallpox cases were treated in tents properly floored, with due regard to drainage, and for heating when necessary, strictly and inflexibly isolated under wise and well guarded precautions. The surgeons and assistant surgeons assigned to such encampments were restricted to these patients.

In the treatment of erysipelas and hospital gangrene, I can recall but a single instance at any one of our hospital posts where a distinct and separate hospital was assigned to all such cases occurring in the hospitals of a post, for the exclusive care and treatment of these cases.

The rule was to treat all such cases just where they occurred, in the same ward where the other wounded were cared for, and this was done with singular success and without marked detriment to the healthy wounds.

One blessing we enjoyed due to the blockade was the absence of sponges, clean rags being substituted for them with telling advantage. The rags could be thoroughly washed as was done, and used over and over again. It is next to impossible to easily if possible at all, to wash an infected sponge so as to render its employment safe again. This fact and the unstinted use of a plentiful supply of pure well or spring water, and the pure condition of the air of the hospital as above explained, were not without their wholesome effect. The healthy wounds were washed very generally with an infusion of red oak bark, a most valuable treatment. They were often stimulated with a brushing over with the tincture of iodine and were always well nigh hermetically sealed by water dressings on which fresh water constantly dripped except when being dressed. The way the cases of erysipelas and the gangrene cases were healed caused them to be almost hermetically sealed also.

I now pass to the single instance in which these two dreaded maladies were treated in a separate and distinct hospital consisting of an encampment of tents. The single instance in my experience was at the post of Griffin, Georgia. Here, at my suggestion, all these cases were sent to me and treated in the tents just mentioned and located within easy reach of my other hospital duties. It is worthy to record here that none of my other numerous wounded patients contributed to this encampment, though I was its surgeon as well. All my infected cases came from the other hospitals of the post, though their surgeons had no contact with this encampment; or came infected from the field of battle because of the tappings of roads or other unavoidable detention in transit.

This opportunity gave me a large practical experience in the treatment of these so much dreaded complications by surgeons in both civil and military life. I can only speak briefly and generally, but I shall hope intelligently, on an occasion like this. When erysipelas had proceeded to the formation of pus, free incisions were made for its ready escape and these openings were syringed with properly diluted chlorinated water solutions, properly weakened tincture of iodine [solutions or solutions of tannic acid, once, twice or thrice daily, according to the severity of the case. The local application found superior to all others was the camphorated oil (not the *linimentum camphorae*), with more or less sugar of lead added occasionally to meet special indications; but usually only the camphorated oil alone freely applied. This proved a cooling salutary and healing evaporating lotion, and could be applied without restriction to any part of the body, even over the eyes when carefully protected.

The internal treatment consisted in giving quinine in pill form in which glycerine was incorporated to facilitate its absorption. These were administered in doses of two grains every one, two, three, or four hours to meet the febrile manifestations, and also for its well known antiseptic properties. The bowels were, of course, carefully looked after. All complications were given their appropriate treatment. Let me note here that the general treatment of the Confederate Hospital Corps was aseptic not antiseptic, on the principle that an ounce of prevention was worth more than a pound of cure. That to prevent the possible diseased movement was better that to permit its occurrence and then strive to overmaster it.

The diet was eggs, milk, concentrated broths, and stimulants to meet the requirements of each case. This treatment gave most satisfactory results; together with an abundance of pure outdoor, fresh air. Occasionally for a short time where pain was a factor to be pre-scribed for, an opiate would be exhibited, say, preferably, gum opium in grain doses every one, two, three, or four hours, or at longer intervals to control this symptom, and given no longer than absolutely required. The gum opium was better tolerated than morphine and did not disturb the stomach or appetite as obtained under morphine.

This treatment, thoroughly enforced in my hands, left nothing to be desired by me, and the local treatment mentioned protected against possible infection to others not so attacked. The best treatment for hospital gangrene was found to be the same internal medication, nourishment and stimulants mentioned for erysipelas, with fresh outdoor air in abundance. These patients were taken out on their bunks and placed in the open air under the shade of trees where they remained during the day time, weather permitting. The local treatment was as follows: In the gangrenous stump, for example, cotton saturated with turpentine short of dripping was pressed into the gangrenous mans, completely plugging it. Over this was bandaged a poultice thus made—pulverized charcoal prepared fresh at the hospital, carrots reduced to a pulp with hot water and flaxseed meal when procurable, but generally cornmeal in suitable proportions. These dressings were changed three or four times during the day and night. It was magical to see how soon the rotten mass would melt away, leaving behind a healthy wound to be subjected to the treatment of such wounds. It is impossible for me to enlarge or be specific in such a paper as I am writing. The healthy wounds were generally treated with solutions of tannin, or tincture of iodine, or of red oak bark infusion with which they were liberally and unstintedly washed as often as each case demanded. The lips of the stump were brought together after thoroughly brushing over their interior parts to be healed with raw turpentine to stimulate the healing process. I say after this treatment the lips were brought in contact with strips of adhesive plaster of that date which would hold to the satisfaction of anyone, when first lightly brushed over with the oil of turpentine. Besides keeping the wound well united it also furthered the healing in a wonderful degree, and no wound thus treated took on gangrene or erysipelas. Over this adhesive dressing cloths were fastened and either saturated with camphorated oil or kept unfailingly wet by the never ceasing water contributed from suspended bottles devised for this purpose—but whichsoever was adopted, it required no failure of the medicated oil or the unceasing supply of water. These stumps were redressed from time to time as required, and whenever this was needed they were syringed out through any inviting aperture with one or the other of the three solutions referred to above, and the same outward application maintained until a complete healing resulted. One more experience and I will conclude this contribution. The best treatment for compound fractures in my experience was to treat them as though they were simple fractures. First, the part was thoroughly cleansed with a free supply of soap and water, then with the oil of turpentine which again was thoroughly removed by ample washing with soap and water, so that not a vestige of the turpentine remained. Now the fracture was bandaged and adjusted precisely as for simple fractures and then starched, the wounds were thus hermetically sealed up. In a large wound, it was brought together with the adhesive strips as above prepared prior to bandaging and adjusting, with an opening left by the strips for the exit from the wound for any accruing discharge. This done, the bandage was applied and starched and the wound otherwise sealed by bandaging. This bandage was not removed until the fracture had united or until the requisite time had elapsed to justify the removal of the splint and bandage. Whenever the bandage showed any soiled spot due to the discharge from the wound, without removing bandage or splint it was thoroughly washed with warm soap and water and then with a weak solution of chlorinated water and again restarched, and this was done as often as a stain appeared or the faintest improper odor obtained. This treatment of sealing up was most perfect and safe in its results. There is a reason, and a most valuable reason for thus treating wounds, as will immediately appear.

Our greatest of all sweeteners and purifiers are fresh air, water, and sunshine, but there is a constituent from which the open wound must be carefully guarded from for any length of time as a rule. Oxygen is the element to which I here allude. It is the active principle of the atmosphere and is destructive in all its effects. Comprising one-fifth of common air, it is all around us for a chance to spring upon and devour something. We gather a basket of luscious peaches and put them out of the way of the children, but we do not outreach the slyest pilferer of them all—the oxygen—and we soon find the fruit covered with the prints of invisible teeth. Black spots appear and we say they are decaying—it is only the oxygen feasting upon them, and in a short time it will devour them, skin and all. To prevent this, we put our fruit in a glass or metal can, heat it to expel the oxygen, seal it up tightly and then it is safe from this chemical plunderer. We open the damper of the stove and the air rushes in, the oxygen immediately attacks the fuel. Each pair of atoms catches up an atom of carbon between them and flies off into the air as carbonic acid. An animal dies. The oxygen is on the alert and the instant the victim expires, and sometimes a little sooner, this agent so anxious to commence, begins by removing that which would soon be an offense to all sensitive nostrils. We accidently cut our finger and soon the unwelcome oxygen begins at the quivering nerve beneath. The keen throb with which an unexpected hollow in a tooth is revealed to us, announces the entrance of this foe at an un guarded breach.

It was the practice of Confederate surgeons and assistant surgeons to hermetically seal up all wounds as soon as practicable, and it was the almost universal adoption of this surgical procedure in all wounded cases that yielded us our splendid results in wound surgery. One word more about that splendid remedy the oil of turpentine, and I will conclude my paper. Applied pure to a healthy stump just amputated it will not only check all bleeding, but soothe the raw surface and immensely stimulate its more certain and rapid healing. It is equally soothing to mucous surfaces, but its contact with the skin is always irritating, as is well known. The other valuable use just alluded to, however, is not so generally known. I should not close without mentioning that our hospitals consisted of such large and commodious buildings as were procurable, as, for instance, school houses, colleges, hotels, court-houses, churches occasionally, stores, and other like buildings suitable for the purpose, and all of which were patriotically tendered for this use. Small and large tents were everywhere employed to meet the wants of house accommodations. Rude, single-story buildings, for hospital use, raised some three or more feet from the ground were also erected at given points in considerable numbers, and were constructed under the thoughtful directions of the Medical Corps, and were marvels of comfort under our trying surroundings, noteworthy for their perfection of ventilation. Apart from the side windows which were ample in number but without sash or glasses, as we could command none, small yet sufficient openings were provided at the floor surface and at the high ceilings and capable of being closed or opened at will. Near the sides of the wall to the right and left of these buildings, one-fourth of these bunks were placed headboard against the sides of these hospitals and the other three-fourths with head boards towards each other in the central space. These buildings were wide enough to allow a broad passageway to the right and left extending through the length of the buildings between the footboard of the walls and centrally located bunks. I will make record at this place, for fear of omitting to do so, that chloroform was out universally accepted anesthetic for all purposes when one was needed, and was found far superior to ether from every point of view, and in all my hospital experience I can recall no death from its employment.

All medical supplies and instruments, and everything else required by us, were made contraband of war in spite of the immense number of prisoners of war held by us, and whose exchange was persistently refused on the part of the United States government. These hospitals were furnished with from forty-eight to sixty-four bunks with well calculated distances between them. They contained but two doors, a large front and a large rear door, and at the rear end two or more small rooms for the necessary hospital use. The bedding and all other material for equipping these bunks and all other washing and bed material were kept by the hospital stewards in separate rooms disconnected from these wards, and the most rigid rules of cleanliness enforced. The laundry work was performed some distance from the hospitals, and the cooking also was done at a proper interval from the sick and the wounded, and these and all else of importance were daily closely inspected and reported upon as stated, by the medical officer of the day.

The subject, my comrades, upon which I have addressed you, and which I now conclude is necessarily, because of its vastness, simply skimmed upon the surface. It teems in all its depths with untold interest and is a harvest field of immeasurable wealth to the possible medical explorer. When Richmond fell into the hands of the enemy, the fire which ensued destroyed the medical buildings of the Confederacy and its contained medical records were consumed. Fortunately our comrade, Medical Director Stout, preserved duplicate copies of the records of his department, and these are yet available for the student of that period in our history. Scattered records of the Trans-Mississippi Department may also be found here and there among the papers of the medical staff who here served during the war. All of the medical records of the Department of Northern Virginia must have been lost during the Richmond fire. The few of us now surviving cannot hope to do more than offer very imperfect sketches, as I have attempted to do in this contribution in honor of the memorable work grandly, ably, and patriotically performed by our dead and living comrades of the splendid medical corps of the great Confederate armies.

April 17, 1902, 623 North Street, Lafayette Square.

Chapter Notes

Chapter 1

1. Chaillé, "Address of Welcome," 375.
2. McLemore, *A History of Mississippi*, 304.
3. "A Complete List of Commanders, Their Adjutants and Brigadier Generals," *Galveston Daily News*, May 22, 1895, 10.
4. Butler, *The Memoirs of Baron Thiébault*.
5. Wicks, *The Italian Exiles in London, 1816–1848*, 296–300.
6. Sage, "Hamilton (also Walker, née Leslie), Lady Mary," 302.
7. Butler, *The Memoirs of Baron Thiébault*.
8. *American Monthly Magazine*, 10 (1897), 541.
9. Duyckinck and Cornell, *The Duyckinck and Allied Families*.
10. Smith, *An Empire of Print*.
11. Gontar, "The King of Royal Street," 72–75.
12. Easby-Smith, *Georgetown University*.
13. *Times-Picayune*, December 25, 1887, 16.
14. Johnson, "Tulane University, The Secret History."
15. Stowe, *A Southern Practice*, 457–458.
16. Helper, *The Impending Crisis of the South*, 406.
17. Ibid., 407–408.
18. Tulane University, "Our History."
19. Tulane University, "History of Tulane University."
20. Mitchell, "On the Medical Department in the Civil War," 1445–1450.
21. Phillips, *Looming Civil War*, 39.
22. Pollard, *The Lost Cause*, 60.
23. Ibid., 61.
24. Ibid.
25. Ibid.
26. Ibid., 129–130.
27. *Richmond Daily Whig*, July 23, 1861.
28. A South Carolinian, *The Confederate*, 24.
29. Farr, "Samuel Preston Moore," 41–56.
30. Purcell, "Samuel Preston Moore," 361–365.
31. Baird, *David Wendel Yandell*, 43.
32. "The Right Man for the Right Place," 403–405.
33. Ward, *Simon Baruch*, 26.
34. Cunningham, *Doctors in Gray*, 37.
35. *Journal of the Congress of the Confederate States of America*, 343.

Chapter 2

1. *Gazette and Sentinel*, April 20, 1861, 2.
2. *Southern Press*, July 10, 1852, 3-4.
3. *Biographical and Historical Memoirs of Louisiana*, 82.
4. *Richmond Examiner*, April 16, 1861, 1.
5. *Gazette and Sentinel*, April 20, 1861, 2.
6. *Bradford Reporter*, March 14, 1861.
7. *New York Herald*, April 17, 1861, 1.
8. *New York Daily Tribune*, April 17, 1861, 4.
9. *New York Herald*, April 30, 1861, 6.
10. Pollard, *The Lost Cause*, 113.
11. Tebault, *Official Historical Report*, 34.
12. Pollard, *The Lost Cause*, 134.
13. Villepigue, "Letter to Captain C.H. Davis," 572.
14. Davis, "Letter to Brig. Gen. John B. Villepigue," 572.
15. Beauregard, "Letter to Maj. Gen. Henry Halleck," 556.
16. Villepigue, "Letter to General Beauregard."
17. Burbank, "Letter to Assistant Adjutant-General Regarding Smallpox in the Exchanged Prisoners," 551–552.
18. Jones, *Contagious and Infectious Diseases*, 398–400.
19. Fortier, *Louisiana*, 767–770.
20. Beauregard, "Letter to Brig. Gen. J.B. Villepigue," 902–903.
21. Beauregard, "Letter to General S. Cooper."
22. Beauregard, "Letter to Brig. Gen. J.B. Villepigue," 902.
23. Sessel, "Our Evacuation of Fort Pillow," 32.
24. Brent, "General Orders, No. 67," 903.
25. Marszalek, "Account of the Siege of Corinth."
26. Cooling, *Fort Donelson's Legacy*.
27. Walker, *Tenth South Carolina Volunteers*.
28. Bragg, "Report to the Adjutant-General C.S. Army," 876.
29. Walker, *Tenth South Carolina Volunteers*.
30. Linden, "General Bragg's Impossible Dream."
31. Tebault, *Compiled Service Records*.
32. Steiner, *Disease in the Civil War*, 39.
33. Gunn, *Gunn's New Domestic Physician*, 342–343.
34. Ibid., 343.
35. Bollet, *Civil War Medicine*, 284.

36. Cozzens, *No Better Place to Die*, 40–47.
37. Walker, *Tenth South Carolina Volunteers*, 87–88.
38. Halleck, "Letter to Major-General Rosecrans, December 4, 1862," 117–118.
39. Sandburg, *Abraham Lincoln*, 6.
40. Walker, *Tenth South Carolina Volunteers*, 95.
41. Halleck, "Letter to Major-General Rosecrans, June 12, 1863," 8.
42. Halleck, "Letter to Major-General Rosecrans, June 11, 1863," 10.
43. Halleck, "Letter to Major-General Rosecrans, June 16, 1863," 10.
44. Rosecrans, "Letter to Major-General Halleck, June 16, 1863," 10.
45. Tebault, *Compiled Service Records*.
46. Elliott, *Doctor Quintard*, 58–61.
47. *Ibid.*, 118.
48. Q. Melton, "History of Griffin," *Griffin Daily News*, May 26, 1972.
49. "Ancestry of the Chief Sponsor," 262–263.
50. "History of Griffin," *Griffin Daily News*, May 26, 1972.
51. Cumming, *Kate*, 263–264.
52. Desmond, *Georgia's Rome*, 49–51.
53. Tebault, "Hospitals of the Confederacy," 499.
54. Goldsmith, *Report on Hospital Gangrene*, 6.
55. Barnes et al., *The Medical and Surgical History of the Civil War*, part 3, vol. 1, 663.
56. *Ibid.*
57. Tebault, "Hospitals of the Confederacy," 504.
58. *Ibid.*
59. Tripler, "Hospital Gangrene," 585–587.
60. Barnes et al., *The Medical and Surgical History of the Civil War*, vol. 3, 824.
61. Tebault, "Hospitals of the Confederacy," 504.
62. Cunningham, *Doctors in Gray*, 62.
63. Fortier, *Louisiana*, 745–746.
64. Watson, *Physicians and Surgeons of America*, 17–18.
65. Tulane University, "Stanford Emerson Chaillé."
66. Chaillé, "Manuscript Collection No. 158."
67. Gunn, *New Domestic Physician*, 643.
68. *Ibid.*, 1024.
69. Tebault, "Hospitals of the Confederacy."
70. *Ibid.*
71. *Ibid.*, 506–507.
72. Chisolm, *A Manual of Military Surgery*, 197.
73. Cunningham, *Doctors in Gray*, 231–233.
74. Chisolm, *A Manual of Military Surgery*.
75. Chisolm, "Conversion of Gun-Shot Wounds," 138.
76. Chisolm, "Why Do Not Gun-Shot Wounds Heal by Quick Union."
77. Myers, *The Children of Pride*, 1699.
78. Mount, *Some Notables of New Orleans*, 180.
79. Myers, *The Children of Pride*, 1394.
80. Tebault, "Ancestry."
81. Daughters of the American Revolution, *History and Reminiscences of Dougherty County*, 24.
82. Tebault, *Compiled Service Records*.
83. Iobst, *Civil War Macon*, 120.
84. Tebault, *Confederate Resources*, 44–50.
85. Porcher, *Resources of the Southern Fields*.
86. Schmidt and Hasegawa, *Years of Change and Suffering*, 118–119.
87. *Charleston Mercury*, September 11, 1861.
88. Tebault, "Hospitals of the Confederacy," 503.
89. Tebault, "Letter to Mrs. Susan Bailey," January 5, 1865.
90. Miller, *Photographic History of the Civil War*, 249.
91. Tebault, "Surgeon General's Report" (1896), 121.
92. Tebault, "Hospitals of the Confederacy."
93. *Ibid.*
94. *Ibid.*
95. *Ibid.*
96. *Ibid.*
97. *Ibid.*
98. *Ibid.*
99. Tebault, "Report of C.H. Tebault," 358.
100. Tebault, "Address by the Surgeon General," 363.
101. Jones, *Medical and Surgical Memoirs*, 655.
102. Barnes et al., *The Medical and Surgical History of the Civil War*, vol. 3, 869.
103. Miller, *Photographic History of the Civil War*, 290.
104. Tebault, *Compiled Service Records*.
105. Williams, *P.G.T. Beauregard*, 256.
106. Basso, *Beauregard, The Great Creole*, 48.
107. Livermore, *Numbers and Losses in the Civil War*.
108. Hacker, "A Census-Based Count of the Civil War Dead," 307–348.

Chapter 3

1. Tebault, "The Drainage System Peculiar to New Orleans," 330.
2. Harris, *Compilation of the Laws of Louisiana*, 66.
3. *Report of the Board of Administrators of the Charity Hospital*, 28.
4. Hinman, "History of Typhus Fever in Louisiana," 1117–1124.
5. Salvaggio, *New Orleans' Charity Hospital*, 46–47.
6. Tulane University, *Catalogue of the Alumni*.
7. Bollet, *Civil War Medicine*, 64–66.
8. *Ibid.*, 67–69.
9. Jones, "Traumatic Tetanus," 1–5.
10. Jasmin, "The Desegregation of a University," 14–19.
11. Powell, *Bring Out Your Dead*, 173.
12. Rush, *An Account of the Bilious Remitting Yellow Fever*.
13. Sternberg, "Yellow Fever and Quarantine," 351–357.
14. Blake, "Yellow Fever," 673–686.
15. Rush, *Medical Inquiries and Observations*, 125.
16. Binger, *Revolutionary Doctor Benjamin Rush*, 150–151.

17. Tebault, "The Drainage System Peculiar to New Orleans," 325–338.
18. Ibid.
19. Ibid.
20. Ibid.
21. Ibid.
22. Ibid.
23. Finlay, "The Mosquito," 601–616.
24. "No Belief in Yellow Fever Germs," *New York Times*, April 27, 1888.
25. "The Late Yellow Fever Epidemic," *New York Times*, November 30, 1878, 8.
26. Espinosa, "Yellow Fever and Cuba," 541–568.
27. United States National Board of Health, *Annual Report of the National Board of Health*, 102.
28. "Dr. Tebault Talks of Fever Prevention," *Lafayette Gazette*, September 25, 1897, 3.
29. Ibid.
30. Ibid.
31. Tebault, "The Parasitic Origin of Phthisis Pulmonalis," 268–277.
32. Pierce, *Yellow Jack*, 103–104.
33. *New Orleans Daily News*, September 5, 1866, 1.
34. Maygarden, *National Register Evaluation of New Orleans Drainage System*, 5.
35. Tebault, "The Drainage System Peculiar to New Orleans," 325.
36. Ibid.
37. Chaillé, *Ocmulgee Hospital Record Book*.
38. *New Orleans Bulletin*, September 14, 1875, front page.
39. *New Orleans Bulletin*, September 30, 1875, 4.
40. Ibid.
41. Wolfe, "Anti-Vaccinationists Past and Present," 430–432.
42. Tebault, "Modified Inoculation" (1866), 36–42.
43. Bossu, "Upon Inoculation with a Mixture of Milk and Variolous Pus," 412.
44. Tebault, "Modified Inoculation" (1866).
45. Tebault, "Modified Inoculation" (1883).
46. Powell, "A Case of Smallpox," 145–149.

Chapter 4

1. Blaine, *Twenty Years of Congress*, 49.
2. Blackburn, "Radical Republican Motivation," 109–126.
3. Thaddeus Stevens, "Restoration vs. Extermination: Views of Hon. Thad. Stevens—An Address Delivered to the Citizens of Lancaster, Sept. 6, 1865," *New York Times*, September 12, 1865.
4. Warmoth, *War, Politics, and Reconstruction*, 39.
5. Wilson, *The Black Codes of the South*, 38.
6. Donald, *Civil War and Reconstruction*.
7. Irwin, "General Order No. 12," 666–667.
8. Hollandsworth, *Pretense of Glory*.
9. *Official Journal of the Proceedings of the Convention for the Revision and Amendment of the Constitution*, 170.
10. Wetta, *The Louisiana Scalawags*, 92.
11. Sheridan, *Personal Memoirs*, 266–267.
12. Hogue, *Uncivil War*, 46.
13. Ibid., 97–106.
14. Haskins, *Pinckney Benton Stewart Pinchback*.
15. Hart, "Semi-Centennial of the 14th September, 1874," 570–658.
16. "Suppression of the Legal Government in Louisiana," *Cincinnati Enquirer*, February 8, 1873.
17. Hogue, *Uncivil War*, 144.
18. Foner, *Reconstruction*, 349.
19. "The Democratic Assassin. Gov. Packard's Attempted Murder," *New York Times*, February 16, 1877.
20. Landry, *The Battle of Liberty Place*, 8.
21. Blaine, *Twenty Years of Congress*, 448.
22. "The Memphis Riots," *Harper's Weekly*, May 26, 1866.
23. Bell, *Revolution, Romanticism, and the Afro-Creole Protest Tradition in Louisiana*.
24. Sheridan, *Personal Memoirs*, 237–240.
25. Wetta, *The Louisiana Scalawags*, 112.
26. *Harper's Weekly*, August 18, 1866.
27. Castel, *The Presidency of Andrew Johnson*.
28. Hogue, *Uncivil War*, 18.
29. Warmoth, *War, Politics, and Reconstruction*, 273–275.
30. Nordhoff, *The Cotton States*.
31. Ibid.
32. *Times-Picayune*, June 30, 1874.
33. Lawson, "The Civil War Union Leagues," 338–362.
34. Foner, *Reconstruction*, 283–286.
35. Wagner, Gallagher, and Finkelman, *Civil War Desk Reference*, 98–103.
36. *Shreveport Comet*, October 1874.
37. *Times-Picayune*, July 1, 1874.
38. *Lafayette Advertiser*, June 10, 1874.
39. Landry, *The Battle of Liberty Place*, 56.
40. Ibid., 58.
41. Ibid., 59.
42. *The Recent Election in Louisiana*.
43. Ibid., 4.
44. Ibid.
45. Warmoth, *War, Politics, and Reconstruction*, vii.
46. Richter, "James Longstreet," 215–230.
47. Ibid.
48. Keith, *The Untold Story of Black Power, White Terror, and the Death of Reconstruction*, 78.
49. "The Riot in Grant Parish," *Daily Picayune*, April 8, 1873.
50. Lane, *The Day Freedom Died*, 90–91.
51. Foner, *Reconstruction*, 437.
52. *Daily Picayune*, April 16, 1873.
53. *Daily Picayune*, April 18, 1873.
54. "The Democratic Conservative Party—The Platform," *Lafayette Advertiser*, August 29, 1874.
55. R. I. Cromwell, *New Orleans Tribune*, April 25, 1867.
56. Warmoth, *War, Politics, and Reconstruction*, 241.
57. Landry, *The Battle of Liberty Place*, 83–86.
58. *Louisiana Affairs*, 801–802.

59. Hart, "Semi-Centennial of the 14th September, 1874," 582.
60. Ibid., 99.
61. Ibid., 632.
62. Landry, *The Battle of Liberty Place*, 169.
63. *Lafayette Advertiser*, September 19, 1874 (article republished from the *Picayune*).
64. Grant, "Proclamation 220."
65. *Daily Picayune*, September 20, 1874.
66. Hart, "Semi-Centennial of the 14th September, 1874," 585.
67. Ibid., 550.
68. Foner, *Reconstruction*, 575.
69. Robinson, *The Stolen Election*, 182–184.
70. Downs, "The Mexicanization of American Politics," 387–409.
71. Woodward, *Reunion and Reaction*.
72. Hair, *Bourbonism and Agrarian Protest*, 16.
73. Landry, *The Battle of Liberty Place*, 228.
74. Ibid., 192–193.
75. "New Orleans Tries to Erase a Symbol," *New York Times*, October 16, 1989.
76. Taylor, *Louisiana Reconstructed*, 206.
77. Foner, *Reconstruction*, 376.
78. *Daily Standard*, September 7, 1867, 1.
79. Cecelski, *The Fire of Freedom*, 211.
80. Tebault, "Official Report."
81. Tebault, *Our City's Problem*.
82. Williams, *Cases Argued and Decided in the Supreme Court*, 455–463.
83. *New Orleans Bulletin*, November 10, 1875.
84. *New Orleans Republican*, November 27, 1875.
85. *St. Landry Democrat*, February 23, 1878.
86. *Times-Picayune*, February 19, 1878, 2.
87. *Weekly Thibodaux Sentinel and Journal of the 8th Senatorial District*, May 11, 1878.
88. *Weekly Thibodaux Sentinel and Journal of the 8th Senatorial District*, April 13, 1878.
89. *New Orleans Democrat*, July 20, 1879, 4.
90. *Acts of the Legislature of the State of Louisiana*.
91. "A Noted Lottery Man Dead," *New York Times*, June 1, 1885.
92. "John A. Morris, Lottery King. History of the Great Louisiana Gambling Concern," *New York Times*, February 11, 1894.
93. Gandolfo, *Metairie Cemetery*, 15.
94. McGinty, *Louisiana Redeemed*, 184–185.
95. *Official Journal of the Proceedings of the Constitutional Convention of the State of Louisiana* (1879), 136–138.
96. Foner, *Reconstruction*, 588.
97. *The Convention of '98*, 14–16.
98. Ibid., 53–60.
99. Wintz, *African American Political Thought*, 30–33.
100. Hair, *Carnival of Fury*, 106–107.
101. *Constitution of the State of Louisiana*, 77–83.
102. Ibid., 114.
103. Ibid., 115–117.
104. O'Connell, "Southern Comfort," 56–63.
105. Brownstein, *Lincoln's Other White House*.
106. J.W. Mapp, "The Civil War: The Origins of Veterans Health Care," U.S. Department of Veterans Affairs, https://www.va.gov/health/NewsFeatures/20110413a.asp.
107. *Official Journal of the Proceedings of the Constitutional Convention* (1898), 19.
108. "The Death of Jefferson Davis," *New York Times*, September 5, 1861.
109. Foster, *Ghosts of the Confederacy*, 73.
110. Gandolfo, *Metairie Cemetery*, 56.
111. "Jeff Davis' Body Exhumed in New Orleans," *Boston Daily Globe*, May 28, 1893.
112. *Times-Picayune*, December 25, 1887.
113. Wier, *Army of Tennessee, Louisiana Division*, 1–7.

Chapter 5

1. Stephens, *A Constitutional View of the War Between the States*, vol. 1, 10.
2. Pollard, *The Lost Cause*.
3. Ibid., 43–44.
4. Pollard, *Black Diamonds*.
5. Ibid., 45.
6. Ibid., 57.
7. Ibid.
8. Pollard, *The Lost Cause Regained*.
9. Davis, *The Rise and Fall of the Confederate Government*.
10. Ransom and Sutch, *One Kind of Freedom*.
11. *Scott v. Sanford*, 60 U.S. 393.
12. Ibid.
13. Vishneski, "What the Court Decided," 373–390.
14. 62 U.S. (21 How.) 506 (1859).
15. Hembree, "The Question of 'Begging.'"
16. Campbell, *The Slave Catchers*, 14.
17. Crallé, *The Works of John C. Calhoun*, 290–313.
18. Spiegel and Suskind, "Uncontrollable Frenzy and a Unique Temporary Insanity Plea."
19. Doyle, *In Memoriam, Edwin McMasters Stanton*, 85.
20. Littell, *Littell's Living Age*, 254.
21. Flower, *Edwin McMasters Stanton*, 89.
22. Marvel, *Lincoln's Autocrat*, 134.
23. McClellan, "George Brinton McClellan Papers," Stanton to McClellan, July 5, 1862; Stanton, "Edwin McMasters Stanton Papers," Stanton to Herman Dyer, May 18, 1862.
24. Stanton, "Order Regarding Telegraphic Communications," 899.
25. Russell, *My Diary North and South*, 338–340.
26. Wilson, "Edward M. Stanton," 234–246.
27. Flower, *Edwin McMasters Stanton*, 310–312.
28. "An Act to Amend the Act Calling Forth the Militia to Execute the Laws of the Union," 280–282.
29. Schruben, "W. Edwin M. Stanton," 150.
30. Tebault, *Surgeon General Tebault's Report* (1902).
31. Caller, *Genealogy of the Descendants of Lawrence and Cassandra Southwick*.
32. Tebault, *Surgeon General Tebault's Report* (1902), 30–31.

33. Duberman, *Charles Francis Adams*.
34. Coulter, *William Montague Browne*, 177.
35. Tebault, *Surgeon General Tebault's Report* (1902).
36. Tebault, *Official Historical Report*.
37. *Ibid*.
38. Prince, "The Passing of the Declaration," 353–364.
39. Tebault, *Official Historical Report*.
40. *Ibid*.
41. Stephens, *A Constitutional View of the War Between the States*, vol. 2, 36.
42. Tebault, *Official Historical Report*.
43. *Ibid.*, 22.
44. *Ibid.*, 26.
45. Hesseltine, *Civil War Prisons*.
46. Atkinson, "John H. Winder."
47. Blakey, *General John H. Winder*.
48. Tebault, "Losses in the Union War," 318.
49. Hoffman, "Circular, Office Commissary-General of Prisoners," 152–153.
50. Levy, *To Die in Chicago*.
51. Halleck, "Letter to E.M. Stanton," 151.
52. *Ibid.*, 151.
53. Hesseltine, *Civil War Prisons*.
54. Speer, *Portals to Hell*, 323–340.
55. "Abstract from Monthly Returns of the Principal U.S. Military Prisons," 989–1004.
56. United States, *Trial of Henry Wirz*, 3–8.
57. Jones, "Failure to Make a Case Against President Davis," 219–222.
58. Stephens, *A Constitutional View of the War Between the States*.
59. Davis, "General Orders, No. 111," 797.
60. Cooper, *In and Out of Rebel Prisons*, vi.
61. Glazier, *The Capture, The Prison Pen, and the Escape*, vi.
62. Geer, *Beyond the Lines*, 3.
63. Levy, *To Die in Chicago*.
64. Hun and Cogswell, "Letter to E.M. Stanton," 588–589.
65. Tebault, "Report of C.H. Tebault," 356–363.
66. Grant, "Letter to Major-General Butler," 606–607.
67. *Ibid.*, 871–872.
68. Davis, *The Rise and Fall of the Confederate Government*.
69. Hitt, "Exchange of Sick Prisoners Discontinued," 538–540.
70. *Ibid.*, 540.
71. Tebault, "Surgeon General's Report."
72. Tebault, "Mortality Statistics of the Prisons During the Civil War," 363–364.
73. Garfield, "Speech of Gen. Garfield at the Andersonville Reunion," 204.

Chapter 6

1. Washington and Chalaron, *Proceedings*, 4.
2. *Ibid*.
3. Jones, "Official Report" (1893), 158.
4. *Ibid.*, 8.
5. Gordon, *Reminiscences*.
6. Breeden, *Joseph Jones, M.D.*
7. Jones, "Official Report" (1892).
8. Jones, "Confederate States Army Medical Corps."
9. "Medical News Items," 540–541.
10. Tebault, "Surgeon General's Report," 121.
11. Hattaway, "The United Confederate Veterans in Louisiana," 24.
12. *Ibid.*, 19.
13. *Minutes of the First Annual Meeting and Reunion*, 2–3.
14. Sons of Confederate Veterans, "Who the SCV Is Today."
15. *Ibid*.

Afterword

1. Roman, *The Military Operations of General Beauregard*, vol. 1, 373.
2. *Times-Picayune*, April 30, 1899.
3. Miller, *Photographic History of the Civil War*, vol. 7, 249.
4. Evans, *Confederate Military History*, 596–599.
5. *Ibid*.
6. *Times-Picayune*, May 26, 1914.
7. Chaillé, "Address of Welcome," 375–376.
8. Foner, *Reconstruction*, 324.
9. McPherson, *The Political History*, 374.
10. Banner, "A Shadow of Secession," 25.
11. United States of America, "Declaration of Independence."
12. Tebault, *Surgeon General Tebault's Report*, 31.
13. Tebault, *Official Historical Report*, 34.
14. *Ibid*.
15. Stephens, *A Constitutional View of the War Between the States*, vol. 2, 36.
16. Peoples, "The Scapegoat of Andersonville."
17. Hesseltine, *Civil War Prisons*, 140, 243.
18. "Execution of Wirz," *Evening Star*, November 10, 1865, 1.
19. Carlson, "White Liar," 21.
20. Pollard, *The Lost Cause*, 752.
21. D.B. Levy, "Confederate Monuments Here to Stay," *Gettysburg Evening Sun*, August 15, 2017.
22. Joshua Zeitz, "Why There Are No Nazi Statues in Germany: What the South Can Learn from Postwar Europe," *Politico Magazine*, August 20, 2017.
23. Neiberg, *The Treaty of Versailles*.
24. *Ibid*.
25. Hanhimäki and Westad, *The Cold War*, 122.
26. Palmer and Wessler, "The Costs of the Confederacy," 58.

Bibliography

Newspapers and Periodicals

American Monthly Magazine (1897–1909)
Boston Daily Globe (1893)
Bradford Reporter (Towanda, PA) (1861)
Charleston Mercury (Charleston, SC) (1861)
Cincinnati Enquirer (1873)
Daily Picayune (New Orleans, LA) (1873–1874)
Daily Standard (Raleigh, NC) (1867)
Evening Star (Washington, DC) (1865)
Frank Leslie's Illustrated Newspaper (1873–1874)
Galveston Daily News (1895)
Gazette and Sentinel (Iberville, LA) (1861)
Gettysburg Evening Sun (Gettysburg, PA) (2017)
Griffin Daily News (Griffin, GA) (1972)
Harper's Weekly (1865–1874)
Lafayette Advertiser (Lafayette, LA) (1874)
Lafayette Gazette (Lafayette, LA) (1897)
New Orleans Bulletin (1875)
New Orleans Daily News (1866)
New Orleans Democrat (1879)
New Orleans Republican (1875)
New Orleans Times-Democrat (1897)
New Orleans Tribune (1867)
New York Daily Tribune (1861)
New York Herald (1861)
New York Times (1861–1989)
Politico Magazine (2017)
Richmond Daily Whig (1861)
Richmond Examiner (1861)
St. Landry Democrat (Opelousas, LA) (1878)
Shreveport Comet (Shreveport, LA) (1874)
Southern Press (1852)
Times-Picayune (New Orleans, LA) (1874–1914)
Weekly Thibodaux Sentinel and Journal of the 8th Senatorial District (Thibodaux, LA) (1878)

Published Sources

"Abstract from Monthly Returns of the Principal U.S. Military Prisons." In *The War of the Rebellion: A Compilation of the Official Records of the Union and Confederate Armies*, ed. United States War Department. Series 2, vol. 8. Washington: Government Printing Office, 1898.

"An Act to Amend the Act Calling Forth the Militia to Execute the Laws of the Union." In *The War of the Rebellion: A Compilation of the Official Records of the Union and Confederate Armies*, ed. United States War Department. Series 3, vol. 2. Washington: Government Printing Office, 1898.

Acts of the Legislature of the State of Louisiana, 1868. No. 25.

"Ancestry of the Chief Sponsor, Miss Corrine Tebault." *Confederate Veteran* 12 (1904): 262–263.

Atkinson, M. "John H. Winder (1800–1865)." In *Encyclopedia Virginia*. Virginia Foundation for the Humanities. Article published April 7, 2016. https://www.encyclopediavirginia.org/Winder_John_H_1800-1865.

Augustine, George. *History of Yellow Fever.* New Orleans: Searcy & Pfaff, Ltd., 1909.

Baird, Nancy Disher. *David Wendel Yandell: Physician of Old Louisville.* Louisville: University Press of Kentucky, 1978.

Banner, James M., Jr. "A Shadow of Secession? The Hartford Convention, 1814." *History Today* 38 (1988): 24–30.

Barkan, Elazar. *The Guilt of Nations: Restitution and Negotiating Historical Injustices.* New York: W.W. Norton & Company, 2000.

Barnes, J.K., et al., eds. *The Medical and Surgical History of the War of the Rebellion.* 6 vols. Washington: Government Printing Office, 1875–1888.

Basso, Hamilton. *Beauregard, The Great Creole.* New York: Charles Scribner's Sons, 1933.

Beauregard, P.G.T. "Letter to Brig. Gen. J.B. Villepigue, May 28, 1862." In *The War of the Rebellion: A Compilation of the Official Records of the Union and Confederate Armies*, ed. United States War Department. Series 1, vol. 10, part 1. Washington: Government Printing Office, 1884. Beauregard, P.G.T. "Letter to General S. Cooper, April 9, 1862." In *The War of the Rebellion: A Compilation of the Official Records of the Union and Confederate Armies*, ed. United States War Department. Series 1, vol. 10, part 1. Washington: Government Printing Office, 1884.

Beauregard, P.G.T. "Letter to Maj. Gen. Henry Halleck, May 20, 1862." In *The War of the Rebellion: A Compilation of the Official Records of the Union and Confederate Armies*, ed. United States War Department. Series 2, vol. 3. Washington: Government Printing Office, 1898.

Bell, C. *Revolution, Romanticism, and the Afro-Creole Protest Tradition in Louisiana 1718–1868.* Baton Rouge: Louisiana State University Press, 1997.

Binger, Carl. *Revolutionary Doctor Benjamin Rush.* New York: W.W. Norton & Company, 1966.

Biographical and Historical Memoirs of Louisiana. Vol. 2. Chicago: The Goodspeed Publishing Company, 1892.

Blackburn, George M. "Radical Republican Motivation: A Case History." *The Journal of Negro History* 54 (1969): 109–126.

Blaine, James G. *Twenty Years of Congress.* Vol. 2. Norwich, CT: The Henry Bill Publishing Company, 1886.

Blake, John B. "Yellow Fever in Eighteenth Century America." *Bulletin of the New York Academy of Medicine* 44 (1968): 673–686.

Blakey, Arch. *General John H. Winder, C.S.A.* Gainesville: University Press of Florida, 1990.

Bollet, Alfred Jay. *Civil War Medicine: Challenges and Triumphs.* Tucson, AZ: Galen Press, Ltd., 2002.

Bossu, M. "Upon Inoculation with a Mixture of Milk and Variolous Pus, to Supersede Vaccination." *Medical Times & Gazette* 199 (April 22, 1854): 412.

Bragg, Braxton. "Report to the Adjutant-General C.S. Army, September 25, 1862." In *The War of the Rebellion: A Compilation of the Official Records of the Union and Confederate Armies,* ed. United States War Department. Series 1, vol. 16, part 2. Washington: Government Printing Office, 1886.

Breeden, James O. *Joseph Jones, M.D.: Scientist of the Old South.* Louisville: University Press of Kentucky, 1975.

Brent, G.M. "General Orders, No. 67, June 11, 1862." In *The War of the Rebellion: A Compilation of the Official Records of the Union and Confederate Armies,* ed. United States War Department. Series 1, vol. 10, part 1. Washington: Government Printing Office, 1884.

Brownstein, Elizabeth. *Lincoln's Other White House: The Untold Story of the Man and His Presidency.* New York: John Wiley, 2005.

Burbank, S. "Letter to Assistant Adjutant-General Regarding Smallpox in the Exchanged Prisoners." In *The War of the Rebellion: A Compilation of the Official Records of the Union and Confederate Armies,* ed. United States War Department. Series 2, vol. 3. Washington: Government Printing Office, 1898.

Butler, A.J. *The Memoirs of Baron Thiébault.* London: Smith, Elder & Co., 1896.

Caller, James M., and M. Ober. *Genealogy of the Descendants of Lawrence and Cassandra Southwick of Salem, Massachusetts.* Salem, MA: J.H. Choate & Co., 1881.

Campbell, Stanley W. *The Slave Catchers: Enforcement of the Fugitive Slave Law, 1850–1860.* Chapel Hill: University of North Carolina Press, 1970.

Carlson, Peter. "White Liar." *American History* 53 (February 2019): 20–21.

Castel, Albert E. *The Presidency of Andrew Johnson.* Lawrence: University Press of Kansas, 1979.

Cecelski, D.S. *The Fire of Freedom: Abraham Galloway and the Slaves' Civil War.* Chapel Hill: University of North Carolina Press, 2012.

Chaillé, S.E. "Address of Welcome by Stanford E. Chaillé, M.D., Ex-Surgeon of the Confederate Army, to the Association of the Medical Officers of the Confederate Army and Navy. New Orleans, La., May 19 1903." *Southern Practitioner* 25 (July 1903): 372–380.

Chaillé, S.E. "Manuscript Collection No. 158." Stuart A. Rose Manuscript, Archives, and Rare Book Library, Emory University, Atlanta, GA.

Chaillé, S.E. *Ocmulgee Hospital Record Book, June 12, 1903.* Emory University, Manuscript Collection #158.

Chaillé, S.E. "The Vital Statistics of New Orleans from 1769 to 1874." *New Orleans Medical and Surgical Journal* 2 (July 1874): 1–37.

Chisolm, J.J. *A Manual of Military Surgery for the Use of Surgeons in the Confederate Army, with an Appendix of the Rules and Regulations of the Medical Department of the Confederate Army.* Columbia, SC: Evans and Cogswell, 1864.

Chisolm, J.J. "Conversion of Gun-Shot Wounds into Incised Wounds as a means of Speedy Cure." *Confederate States Medical and Surgical Journal* 1 (September 1864): 138.

Chisolm, J.J. "Why Do Not Gun-Shot Wounds Heal by Quick Union." *Richmond Medical Journal* 3 (1867): 313–319.

Constitution of the State of Louisiana. Adopted in Convention at the City of New Orleans, May 12, 1898.

The Convention of '98. A Complete Work on the Greatest Political Event in Louisiana History and a Sketch of the Men Who Composed it Together with a Historical Review of the Conventions of the Past and the General Assembly which Called. New Orleans: William E. Myers, 1898.

Cooling, B. Franklin. *Fort Donelson's Legacy: War and Society in Kentucky and Tennessee, 1862–1863.* Knoxville: University of Tennessee Press, 1997.

Cooper, A. *In and Out of Rebel Prisons.* Oswego, NY: R.J. Oliphant, 1888.

Coulter, E.M. *William Montague Browne.* Athens: University of Georgia Press, 2010.

Cozzens, P. *No Better Place to Die: The Battle of Stones River.* Champaign: University of Illinois Press, 1990.

Crallé, Richard K., ed. *The Works of John C. Calhoun.* Vol. 6. Columbia, SC: A.S. Johnston, 1851.

Cumming, K., and R.B. Harwell. *Kate: The Journal of a Confederate Nurse.* Baton Rouge: Louisiana State University Press, 1998.

Cunningham, H.H. *Doctors in Gray.* Baton Rouge: Louisiana State University Press, 1960.

Daughters of the American Revolution, Georgia State Society, Thronateeska Chapter, Albany. *History and Reminiscences of Dougherty County, Georgia.* Albany, GA: Herald Publishing Company, 1924.

Davis, C.H. "Letter to Gen. John B. Villepigue, May 21, 1862." In *The War of the Rebellion: A Compilation of the Official Records of the Union and Confederate Armies,* ed. United States War Department. Series 2, vol. 3. Washington: Government Printing Office, 1898.

Davis, J. "General Orders, No. 111." In *The War of the Rebellion: A Compilation of the Official Records of the Union and Confederate Armies,* ed. United States War Department. Series 2, vol. 5. Washington: Government Printing Office, 1899. Davis, J.

The Rise and Fall of the Confederate Government. New York: D. Appleton & Co., 1881.

Desmond, J.R. *Georgia's Rome: A Brief History*. Atlanta, GA: The History Press, 2008.

Donald. H.D. *Civil War and Reconstruction*. New York: W.W. Norton & Company, 2001.

Downs, Gregory P. "The Mexicanization of American Politics: The United States' Transnational Path from Civil War to Stabilization." *American Historical Review* 117 (April 2012): 387–409.

Doyle, John B. *In Memoriam, Edwin McMasters Stanton, His Life and Work*. Steubenville, OH: Joseph B. Doyle, 1911.

Duberman, Martin. *Charles Francis Adams, 1807–1886*. Palo Alto, CA: Stanford University Press, 1968.

Duncan, J.K. "Report of Brig. Gen. Johnson K. Duncan, C.S. Army, of the Bombardment and Surrender of Forts Jackson and Saint Philip, April 30, 1862." In *The War of the Rebellion: A Compilation of the Official Records of the Union and Confederate Armies*, ed. United States War Department. Series 1, vol. 16. Washington: Government Printing Office, 1886.

Duyckinck, Whitehead Cornell, and John Cornell. *The Duyckinck and Allied Families—Being a Record of the Descendants of Evert Duyckinck who Settled in New Amsterdam, now New York, in 1638*. New York: Tobias A. Wright, 1908.

Easby-Smith, James Stanislaus. *Georgetown University in the District of Columbia, 1789-1907*. New York: The Lewis Publishing Co., 1907.

Elliott, S.D., ed. *Doctor Quintard, Chaplain CSA and Second Bishop of Tennessee*. Baton Rouge: Louisiana State University Press, 2003.

Espinosa, Mariola. "Yellow Fever and Cuba." *Journal of Southern History* 72 (2006): 541–568.

Evans, Clement Anselm. *Confederate Military History: A Library of Confederate States History*. Vol. 10. Atlanta, GA: Confederate Pub. Co., 1899.

"A Fair Sponsor for the South." *The Washington Times* May 29, 1904, 10.

Farr, Warner Dahlgren. "Samuel Preston Moore: Confederate Surgeon General." *Civil War History* 41 (1995): 41–56.

Finlay, Carlos. *Carlos Finlay and Yellow Fever*. New York: Oxford University Press, 1940.

Finlay, Carlos. "The Mosquito Hypothetically Considered as an Agent in the Transmission of Yellow Fever Poison." Translated by Rudolph Matas. *New Orleans Medical and Surgical Journal* 9 (1881): 601–616.

Flower, Frank Abial. *Edwin McMasters Stanton: The Autocrat of Rebellion, Emancipation, and Reconstruction*. Boston: George M. Smith & Co., 1905.

Foner, Eric. *Reconstruction: America's Unfinished Revolution 1863-1877*. New York: Harper & Row, 1988.

Fortier, Alcée, ed. *Louisiana: Comprising Sketches of Parishes, Towns, Events, Institutions, and Persons, Arranged in Cyclopedic Form*. Vol. 3. New Orleans: Century Historical Association, 1914.

Fossier, A.E. "History of Medicine in New Orleans from Its Birth to the Civil War." *Annals of Medical History*, n.s., 6 (1934): 320–352, 427–447.

Foster, Gaines M. *Ghosts of the Confederacy: Defeat, the Lost Cause, and the Emergence of the New South, 1865 to 1913*. New York: Oxford University Press, 1987.

Gandolfo, Henri. *Metairie Cemetery, An Historical Memoir*. New Orleans: Stewart Enterprises, Inc., 1998.

Garfield, James. "Speech of Gen. Garfield at the Andersonville Reunion at Toledo, Ohio, October 3, 1879." In *Prison Life in Dixie*, by Sergeant Oats. Scituate, MA: Digital Scanning, Inc., 1999. First published 1880 by Central Book Concern (Chicago).

Geer, J.J. *Beyond the Lines or A Yankee Prisoner Loose in Dixie*. Philadelphia: J.W. Daughaday, 1864.

Glazier, W.W. *The Capture, The Prison Pen, and the Escape*. New York: R.H. Ferguson & Co., 1870.

Goldsmith, M. *A Report on Hospital Gangrene, Erysipelas, and Pyaemia, as Observed in the Departments of the Ohio and the Cumberland*. Louisville, KY: Bradley & Gilbert, 1863.

Gontar, Cybele. "The King of Royal Street—W.G. Tebault and the Poetry of Furniture." *Louisiana Endowment for the Humanities* (Winter 2015–16): 72–75.

Gordon, John B. *Reminiscences of the Civil War*. New York: Charles Scribner's Sons, 1903.

Grant, U.S. "Letter to Major-General Butler, August 18, 1864, Regarding Prisoner Exchanges." In *The War of the Rebellion: A Compilation of the Official Records of the Union and Confederate Armies*, ed. United States War Department. Series 2, vol. 7. Washington: Government Printing Office, 1899.

Grant, U.S. "Proclamation 220—Law and Order in the State of Louisiana." In *The American Presidency Project*, edited by Gerhard Peters and John T. Woolley. https://www.presidency.ucsb.edu/node/204002.

Gunn, John C. *Gunn's New Domestic Physician*. Cincinnati: Moore, Wilstach, Keys & Co., 1862.

Hacker, J.D. "A Census-Based Count of the Civil War Dead." *Civil War History* 57 (2011): 307–348.

Hair, William I. *Bourbonism and Agrarian Protest: Louisiana Politics, 1877-1900*. Baton Rouge: Louisiana State University Press, 1969.

Hair, William I. *Carnival of Fury: Robert Charles and the New Orleans Race Riot of 1900*. Baton Rouge: Louisiana State University Press, 1976.

Halleck, H.W. "Letter to E.M. Stanton, May 19, 1864." In *The War of the Rebellion: A Compilation of the Official Records of the Union and Confederate Armies*, ed. United States War Department. Series 2, vol. 7. Washington: Government Printing Office, 1899. Halleck, H.W. "Letter to Major-General Rosecrans, December 4, 1862." In *The War of the Rebellion: A Compilation of the Official Records of the Union and Confederate Armies*, ed. United States War Department. Series 1, vol. 20, part 2. Washington: Government Printing Office, 1887.

Halleck, H.W. "Letter to Major-General Rosecrans, June 11, 1863." In *The War of the Rebellion: A Compilation of the Official Records of the Union and Confederate Armies*, ed. United States War Department. Series 1, vol. 23, part 1. Washington: Government Printing Office, 1889.

Halleck, H.W. "Letter to Major-General Rosecrans, June 12, 1863." In *The War of the Rebellion: A Compilation of the Official Records of the Union and Confederate Armies*, ed. United States War Department. Series 1, vol. 23, part 1. Washington: Government Printing Office, 1889.

Halleck, H.W. "Letter to Major-General Rosecrans, June 16, 1863." In *The War of the Rebellion: A Compilation of the Official Records of the Union and Confederate Armies*, ed. United States War Department. Series 1, vol. 23, part 1. Washington: Government Printing Office, 1889.

Hanhimäki, J.M., and O.A. Westad, eds. *The Cold War: A History in Documents and Eyewitness Accounts*. New York: Oxford University Press, 2004.

Harris, T.S. *Compilation of the Laws of Louisiana Relating to the Public Schools*. Baton Rouge, LA: The New Advocate, 1909.

Hart, W.O., A.W. Robinson, J.A. Renshaw, and B.F. Jonas. "Semi-Centennial of the 14th September, 1874." *The Louisiana Historical Quarterly* 7 (1924): 570–658.

Haskins, James. *Pinckney Benton Stewart Pinchback*. New York: Macmillan, 1973.

Hattaway, Herman. "The United Confederate Veterans in Louisiana." *Louisiana History: The Journal of the Louisiana Historical Association* 16 (1975): 24.

Helper, Hinton R. *The Impending Crisis of the South: How to Meet It*. New York: A.B. Burdick, 1860.

Hembree, Michael F. "The Question of 'Begging': Fugitive Slave Relief in Canada, 1830–1865." *Civil War History* 37 (1991): 314–327.

Hesseltine, William. *Civil War Prisons: A Study in War Psychology*. Columbus: Ohio University Press, 1998.

Hinman, E.H. "History of Typhus Fever in Louisiana." *American Journal of Public Health* 26 (1936): 1117–1124.

Hitt, V.G. "Exchange of Sick Prisoners Discontinued." *Southern Practitioner* 31 (1909): 538–540.

Hoffman, W. "Circular, Office Commissary-General of Prisoners, July 7, 1862." In *The War of the Rebellion: A Compilation of the Official Records of the Union and Confederate Armies*, ed. United States War Department. Series 2, vol. 4. Washington: Government Printing Office, 1898.

Hogue, James K. *Uncivil War: Five New Orleans Street Battles and the Rise and Fall of Radical Reconstruction*. Baton Rouge: Louisiana State University Press, 2006.

Hollandsworth, J.G. *Pretense of Glory: The Life of General Nathaniel P. Banks*. Baton Rouge: Louisiana State University Press, 1998.

Hun, T., and M.F. Cogswell. "Letter to E.M. Stanton, May 10, 1863, Regarding the Deplorable Conditions of the Hospitals Containing Rebel Prisoners." In *The War of the Rebellion: A Compilation of the Official Records of the Union and Confederate Armies*, ed. United States War Department. Series 2, vol. 5. Washington: Government Printing Office, 1899.

Iobst, R.W. *Civil War Macon: The History of a Confederate City*. Macon, GA: Mercer University Press, 2009.

Irwin, R.B. "General Order No. 12." In *The War of the Rebellion: A Compilation of the Official Records of the Union and Confederate Armies*, ed. United States War Department. Series 1, vol. 15. Washington: Government Printing Office, 1886.

Jasmin, A.D. "The Desegregation of a University." *Tulane Magazine* (September 2013): 14–19.

Johnson, S., and M. DeMocker. "Tulane University, The Secret History." Tulane University. https://www2.tulane.edu/news/tulanian/the_secret_history.cfm (accessed November 28, 2018).

Jones, J. William. "Failure to Make a Case Against President Davis." *Southern Historical Society Papers* 1 (1876): 219–222.

Jones, Joseph. "Confederate States Army Medical Corps." *The Medical News*, April 26, 1890.

Jones, Joseph. *Contagious and Infectious Diseases*. Baton Rouge, LA: Leon Jastremski, 1884.

Jones, Joseph. *Medical and Surgical Memoirs, 1855–1876*. Vol. 1. New Orleans: Clarke and Hofeline, 1876.

Jones, Joseph. "Official Report." *The Saint Louis Medical and Surgical Journal* 61 (September 1893): 158.

Jones, Joseph. "Official Report of Joseph Jones, M.D., of New Orleans, Louisiana, Surgeon-General United Confederate Veterans, Concerning the Medical Department of the Confederate Army and Navy." In *Minutes of the Third Annual Meeting and Reunion of the United Confederate Veterans*. New Orleans: Hopkins' Printing Office, 1892.

Jones, Joseph. "Traumatic Tetanus." *Confederate States Medical and Surgical Journal* 1 (1864): 1–5.

Journal of the Congress of the Confederate States of America, 1861–1865. Vol. 2. Washington: Government Printing Office, 1904.

Keith, L. *The Untold Story of Black Power, White Terror, and the Death of Reconstruction*. New York: Oxford University Press, 2007.

Kelly, Howard A. *Walter Reed and Yellow Fever*. Baltimore, MD: Medical Standard Book Co., 1906.

Landry, Stuart O. *The Battle of Liberty Place*. Gretna, LA: Pelican Publishing Co., 2000.

Lane, C. *The Day Freedom Died: The Colfax Massacre, the Supreme Court, and the Betrayal of Reconstruction*. New York: Henry Holt and Co., 2008.

"The Last Roll, In Memoriam, Dr. Christopher Hamilton Tebault." *Confederate Veteran* 22 (August 1914): 372–373.

Lawson, Melinda. "The Civil War Union Leagues and the Construction of a New National Patriotism." *Civil War History* 48 (2002): 338–362.

Levy, George. *To Die in Chicago*. Gretna, LA: Pelican Publishing Co., 1999.

Linden, Frank van der. "General Bragg's Impossible Dream: Take Kentucky." *Civil War Times* 1 (November/December 2006): 21–25.

Littell, E. *Littell's Living Age*. Series 3, vol. 17. Boston: Littell, Son and Company, 1862.

Livermore, Thomas L. *Numbers and Losses in the Civil War in America, 1861–65*. Cambridge, MA: Riverside Press of Houghton, Mifflin and Company, 1901.

Louisiana Affairs. Report by the Select Committee on that Portion of the President's Message Relating to the Conditions in the South. 43rd Congress, House of Representatives. Report 261, Part 3. Washington: Government Printing Office, 1875.

Mapp, J.W. "The Civil War: The Origins of Veterans Health Care." U.S. Department of Veterans Affairs, https://www.va.gov/health/NewsFeatures/20110413a.asp.

Marszalek, John F. "Account of the Siege of Corinth." *Civil War Times* February 2006.

Marvel, William. *Lincoln's Autocrat: The Life of Edwin Stanton*. Chapel Hill: University of North Carolina Press, 2015.

Maygarden, B.D., et al. *National Register Evaluation of New Orleans Drainage System, Orleans Parish, Louisiana*. New Orleans: Earth Search, Inc., 1999.

McClellan, George Brinton. "George Brinton McClellan Papers, 1898–1823." Manuscript Division, Library of Congress, Washington, DC. http://hdl.loc.gov/loc.mss/eadmss.ms010155.

McGinty, Garnie W. *Louisiana Redeemed: The Overthrow of Carpet-Bag Rule 1876–1880*. New Orleans: Pelican Publishing, 1941.

McLemore, Richard Aubrey. *A History of Mississippi*. Vol. I. Jackson: University of Mississippi Press, 1973.

McPherson, Edward. *The Political History of the United States of America During the Period of Reconstruction*. Washington: James J. Chapman, 1880.

"Medical News Items, Joseph Jones, M.D." *New Orleans Medical and Surgical Journal* 23 (March 1896): 540–541.

Miller, Francis T. *The Photographic History of the Civil War in Ten Volumes*. New York: The Review of Reviews Co., 1911.

Minutes of the First Annual Meeting and Reunion of the United Confederate Veterans. New Orleans: Hopkins' Printing Office, 1891.

Mitchell, S.W. "On the Medical Department in the Civil War." *Journal of the American Medical Association* 62 (1914): 1445–1450.

Mount, M.W. *Some Notables of New Orleans: Biographical and Descriptive Sketches of the Artists of New Orleans, and Their Work*. New Orleans: May M. Mont, 1896.

Myers, R.M., ed. *The Children of Pride: A True Story of Georgia and the Civil War*. New Haven, CT: Yale University Press, 1972.

Neiberg, Michael S. *The Treaty of Versailles: A Concise History*. New York: Oxford University Press, 2017.

Nordhoff, C. *The Cotton States in the Spring and Summer of 1875*. New York: D. Appleton & Company, 1876.

O'Connell, Kim. "A. Southern Comfort." *America's Civil War* 25 (2012): 56–63.

Official Journal of the Proceedings of the Constitutional Convention of the State of Louisiana. New Orleans: Jas. H. Cosgrove, 1879.

Official Journal of the Proceedings of the Constitutional Convention of the State of Louisiana Held in New Orleans, Tuesday, February 8, 1898. New Orleans: H.J. Hearsey, Printer to the Convention, 1898.

Official Journal of the Proceedings of the Convention for the Revision and Amendment of the Constitution of the State of Louisiana. New Orleans: W.R. Fish, Printer to the Convention, 1864.

"The Orleans Cadets." *Confederate Veteran* 29 (1921): 207–208.

Palmer, Brian, and Seth F. Wessler. "The Costs of the Confederacy." *Smithsonian Magazine* 49 (December 2018): 56–63.

Peoples, Morgan. "The Scapegoat of Andersonville: Union Execution of Confederate Captain Henry Wirz." *North Louisiana Historical Association Journal* 11 (Fall 1980): 3–18.

Peyton, H.E. "Official Synopsis of Exchange of 200 Prisoners to General Beauregard." In *The War of the Rebellion: A Compilation of the Official Records of the Union and Confederate Armies*, ed. United States War Department. Series 2, vol. 3. Washington: Government Printing Office, 1898.

Phillips, Jason. *Looming Civil War: How Nineteenth-Century Americans Imagined the Future*. New York: Oxford University Press, 2018.

Pierce, J.R., and J. Writer. *Yellow Jack: How Yellow Fever Ravaged America and Walter Reed Discovered Its Deadly Secrets*. New York: John Wiley and Sons, 2005.

Pollard, Edward A. *Black Diamonds Gathered in the Darkey Homes of the South*. New York: Pudney & Russell, 1859.

Pollard, Edward A. *The Lost Cause—A New Southern History of the War of the Confederates*. New York: E.B. Treat & Company, 1867.

Pollard, Edward A. *The Lost Cause Regained*. New York: G.W. Carleton & Co., 1868.

Porcher, F.P. *Resources of the Southern Fields and Forests, Medical, Economical, and Agricultural: Being also a Medical Botany of the Confederate States, with Practical Information on the Properties of Trees, Plants, and Shrubs*. Charleston, SC: Evans & Cogswell, 1863.

Powell, J.H. *Bring Out Your Dead: The Great Plague of Yellow Fever in Philadelphia in 1793*. Philadelphia: University of Pennsylvania Press, 1949.

Powell, W.B. "A Case of Smallpox—Modified Inoculation in the Family of Patient." *Gaillard's Medical Journal* 36 (1883): 145–149.

Preston, W. "Report of Col. William Preston, Aide-de-Camp to General Johnston." In *The War of the Rebellion: A Compilation of the Official Records of the Union and Confederate Armies*, ed. United States War Department. Series 1, vol. 10, part 1. Washington: Government Printing Office, 1884.

Prince, Leon C. "The Passing of the Declaration." *The Arena* 25 (1901): 353–364.

Purcell, P.N., and Hummel, R.P. "Samuel Preston Moore: Surgeon-General of the Confederacy." *American Journal of Surgery* 164 (1992): 361–365.

Ransom, Roger L., and Richard Sutch. *One Kind of Freedom: The Economic Consequences of Emancipation*. 2nd ed. New York: Cambridge University Press, 2001.

The Recent Election in Louisiana. House of Representatives, 44th Congress. Report 156, Part 2, February 1, 1877.

Report of the Board of Administrators of the Charity Hospital to the General Assembly of the State of Louisiana, 1898. New Orleans: Democrat Print, 1898.

Richter, William L. "James Longstreet: From Rebel to Scalawag." *Journal of Louisiana History* 11 (1970): 215–230.

"The Right Man for the Right Place." *American Medical Times* 2 (June 22, 1861): 403–405.

Robinson, L. *The Stolen Election: Hayes versus Tilden—1876*. New York: Tom Doherty Associates, 2001.

Roman, Alfred. *The Military Operations of General Beauregard*. New York: Harper & Brothers, 1884.

Rosecrans, W.S. "Letter to Major-General Halleck, June 16, 1863." In *The War of the Rebellion: A Compilation of the Official Records of the Union and Confederate Armies*, ed. United States War Department. Series 1, vol. 23, part 1. Washington: Government Printing Office, 1889.

Rush, Benjamin. *An Account of the Bilious Remitting Yellow Fever, as it Appeared in the City of Philadelphia in the Year 1793*. Philadelphia: Thomas Dobson, 1794.

Rush, Benjamin. *Medical Inquiries and Observations*. Vol. 1. Philadelphia: Thomas Dobson, 1794.

Russell, William Howard. *My Diary North and South*. Boston: T.O.H.P. Burnham, 1863.

Sage, Lorna, ed. "Hamilton (also Walker, née Leslie), Lady Mary." In *The Cambridge Guide to Women's Writing in English*. London: Cambridge University Press, 1999.

Salvaggio, John E. *New Orleans' Charity Hospital: A Story of Physicians, Politics, and Poverty*. Baton Rouge: Louisiana State University Press, 1992.

Sandburg, Carl. *Abraham Lincoln: The War Years*. Vol. 2. New York: Harcourt, Brace & Company, 1939.

Schmidt, J.M., and G.R. Hasegawa, eds. *Years of Change and Suffering: Modern Perspectives on Civil War Medicine*. Roseville, MN: Edinborough Press, 2009.

Schroeder-Lein, G.R. *The Encyclopedia of Civil War Medicine*. Armonk, NY: M.E. Sharpe, 2008.

Schruben, Francis. "W. Edwin M. Stanton and Reconstruction." *Tennessee Historical Quarterly* 23 (1964): 150.

Sessel, Edwin H. "Our Evacuation of Fort Pillow." *Confederate Veteran* 6 (1898): 32.

Sheridan, P.H. *Personal Memoirs of P.H. Sheridan*. Vol. 2. New York: Charles L. Webster & Company, 1888.

Smith, Steven Carl. *An Empire of Print: The New York Publishing Trade in the Early American Republic*. University Park, PA: Penn State University Press, 2017.

Sons of Confederate Veterans. "Who the SCV Is Today." http://www.scv.org/new/.

A South Carolinian. *The Confederate*. Mobile, AL: S.H. Goetzel & Co., 1863.

Speer, L.R. *Portals to Hell: Military Prisons of the Civil War*. Mechanicsburg, PA: Stackpole Books, 1997.

Spiegel, A.D., and P.B. Suskind. "Uncontrollable Frenzy and a Unique Temporary Insanity Plea." *Journal of Community Health* 25 (April 2000): 157–179. Stanton, E.M. "Edwin McMasters Stanton Papers: Correspondence, 1831–1870." Manuscript Division, Library of Congress, Washington, DC. https://www.loc.gov/collections/edwin-mcmasters-stanton-papers/.

Stanton, E.M. "Order Regarding Telegraphic Communications." In *The War of the Rebellion: A Compilation of the Official Records of the Union and Confederate Armies*, ed. United States War Department. Series 3, vol. 1. Washington: Government Printing Office, 1899.

Steiner, Paul E. *Disease in the Civil War*. Springfield, Ill: Charles C. Thomas, Publisher, 1968.

Stephens, Alexander H. *A Constitutional View of the Late War Between the States: Its Causes, Character, Conduct and Results*. Philadelphia: National Publishing Company, 1868.

Sternberg, George M. "Yellow Fever and Quarantine." *Public Health Papers and Reports* 6 (1880): 351–357.

Stowe, S.M. *A Southern Practice: The Diary and Autobiography of Charles A. Hentz, M.D.* Charlottesville: University Press of Virginia, 2000.

Taylor, J.G. *Louisiana Reconstructed, 1863–1877*. Baton Rouge: Louisiana State University Press, 1984.

Tebault, C.H. "Address by the Surgeon General, U.C.V." *Confederate Veteran* 8 (1900): 362–367.

Tebault, C.H. *Compiled Service Records, 10th South Carolina Infantry*. South Carolina Department of Archives and History, Columbia, SC, Reels CW 171, 780.

Tebault, C.H. "Confederate Resources." *Southern Practitioner* 24 (January 1902): 44–50. Tebault, C.H. "The Drainage System Peculiar to New Orleans. Its Demonstrated Possibilities and Its Bearing When Properly Enforced Upon the General Health of the City Under a Most Crucial Test." *Gaillard's Medical Journal* 49 (1889): 325–348.

Tebault, C.H. "Hospitals of the Confederacy." *Southern Practitioner* 24 (1902): 499–509.

Tebault, C.H. "Letter to Mrs. Susan Bailey, Jan. 5, 1865." New Orleans Historical Society.

Tebault, C.H. (misspelled "Tibault"). "Losses in the Union War." *Southern Historical Papers* 40 (1915): 318.

Tebault, C.H. "Modified Inoculation." *Gaillard's Medical Journal* 36 (1883): 18–22.

Tebault C.H. "Modified Inoculation." *New Orleans Medical and Surgical Journal* 19 (July 1866): 36–42.

Tebault, C.H. "Mortality Statistics of the Prisons During the Civil War." *The Sanitaeian, a Monthly Magazine Devoted to the Preservation of Health, Mental and Physical Culture* 41 (1898): 363–364.

Tebault, C.H. *Official Historical Report, 11th Annual Meeting and Reunion of the U.C.V.* New Orleans: Hopkins' Printing Office, 1902.

Tebault, C.H. "Official Report." From the *United Confederate Veterans Reunion Official Souvenir, 13th Annual Reunion*. New Orleans: Hopkins' Printing Office, 1903.

Tebault, C.H. *Our City's Problem. Her Property, Real and Personal, Confiscated by Taxation in Ten Years. What She Owes and What She Does Not Owe*. New Orleans: Franklin House, 1877.

Tebault, C.H. "The Parasitic Origin of Phthisis Pulmonalis." *Gaillard's Southern Medicine* (June 1905): 268.

Tebault, C.H. "Report of C.H. Tebault, M.D., Surgeon General to the United Confederate Veterans at the Reunion at Louisville, Ky., May 30-June 2, 1900." *Confederate Veteran* 8 (August 1900): 356–363.

Tebault, C.H. "Surgeon General's Report." *Minutes of the Sixth Annual Meeting and Reunion of the United Confederate Veterans. Richmond, VA, June 30-July 2, 1896.* New Orleans: Hopkins' Printing Office, 1897, 121–125.

Tebault, C.H. *Surgeon General Tebault's Report, New Orleans, La., February 10th, 1902.* New Orleans: Hopkins' Printing Office, 1903.

Tebault, S.B. "Ancestry of Mrs. C. Hamilton Tebault, Louisiana State Regent, D.A.R." New Orleans Genealogy Society.

Tripler, C.S. "Hospital Gangrene: A Lecture Delivered to Prof. Blackman's Class at the Medical College of Ohio, Session of 1860-1861." *The Cincinnati Lancet and Observer* 6 (October 1863): 585–587.

Trombold, John M. "Gangrene Therapy and Antisepsis Before Lister: The Civil War Contributions of Middleton Goldsmith of Louisville." *The American Surgeon* 77 (2011): 1138–43.

Trotter, Michael C. "G.H. Tichenor, MD, and His Antiseptic Solution: The Mississippi Years—Part 1 of 2." *Journal of the Mississippi State Medical Association* 53 (2012): 88–92.

Tulane University. *Catalogue of the Alumni from 1834 to 1901, Inclusive, of the Medical Department of the Tulane University of Louisiana.* New Orleans: L. Graham & Sons, Ltd., 1901.

Tulane University. "History of Tulane University." http://www.tulane.edu/~matas/historical/medschool/founders.htm (accessed November 9, 2018).

Tulane University. "Our History." https://admission.tulane.edu/history (accessed November 9, 2018).

Tulane University. "Stanford Emerson Chaillé—Distinguished Tulane Medical and Public Health Faculty and Tulane Health Sciences Alumni." https://libguides.tulane.edu/famousalumni (accessed April 4, 2018).

United States, 40th Congress, House of Representatives. *Trial of Henry Wirz.* Ex. Doc. No. 23. Washington: Government Printing Office, 1866.

United States National Board of Health, ed. *Annual Report of the National Board of Health, 1880.* Washington: Government Printing Office, 1881.

United States of America. "Declaration of Independence." http://www.ushistory.org/declaration/document/.

Villepigue, J.B. "Letter to Captain C.H. Davis, May 20, 1862." In *The War of the Rebellion: A Compilation of the Official Records of the Union and Confederate Armies*, ed. United States War Department. Series 2, vol. 3. Washington: Government Printing Office, 1898.

Villepigue, J.B. "Letter to General Beauregard, May 22, 1862." In *The War of the Rebellion: A Compilation of the Official Records of the Union and Confederate Armies*, ed. United States War Department. Series 2, vol. 3. Washington: Government Printing Office, 1898.

Vishneski, John. "What the Court Decided in 'Dred Scott v. Sandford.'" *The American Journal of Legal History* 32 (1988): 373–390.

Wagner, M.E., G. Gallagher, and P. Finkelman, eds. *Civil War Desk Reference.* New York: Simon & Schuster, 2002.

Walker, C.I. *Rolls and Historical Sketch of the Tenth South Carolina Volunteers.* Charleston, SC: Walker, Evans & Cogswell, 1888.

Ward, Patricia Spain. *Simon Baruch, Rebel in the Ranks of Medicine, 1840-1921.* Tuscaloosa: University of Alabama Press, 1994.

Warmoth, Henry Clay. *War, Politics, and Reconstruction: Stormy Days in Louisiana.* New York: Macmillan, 1930.

Washington, F.S., and J.A. Chalaron. *Proceedings of the Convention for Organization and Adoption of the Constitution of the United Confederate Veterans.* New Orleans: Hopkins' Printing Office, 1891.

Watson, Irving A., ed. *Physicians and Surgeons of America—A Collection of Biographical Sketches of the Regular Medical Profession.* Concord, NH: Republican Press, 1896.

Wetta, Frank J. *The Louisiana Scalawags.* Baton Rouge: Louisiana State University Press, 2012.

Wicks, Margaret Campbell Walker. *The Italian Exiles in London, 1816-1848.* Freeport, NY: Books for Libraries Press Inc., 1937.

Wier, J.J. *Army of Tennessee, Louisiana Division: The Association and Tumulus.* Lafayette, LA: Center for Louisiana Studies, University of Southwestern Louisiana, 1999.

Williams, Harry T. *P.G.T. Beauregard, Napoleon in Gray.* Baton Rouge: Louisiana State University Press, 1955.

Williams, S.K. *Cases Argued and Decided in the Supreme Court of the United States.* Rochester, NY: The Lawyers Co-Operative Publishing Company, 1885.

Wilson, Henry. "Edward M. Stanton." *The Atlantic Monthly* 25 (February 1870): 234–246.

Wilson, Theodore B. *The Black Codes of the South.* Tuscaloosa: University of Alabama Press, 1965.

Wintz, Cary D. *African American Political Thought, 1890-1930: Washington, DuBois, Garvey.* New York: M.E. Sharpe, Inc., 1996.

Wolfe, Robert M., and Lisa K. Sharp. "Anti-Vaccinationists Past and Present." *British Medical Journal* 325 (2002): 430–432.

Woodward, C. Vann. *Reunion and Reaction: The Compromise of 1877 and the End of Reconstruction.* London: Oxford University Press, 1991.

INDEX

Numbers in ***bold italics*** indicate pages with illustrations

A.B. Griswold & Co. 95
Abbeville, MS 23
Abell, Judge Edmund 74
Aberdeen, MS 167
abolitionists 15–17, 76, 79, 112, 115, 120, 146
acroia 169
Adams, Charles Francis 122
Adams, John Quincy 121, 122, 124
Aedes aegypti mosquito 36; *see also* mosquitoes
air, therapeutic value of 35, 37, 42, 43, 58, 166, 172–175
Alabama 10, 28, 101, 168; secession of 16
Albany, GA 39, 40, 143, 167
Alexander, PA 11
Allegheny City Penitentiary, PA 128
Allen, C.H. 86
allspice 169
aloes 169
Alton, IL, prison 19, 20, 128
Amelia (brig) 7
American Hemlock 40
The American Medical Times 13
American Public Health Association 52
American Revolution 6, 39, 141
American Tobacco Company 144
amputations 44, 176
Anderson, Maj. Robert 16, 118, 125
Andersonville Prison 112, 126–131, ***132***, 133–135, 147, 148
Andover, MA 35
Andress, F.M. 86
Annan, A.H. 144
antimony 40
antiphlogistics 38
antiseptics 36, 37, 61, 62, 107, 174
Antoine, C.C. 85
April 16 Armistice 44
Arent, David ***107***
Arkansas 10
Army of Northern Virginia tumulus 107, ***108***
Army of Tennessee 31, 33, 35, 41, 134, 141, 142; tumulus 111, 143, 144, ***145***; *see also* Society of the Army of Tennessee
Army of the Cumberland 26
artillery 17, 18, 23, 24, 26, 28, 43, 86, 122
asafoetida 169
assassination, threats of 68, 71
assistant surgeons 11, 13, 41, 43, 171, 173, 175
Association of Medical Officers of the Army and Navy of the Confederacy 41, 144, 155, 167, 170
asthma, treatment 170
Athens, GA 167
Atlanta, GA 31, 33, 35, 39, 167
Atlanta Exposition 38
The Atlantic Monthly Magazine 119
Augusta, GA 49, 167
auscultation 48, 49
Austen, Jane 6

bacteriology 55
Bailey, Annie Tinsley 32
Bailey, David Jackson 32, 38, 39, 142
Bailey, Robert 39
Bailey, Sallie Bradford 32, 38, 39
Bailey, Susan 40
Bailey-Tebault House ***32***, 38
Baird, Gen. Absalom 120
Baker, Gov. Joshua 81
Bakewell, Rev. A. Gordon 144
balsam of Peru 37
Baltimore, MD 39, 54, 97
bandaging 32, 175; *see also* wound dressings, water
Bank of Louisiana 6, 142
Banks, Gen. Nathaniel 67; General Order No. Twelve 68
Barksdale, Gen. Allen ***107***
Barnes, Gen. Joseph K. 127, 134
Barton, Dr. Edward Hall 52, 161, 163
baths, public 61
Baton Rouge, LA 15, 85
Battle of Antietam 151
Battle of Atlanta 32
Battle of Bull Run (Manassas) 12; second Battle of Bull Run 25
Battle of Fredericksburg 28
Battle of Gettysburg 29, 30, 38, 82, 113, 117, 150, 151
Battle of Jonesboro 32
Battle of Liberty Place 5, 80, 85, 86, ***87***, 88–92, 141, 144, 146, 149, 151
Battle of Liberty Place Monument 90, ***91***, 153
Battle of Pea Ridge 20, 21
Battle of Shiloh 23, 110
Battle of Stones River 28
Battle of the Crater 65
battlefields 172; post war 135, 149, 151
bayous 60, 163
beans 27
"Beast" Butler 133; *see also* Butler, Gen. Benjamin
Beauregard, Laure 144
Beauregard, Gen. P.G.T. 2, 5, 19, 20, ***21***, 22, 44, 144, 145; association with lottery 96, 97; attack on Fort Sumter 16, 125
Beauvoir 151; *see also* Davis, Pres. Jefferson
beeswax 40, 170
Behan, Gen. W.J. ***107***, 144
belladonna 169
Belle Isle prison, VA 129, 130
Benevolent Association of the Army of Tennessee 111
Berkshire Medical Institution 7
Berrian, Dr. J.A.A. 7
Black, Justice Jeremiah Sullivan 114, 117, 120, 122, 147
Black Codes 66, 69, 76, 77, 78, 101
Black Leagues 78, 79; *see also* Union Leagues
black vomit 52, 54, 164; *see also* yellow fever symptoms
Blaine, Hon. James G. 65
Blanchard, Gov. Newton C. 144
bleeding, as therapy 51
blistering, as therapy 51
Block, John T. ***107***

blockade 40, 43
blockade runner 2, 40, 167
Bloom, Dr. J.D. 144
Blow, Peter 115
board of health 61, 103, 141
Boerne prison, TX 129
Bohrman, Martin 144
Bollet, Dr. Afred J. 48
Bolton, Dr. James 137
Bonaparte, Napoleon 6, 141
Boston, MA 9, 110
Bouchacourt, Dr. M. 63, 155
bougies 169
Boylan, Thomas N. 94, 95
Boyle, Rev. F.E. 130
Brachet, Dr. M. 63, 155
Bradford, Gov. William 6, 39, 142
Bragg, Gen. Braxton 24, **25**, 26, 29, 30, 31, 33; Tennessee Campaign 2, 28
Brazil 55
Breaux, Judge Arsenne 144
Breckenridge, Dr. Robert J. 137
bribery 96, 97, 98
Brickell, Dr. Daniel Warren 62, 94, 143, 144
Brown, H.T. **107**
Brown, John 15
Bruns, Dr. J. Dickinson 143, 144
Bryan, William Jennings 100, 101
Buchanan, Pres. James 6, 114, 117–119
Buell, Maj. Gen. Don Carlos 25, 26
Burbank, Lt. Col. S. 21
Burgess, Dr. D.M. **56**
Burnside, Gen. Ambrose 28
Butler, Gen. Benjamin 67, 92, 118, 130, 132; *see also* "Beast" Butler
butterfly weed 40

Cahaba prison, AL 129
Cairo, KY 18
Caldwell, Rev. John 144
Calhoun, GA 143
Calhoun, John C. 112, 116
calomel 169
Cameron, Simon 119
Camp Butler prison, IL 128
Camp Chase prison, OH 128
Camp Douglas prison, IL 127, 128, 131, **133**, 148
Camp Ford prison, TX 129
Camp Groce prison, TX 129
Camp Milner 31
Camp Morton prison, IN 128
Camp Stephens 31
Camp Walker 97
camphorated oil 34, 174, 175
camps, Confederate veterans 136
Canada 116
canals, New Orleans 54, 163, 166
candles 40, 170

carbolic acid 59; street disinfection with 61, 62
Carolina hipps 40
carpetbaggers 3, 67, 71, 72, 77, 79–81, 89, 96, 146, 148
Carrington, Dr. W.A. 137
carrots 35, 174
Carter, Dr. L. 157, 158
Carter, Howell **107**
Castle Pinckney prison, SC 129
Castle Thunder prison, VA 129
Castleman, T.W. **107**
catechu 169
cathartics 169
cats, feral 60
cavalry 12, 29, 31, 39, 43, 44, 83, 122
cellulitis 34
cemeteries 60, 150, 163
cesspools 33, 60
Chaillé, Dr. Stanford E. 35, 39, 44, 50, 55, **56**, **59**, 61, 144
chamomile 169
charcoal 35, 36, 174
Charity Hospital 8, 11, 21, 22, 46, **47**, **48**, 52, 98, 141, 143, 144, 155
Charleston, SC 2, 5, 7, 16, 40, 78, 118, 125, 142, 167, 168; prison 129
The Charleston Courier 170
Charlotte, NC 167; prison 129
charpie 36; *see also* lint bandages
Chattanooga, TN 28, 137
Chief Sponsor for the South 39, 138
Chisolm, Dr. John Julian 38
chlorination, of water 34, 62, 174
chloroform 86, 167
cholera 7, 8, 46, 48, 50
Choppin, Dr. Samuel Paul 59, 86, 137
The Cincinnati Enquirer 70
cisterns 52, 159
citizenship, black 67, 105, 101
Civil Rights Act of 1866 70
Civil War, responsibility for 112, 114, 124, 146, 147
Clemenceau, French Pres. Georges Eugène Benjamin 150, 151
Clements, Thomas **107**
Cleveland, TN 27, 30–32, 143
climate, New Orleans 7, 52, 53, 161, 162, 165
Cobb, Gen. Howell 130
Cogswell, Dr. Mason 132, 148
colchicum 169
Colfax, LA 82
Colfax Massacre 82–85
colocynth 169
Colonial Dames of America 39, 142
Columbia, TN, prison 129
columbo quassia 168
Columbus, GA 33, 167

Columbus, MS 28, 167
Columbus, SC 167
Committee on Contested Elections 98
Committee on Military Affairs 14
Compromise of 1877 90, 92, 98
Confederacy, leaders of 65, 71, 150, 151
Confederate Congress 14
Confederate General Hospital 49
Confederate Memorial Hall Museum **105**
Confederate monuments 2, 4, 103, 135, 146, 149–153
Confederate resources 40, 15, 167, 168, 173
The Confederate States Medical and Surgical Journal 38
The Confederate Veteran 3, 141, 144
Confederate veterans 65, 113, 119, 141; black 139; disenfranchisement of 67, 68, 72; old soldiers' home 103, 136–138
conium 169
Connecticut 10, 116, 146
Constitutional Conventions, Louisiana 67, 93–95; 1864 66, 68, 72–75; 1868 50, 71, 146; 1874 85; 1879 98; 1898 59, 96, 100–104, 141–144
contraband 43, 68, 134, 167, 176
contract surgeons 33, 41, 171
Copeland, W.B. 118
Corinth, MS 19, 23, 24, 143
corks 169
corn 26
Cornelson, Jr. Dr. George H. 144
cornmeal 35, 37
coughs, treatment for 36
Coupland, Rev. Robert S. 144
Covey, Dr. E.N. 137
cowpox 37, 63
Crawcour, Dr. I.L. 52, 164
creolization 162; *see also* yellow fever, immunity from
Crescent City 52, 61, 161, 164; *see also* New Orleans
Crescent City White League 78–80, 85–87, 146
Cuba 40, 167; *see also* Havana
cucumbers 27
Cumberland River 18
Cummings, Kate 23, 33
Cutler, King 74

Dallas, TX 37, 120, 171
dandelion 40
Danville, VA 167
Danville prison, VA 129
Darby, Dr. J.T. 137
Daughters of 1812 39

Daughters of the American Revolution 39, 141, 142, 152
Davis, Commodore Charles H. *19,* 20
Davis, Pres. Jefferson 12, 16, 26, 50, 59, 67, 113, 123, 130, 133, 134, 148, 149; reinterment of 2, 5, 107–111; see also Beauvoir
Davis, Varina 109
Davis, Winnie 109
debt, bonded 59, 82, 84, 88, 93–98
Declaration of Independence 51, 115, 124, 142, 146
dehydration 27
de la Vergne, Hugues 144
Delaware 10
DeLeon, Dr. D.C. 13
Democrat Party 5, 16, 17, 32, 68, 71, 77, 83, 89, 149
Democratic Convention of Louisiana (1865) 66; (1872) 69
Democrats 94, 142
Demoruelle, Joseph *107*
Denis, Henry 144
dentistry 103
"deobstruent" 36
diarrhea 27, 53, 162, 170
Dickinson College 124
diet 34, 36, 42, 156, 174
digitalis 169
discrimination 67, 127
disease epidemics 8, 33, 46, 59, 162, 165; see also yellow fever, epidemics
disenfranchisement of black voters 100–104, 107, 149, 151
The Dispensatory of the United States 11
dissection 9
diuretics 35, 169
dogs, feral 60
Donaldsonville, LA 6
Dostie, Anthony Paul 73, 74
Dowler, Dr. Bennet 53, 161, 164
Doyle, Alexander 110
drainage ditches, New Orleans 54, 155, 166
drainage system, New Orleans 159, 163, 166; districts 160
Dred Scott Decision 114, 125, 146, 147; see also Scott, Dred
druggists 167, 168
drugs 40, 42, 103, 167, 172; see also medicines
Ducros, Col. M.T. *107*
Dugas, H. *107*
Duke, David 90
Duncan, Stephen 92
Dupree, George 86
Durell, Edward H. 70, 71
Duyckinck, Evert 6, 39
Duyckinck, Sarah 6
dysentery 23, 26, 27, 31, 32, 133
dyspepsia 169

Early, Gen. Jubal Anderson 96, 97, 112
economic depression in the South, post war 49, 65, 90, 92, 98, 113, 149; see also Reconstruction
education, medical 9–11, 46
8th Louisiana Regiment 107
elm bark 36
Elmira, NY, prison 128
Emancipation Proclamation 67, 104
Emerson, Dr. John 114
emetics 27
Emily B. Souder (steamship) 55
ergot 169
eruptive fever 33, 58
erysipelas 33, *34,* 35, 37, 156, 173–175
escharotic 169
Eshleman, Col. B.F. *107*
Estopinal, Gen. Albert 144
ether 167
Eufaula, AL 167
Evans, Gen. Clement A. 5
Eve, Dr. Paul F. 137
Ewing, Robert 144
examinations, surgeon 11, 33, 172; see also Medical Boards

Fair Ground No. 2 Hospital 35
Fayetteville, NC 167
federal forts, seizure of 16
Felder, Hon. J.M. 170
Fenner, Dr. Darwin 52, 161
fevers 33–35, 50, 57, 58, 159, 170
Finlay, Dr. Carlos 54, 58
Finlay, T.B. *107*
first grade teaching certificate 46
1st Mississippi Cavalry 107
Fitzpatrick, Mayor John 144
5th Military District 44, 69, 76
5th New Hampshire Infantry 45
5th West Virginia Cavalry 11
flaxseed 35, 169, 174
Flood, Edward 86
Florida 89, 158
Floyd House Hospital 39, 157; see also Ocmulgee Hospital
Flynn, George W. 144
Foard, Dr. A.J. 40
Foard, Dr. Louis D. 137
Folly Island, SC 7
fomites 51, 61, 64, 164, 165
Food and Drug Administration 103
Foote, Flag Officer Andrew H. 18
foraging 42, 172
Ford, Dr. A.J. 137
Ford, Dr. Sample 11
formaldehyde 9
Fort Delaware prison, DE 128
Fort Donelson 17, 18, 23, 128
Fort Henry 17, 18, 23

Fort Lafayette prison, NY 128
Fort McHenry prison, MD 128
Fort Mifflin prison, PA 128
Fort Moultrie 118
Fort Philip 61, 164
Fort Pickens prison, FL 128
Fort Pillow 17–21, 23, 37
Fort Pillow Massacre 65, 83
Fort Sumter 15–17, 118, 122, 124, 147
Fort Warren prison 128
Fort Wood prison, NY 128
Foster, Gov. Murphy J. 100
4th Louisiana Battalion 69
Fourteen Points, Woodrow Wilson's 150
fractures, compound 175
freedmen 3, 65–69, 71, 73, 76–78, 82
Freedmen's Bureau 73, 118
Fremaux, Col. L.J. *107*
Fugitive Slave Act of 1850 15, 116, 147
Fulton, TN 24

Gaillard's Medical Journal 64, 159
Galliard, Dr. E.S. 137
Gallion, Dr. Z.T. 64
Galloway, Abraham 92
Galveston, TX 40, 167
The Galveston Daily News 62
Gamble, Dr. C.B. 158
gambling 96
gangrene 37, 156, 175; see also hospital gangrene
Gannon, John J. 144
garbage 55, 60, 61, 163
Garfield, Pres. James Abram 114, *118,* 120, 134; assassination of 118
Garrison, William Lloyd 15
gastritis 36
Gauche, C. Taylor 144
General Order No. 111, Pres. Davis' 130
Georgetown College 6
Georgia 10, 39, 92, 111, 137, 142, 157, 168; secession of 16, 32
Georgia Secession Convention 32
germ theory 36, 54, 55, 59
Germany 3, 150, 151
Gessner, Dr. Hermann B. 144
Gibbes, Dr. Robert 137
Gibson, Dr. Charles Bell 137
Gilmore, J.Y. *107*
Glasgow, KY 25
glycerine 174
Glynn, Gen. John *107*
Golden Age (steamship) 24
Goldsboro, NC 167
Gordon, Gen. George W. 5
Gordon, Gen. John B. 5, 111, 136–139

Grand Army of the Republic (GAR) 136
Grant, Ulysses S. 18, 26, 69–71, 88–90, 132, 133; capture of Fort Henry 17; siege of Vicksburg 28
Grantland, Mary Susan 39
Grantland, Hon. Seaton 32, 39, 142
Gratiot Street prison, MO 128
Great Britain 122
Greeley, Horace 12
Greensboro, NC 44
Greenville, SC 167
Griffin, GA 31–33, 36, 38, 40, 143, 173
Griffith, David W. 77
guaiacum 169
Guild, Dr. L. 137
Guion, Lewis 144
Guion, Walter 144
Guiteras, Dr. J. **56**
gum Arabic 169
gunboats, associated with yellow fever 51–53, 161–165
gunboats, Union 18, 19
Gunn, Dr. John C. 36
Gunn's New Domestic Physician 27, 36

Haas, Col. Alex M. **107**
Habersham, Dr. S.E. 137
Hacker, David 45
Hahn, Michael 74
Hall, Caroline 6
Hall, Col. Christopher 141, 142
Hall, Hon. Luther E. 144
Halleck, Gen. Henry W. 20, 26, 28, 29, **30**, 127, 128
Hamilton, Alexander 6
Hamilton, George R. 6
Hamlin, Dr. Charles 64
Harper, Howard V. 143
Harper's Weekly 72, 75, 81, 131
Harral, J.A. 144
Harris, Dr. Elisha 52, 160, 161
Harrison, Dr. John Hoffman 8
Harrod, Maj. B.M. 159
Hart, William Octave 144
Hartford Convention 146, 147
Hart's Island prison, NY 128
Harvard College 35, 48
Hatchie Island 21, 22, 64
Havana, Cuba 55; *see also* Cuba
Hawkins, William H. 27
Hayes, Rutherford B. 89, 90, 98
Health Insurance Portability and Accountability Act (HIPA) 103
Heller, Rev. Max 144
Henry Clay Statue 84, **85**, 86
Hentz, Charles 9
Herndon, Dr. Dabney 157
heroic medicine 51
Hicks, Dr. Braxton 58

Higgins, Thomas **107**
Hill, James D. 144
Hill, Samuel Van Dyke 30, 32
Hitchcock, Gen. Ethan A. 133
Hitt, Dr. V.G. 133, 134
Hoffman, Col. William 127, 128
Hollywood Cemetery, Richmond 107
Holmes, Oliver Wendell 48
hop yeast 36
hospital gangrene 33, 35, 36, 173, 174; mortality 35
hospital stewards 13, 43, 176
hospitals, Confederate 5, 22, 33, 39, 41–44, 49, 127, 128, 137, 138, 155–157, 171–177
hospitals, inspection of 33, 42, 172
House of Burgesses 39
house painting, as sanitation method 61
Howard, Charles T. **97,** 98, **99,** 105
Howard, Frank T. 105
Huard, Dr. L.O. 53, 164
Huguenots 142
Hun, Dr. Thomas 132, 148
Hunt, Carlton 144
Hunt, Dr. Thomas 7, **8**, 11
Huntsville, AL 167
hygiene, household 61, 161

Illinois 10, 114
illiteracy 10, 67, 72, 76, 77; as reason for disenfranchisement of blacks 100, 101
immigrants 10, 46
Indiana 10
Indians, American as slaves 121
infantry 23, 24, 31, 43, 122; scouts 83
infections 9, 19, 22, 33, 36, 38, 50, 51, 54, 61, 63, 64, 156, 164, 165, 174
inflammation 38, 159
inoculations 37; *see also* modified inoculations
insects, as disease vectors 51
iodine, tincture of 34, 36, 173, 174
Ipecacuanha 27, 40, 169
Irby, W.R. 144
Island No. 10 17, 18

Jackson, Andrew 100, 146
Jackson, Gen. Thomas "Stonewall" 96, 107, 108, 113
Jackson, MS 167
Jackson Square, New Orleans 86
jalap 168
Jefferson, Thomas 100, 101, 146
Jefferson Medical College 9
Jenner, Dr. Edward 64
J.H. Hancock (steamer) 53, 164
Jim Crow Laws 76, 77, 101, 149

Johnson, Pres. Andrew 65, 66, 75, 119, 120, 130; impeachment of 65, 76, 117
Johnson's Island prison, OH 128
Johnston, Gen. Albert Sidney 23, **110,** 145
Johnston, Gen. Joseph E. 29, 44, 130, 156
Johnston, William P. 50
Jones, Dr. Edward 144
Jones, Rev. John 39
Jones, Dr. Joseph 22, 43, 49, 50, 64, 136–138

Kellogg, Gov. William P. 68, 69, 71, 82, 83, 85–89
Kelly, Capt. J.B. 95
Kennedy, Gen. John B.G. 17
Kentucky 10, 13, 24–26, 124, 143
Key, Francis Scott 117
Key, Phillip Barton 117
"King of Royal Street" 6; *see also* Tebault, William Gartley
kino 169
Knights of the White Camelia 77, 89
Knoxville, TN 26, 27
Kruttschnitt, Ernest B. 100, 101
Ku Klux Klan 2, 3, 76, 77, **81,** 89, 149
Kursheedt, Lieutenant E.I. **107**

Lafaye, E.E. 144
Lafayette, Gen. Marie-Joseph Paul Yves Roch Gilbert du Motier 6, 141
The Lafayette Advertiser 79
The Lafayette Gazette 55
Lafayette parish, New Orleans 79
Lafayette Square, New Orleans 85, 95, 139, 142, 177
Lake Pontchartrain 60, 163
Lancaster, PA 66
Landry, Stuart 90
Larendon, Charles A. 144
laudanum 169
Lauzer, Dr. A. Martin 158
laxatives 35
lead, sugar of 40, 174
Lee, Gen. Robert E. 82, 96, 113, 149, 153
Lee, Gen. Stephen Dill 5, 39, 139
LeGardeur, Gustave 86
Leibrook, F. 94
LeMonnier, Dr. Y.R. 144
Letterman Jonathan 33
Leucht, Rev. I.L. 144
Lewis, Dr. Ernest E. 144
Libby Prison 112, 129, 130
The Liberator 15
lice, body 46
Ligon's Warehouse prison, VA 129
Lincoln, Pres. Abraham 15 28,

Index

65, 90, 104, 105, 117, 121–125, 151; assassination of 66, 119; call for 75,000 troops 12, 16, 147
lint bandages 32; *see also* charpie
Little Rock, AK, prison 128
Livermore, Thomas 45
Logan, Dr. Samuel 86
Longstreet, Gen. James 82, 86, 87, 113
Lookout Mountain 30, 31
The Lost Cause 12, 81, 96, 112, 124, 132, 146–149, 153; doctrine 3, 113, 122, 138, 139, 146, 149, 152
Louisiana 10, 16, 44, 67–71, 73, 83, 88, 89, 100, 141
Louisiana Board of Health 59
Louisiana Lottery Company 96–98, 141; *see also* Louisiana State Lottery
Louisiana Purchase 147
Louisiana State Legislature 96, 144
Louisiana State Lottery 96, 97, 105; *see also* Louisiana Lottery Company
Louisiana State Regent 39
Louisville, KY 25, 26; prison 128
Louisville and Nashville Railroad 25
Louisville Medical Institute 9
Lyman, Col. W.R. *107*
Lynchburg, VA 167

Mackall, Brig. Gen. William Whann 18
Macon, GA 21, 22, 39, 40, 44, 143, 156–159, 167; prison 129
Macon and Western Railroad 31
Maine 10, 65, 71, 116
malaria 52, 62, 162
Mancel, Henry *56*
Manson, Dr. O.F. 137
Marr, Robert H. 84–86, 144
Marshall, Sec. of State George 150
Marshall Plan 150
Maryland 10
Massachusetts 6, 10, 116, 120, 146; secession threat 113; slavery in 120, 121
Matas, Rudolph *56*
Materia Medica 40, 168
Mauberret, Victor 144
May, Eugene 57
McClellan, Gen. George B. 26, 117, 119
McConnel, James 98
McCown, Maj. Gen. John P. 17
McCullom, E. *107*
McEnery, Gov. John 69, 70, 82, 84–87
McIntyre, Thomas 86
McKee, Dr. W.F. 144

McLean Barracks prison, OH 128
McLellan, Alden 144
measles 34
Mechanics Institute, New Orleans 73–75
The Medical and Surgical History of the War of the Rebellion 34, 44
Medical Boards 13, 14, 41, 171; *see also* examinations, surgeon
Medical College of Louisiana 6–8, 11, 17, 46–48, 53, 141, 143, 146; *see also* University of Louisiana
Medical College of Virginia 13
medical corps of the Confederate army & navy 12, 13, 41, 138
medical director in the field 42, 171
medical director of the hospitals 41, 171
medical director of the post 41, 52, 161
medical history, Confederate 45, 138
medical instruments 42, 43, 134, 172, 176
medical preparations for war 11, 13
medical service, Confederate 39, 41, 43
medical supplies 39, 43, 176
medicines 1, 35, 37, 41, 57, 103, 114, 133, 134, 168; southern plant substitutes 168–170; *see also* drugs
Memorial Hall, New Orleans 103, *105*, 107, 109
Memphis, TN 18, 23, 24, 167; riots of 1866 73
mercuric chloride 40; *see also* calomel
mercury 40
Meridian, MS 167; prison 129
Metairie Cemetery 97–99, 107–111, 144, 145, 152
Metairie Jockey Club 97
Metairie racecourse 97
metropolitan police 2, 82, 84–87, 90, 91, 151; *see also* police
Mexican American War 110, 127
Mexico 55, 167
mezereon 169
miasmas 33, 42, 50, 51, 54, 58–61, 163, 165
Michigan 10, 116
microscope 48
militia, Louisiana State 68, 72, 82, 88
Millen prison, GA 129
Miller, Francis Trevelyan 18, 41
Miller, W. *107*
minimum wage 71
Mississippi 5, 10, 44, 76, 109; secession of 16

Mississippi (steamer) 84
Mississippi Cavalry 107
Mississippi River 17–21, 26, 52, 54, 60, 166
Missouri 10, 104, 115
Mobile, AL 2, 40, 44, 167
modified inoculations 21, 22, 63, 64, 142, 143, 155, 157–159; *see also* inoculations
money, Confederate 44, 71
Monroe, Mayor John F. 72–74, 144
Montgomery, AL 12, 167
Moore, Dr. Samuel Preston 13, 14, 41, 137
Morine, H.A. 144
The Morning Chronical 144
morphine 35, 167, 174
Morris Island prison, SC 128
mortality, New Orleans 162, 163, 165
mosquitoes 51, 54, 58, 59, 62; *see also* Aedes aegypti mosquito
motherwort 40, 169
Mulford, Maj. John Elmer 133, 134
Munfordville, KY 25
Murfreesboro, TN 26–31, 143
myrrh, tincture of 36, 37
myrtle 40

Napoleonville, LA 6
Nashville, TN 13, 18, 28; prison 129
Nashville and Chattanooga Railroad 26
Natchez, MS 35
Naval Hospital, New Orleans 51, 162, 164, 165
Nazi Party 150
Nebraska 100
New England Anti-Slavery Society 15
New Hampshire 10, 44
New Jersey 10
New Madrid, MO 18
New Orleans 15, 40, 44, 46, 54, 65, 67, 76, 80, 87, 89, 90, 92, 97, 141, 143, 160, 167; fall of 11; drainage system 51, 59–61; prison 129; Union occupation of 52, 54, 68, 160–162, 165, 166; *see also* Crescent City
New Orleans Board of Health 59, 62, 143
The New Orleans Bulletin 61
New Orleans City Hall 109
New Orleans Cotton Exchange 144
New Orleans Custom House 71, 86
New Orleans Light Horse 35
The New Orleans Medical and Surgical Journal 52, 63, 143, 155

Index

The New Orleans Medical News 62
New Orleans Pacific Railway 94
New Orleans Railway & Light Company 144
New Orleans Riots of 1866 73, 74, **75**, 120, 149
New Orleans School of Medicine 94
New Orleans Stock Exchange 144
The New Orleans Times-Democrat 57
New York 9, 10, 116, 124, 125, 147, 168; New York City 6, 39, 51, 163
The New York Herald 16
New York Times 12, 109
The New York Tribune 12, 84
Newman, Harold W. 144
Newport News prison, VA 129
newspapers 10, 16, 119, 136, 146, 148; inflaming passions 74, 78, 79, 82, 84, 149
Nicholls, Gov. Francis T. 98
Nichols, Dr. William Charles 30, 31
night soil 60
1906 Pure Food and Drugs Act 103
19th South Carolina Volunteers 27
Norfolk, VA 6, 125, 141, 147
North Carolina 10, 76, 92, 128, 168
northern attitudes for war 12
Nott, George W. 144
Nugent, James 98
nurses 23, 33, 36, 38, 43, 156, 171, 172

oath of allegiance 68, 72
Ocmulgee Hospital 21, 22, 35, 156; *see also* Floyd House Hospital
Ocmulgee River 39
Ogden, Fred N. 80
Ohio 10, 116
Ohio Penitentiary, OH 129
Ohio River 18, 25
Old Capital Prison, DC 129, 130
Old Soldiers' Home for U.S. Army Veterans 104
olive oil 169
Opelousas, LA 77
opium 27, 35, 40, 43, 86, 167, 169, 174
Orleans Cadets 107
Ould, Col. Robert 133, 134
oxygen, effects on wound healing 37, 175

Packard, Gov. Stephen B. 68, 71
Paris Peace Conference 150
patient confidentiality 103

patriotism, northern 17
patriotism, southern 16
Penn, Lieutenant Gov. D.B. 85
Pennsylvania 10, 92, 117, 124
Pensacola, FL 2, 40, 167
pensions: Confederate veterans 2, 5, 103, 136, 138; Union veterans 104
Pequot Indians 121
percussion 48
persimmon beer 170
personal liberty laws 116
Peters, A.J. 144
Petersburg, VA 167
Phelps, John 98
Philadelphia, PA 9, 39, 50, 168
Philadelphia Academy of Fine Arts 38
The Philadelphia Press 12
Phillips, A.B. 86
Phillips' Academy 35
Pillow, Brig. Gen. Gideon Johnson 18
Pilsbury, Mayor Edward 94
Pinchback, Gov. Pinckney Benton Stewart 68, 69, **70**, 96
pink root 169
Pittsburgh, PA 118
Pittsfield, MA 7
plague 50
pleurisy root 40
pneumonia 34
Point Lookout prison, MD 129
police 3, 72–78, 94, 95, 174; *see also* Metropolitan Police
Polk, Gen. Leonidas 30
poll taxes 92
Pollard, Edward 12, 112, 113, 148, 149; *Black Diamonds in the Darkey Homes of the South*, 112; *The Lost Cause* 12, 112; *The Lost Cause Regained* 113
Pope, Gen. John 18
Pope, Susan G. 31
population of New Orleans 80, 163
Porcher, Dr. Francis 40, 168
poultices 35, 36
Premium Bond Act 105 93
Presbyterian Hospital of New Orleans 53
presidential election of 1876 89
Prince, Leon 124
prison deaths 126, 134, 148
prisoner exchanges 19, 20, 43, 113, 126, 130–134, 173
prisoners of war 19–22, 33, 43, 74, 112, 113, 126–128, 143, 146, 148, 173, 176; Confederate treatment of 113, 125, 130, 134, 143, 146, 147, 173; Union treatment of 127, 173
prisons: Confederate 43, 45, 131, 133, 148; Confederate, medical care of inmates 127, 132, 134; Union 20, 128, 134

privies 60, 61, 163
Proclamation 220—Law and Order in the State of Louisiana 88
propaganda 15, 148
Provisional Confederate Congress 12
puerperal peritonitis 33
purging, as therapy 51
pus 34, 35, 38, 63, 64, 174; laudable 38
pyroligneous acid 36, 37

quarantines, yellow fever 50–53, 55, 59–62, 161, 164, 165
quinine 34, 56, 167, 169, 170, 174
Quintard, Charles **31**
Quintard Hospital 30–33, 39
Quitman, John A. 5

rabies 60
race riots 73
racism 3, 50, 65, 66, 82, 90, 92, 100, 112
Radical Republicans 66, 67, 73, 75, 76, 92, 117–119, 146, 151
rainfall, New Orleans 159, 160, 163, 166
Raleigh, NC 92, 167
Raleigh Prison Barracks 128, 129
Ramsay, Dr. S.A. 137
rape of white women, reports of 83, 86, 149
Raspier, Thomas C. 144
rattlesnake bite, treatment 169
Real Estate and Taxpayers' Union 92, 94–96, 141, 143
Reconstruction 3, 44, 67–69, 75, 78, 79, 83, 89, 107, 114, 117, 119, 122, 124, 146, 148; end of 90, 92; military districts 67; military rule 3, 44, 60, 61, 65, 67, 81, 89, 149, 164; taxation under 2, 5, 65, 67, 92–96, 141, 143
red oak bark 173
Reed, Dr. Walter 58
Rees, Dr. Paul 144
Renaud, J.K. **107**
Republican administration 86
Republican party 105, 115
Republican platform 92
Republicans 16, 66, 68, 71, 73, 82, 89, 98, 118, 136; black 16, 94
Returning Board 69, 70, 82
rheumatism, treatment 170
Rhode Island 10, 116, 124
rhubarb 167
Richardson, Dr. B. Ward 58
Richmond, VA 2, 5, 12, 16, 41, 107, 126, 155, 167; fires 2, 137, 176, 177; prison 129
The Richmond Daily Whig 12
The Richmond Examiner 12
The Richmond Times 126
Rickettsia 46; *see also* typhus

Index

Ricks, A.G. 144
riverboats 165
robberies 86
Robert, Dr. M. 63, 155
Rock Island prison, IL 129
Rodman, Judge 141
Rogers, William O. 50
Rome, GA 33, 167
Roosevelt, Theodore 142
Roper, Thomas 1
Roper Hospital prison, SC 129
Rosecrans, Gen. William S. 26–28, **29**, 30
Royster, T.J. **107**
rubefacient 35
Rush, Benjamin 50, **51**
Russia 119
Rutland, W.R. 82
Rutledge, John 142

St. Louis, MO 114
Salisbury prison, NC 129, 130
Sally, T.O. 94
Sanitary Commission, New Orleans 52, 161
Sanitary Commission, U.S. 132
sanitary police 52, 53, 61, 161–164
sanitation 2, 23, 27, 36, 51, 54, 59–61 103, 160–162, 165, 166
Santana, Charles **107**
sarsaparilla 169
Savannah, GA 2, 40, 167; prison 129
Savory and Moore 1
scalawags 3, 67, 71–73, 79, 82, 146
Schade, Louis 130
Schmidt, Fred 144
School Board, New Orleans 100
school integration 50, 67, 71
schools, public 92, 98, 100, 101; rural 10
Scott, Dred 15, 104, **114**, 115; *see also* Dred Scott Decision
Scott, Gen. Winfield 119, 122
secession 15, 17, 113, 117, 118, 121, 124, 146, 147
second grade teaching certificate 46
2nd Louisiana Infantry 107
2nd Military District, Reconstruction 76
Seddon, Gen. James A. 130
segregation 50, 71, 77
Selma, AL 167
senna 169
septic shock 43, 35
Sessel, Edwin 23
Sessume, Bishop Davis 144
7th Louisiana Infantry 136
sewage 36, 55, 59–62, 163
Seward, William 105, 119, 122, 147
Shaddock, M.E. **107**

Sheridan, Gen. Philip H. 26, 28, 44, 69, 73, 74, 113
Sherman, Gen. William Tecumseh 28, 44, 113, 133
Ship Island prison, MS 129
Sickles, Gen. Daniel E. 117, 118
Sickles, Teresa Bagioli 117
Simonds, J.C. 52, 161
Sims, W. Gilmore 170
Sisters of Charity 11, 47
slaughterhouses 59, 61, 163
slave revolts 78, 79, 130, 131
slavery 2, 3, 9, 44, 66, 76, 84, 92, 104, 112, 116, 122, 124, 146, 148; as benign institution 15, 112, 113, 122, 148, 151
slaves 67, 68, 72, 73, 77, 79, 92, 105, 121, 151; lack of rights 115; runaway 116, 117; trade 65
smallpox 7, 19–21, **22**, **34**, 37, 42, 46, 50, 53, 61, 142, 155–158, 162–165, 173; *see also* variola
Smith, Dr. Howard 86
Smith, Maj. Gen. Kirby 25
The Smithsonian Magazine 151
Smythe, Dr. John 52, 164
Society of the Army of Tennessee 97; *see also* Army of Tennessee
soldiers, black 65, 130, 131
Soldiers Home of the State of Louisiana 103
Sommerville, Judge Walter B. 144
Sons of Confederate Veterans (SCV) 112, 139
Sons of Union Veterans of the Civil War (SUVCW) 136, 139
Soule, Col. George 144
Soule College, New Orleans 144
South Carolina 5, 10, 17, 44, 76, 89, 111, 112, 118, 124, 125, 142, 147, 169, 170; secession of 15, 16
southern attitudes for war 12
The Southern Historical Society 96
The Southern Journal of Medicine 62
The Southern Practitioner 167, 171
The Southern Recorder 141
Southwestern Railroad 30
Southwick, Cassandra 121
Southwick, Daniel 120
Southwick, Provided 121
Southwick Lawrence 121
Spanish American War 58, 135
Spanish flies 168
Spartanburg, SC 167
sponges, surgical 40, 86, 173
spurious vaccinations 156
stables 61, 163
Standifer, Col. T.C. **107**
Stanton, Secretary of War Edwin McMasters 29, 75, 76, 114, **117**, 118–120, 127, 134

"Star-Spangled Banner" 117
State House, New Orleans 86
states' rights 3, 15, 17, 112, 113, 124, 125, 137, 149
Statesville, NC 167
Stephens, Vice Pres. Alexander H. 16, 112, 125, 130, 147; *A Constitutional View of the War Between the States* 125
sterilization 40
Sternberg, Dr. George M. 54, 55, **56**, 58
sternutatory 169
stethoscope 48, 49
Stevens, Hon. Thaddeus 66
Stevenson, AL 26
Stone, Dr. Warren **7**, 8, 11, 59, 143
Stout, Dr. Samuel H. 32, 33, 39, 41, 171, 176
Stowe, Harriet Beecher 15; *Uncle Tom's Cabin* 15, 116
street cleaning 59–61, 163, 166; street paving 36, 61
streptococcus bacteria 33
students, medical 11, 47
suffrage, black 66, 82, 149
sugar trade 5, 23, 65, 144
Sullivan, D.S. **107**
Sumner, Hon. Charles 66, 105, 117, 119
sunshine, therapeutic value of 37, 42, 54, 166, 172, 175
Surgeon General of the Confederate States 13, 33, 40, 41, 168
Surgeon General of the United Confederate Veterans 2, 5, 22, 39, 62, 111, 120, 132, 136–138, **139**, 142, 146, 155
Surgeon General of the United States 14, 127
surgeon in charge of the hospital 42
surgeon of the post 42, 158
surgeons 11, 13, 27, 41, 133, 134, 171, 173, 175; qualifications of 13
surgical incisions 33
Synodical College 31, 33
syphilis 156

Taney, Chief Justice Roger B. 114–116
tannic acid 34, 169, 174
tax, progressive income 71
Taylor, Zachary 5
Tebault, Amanda **152**
Tebault, B. Rutledge 6, 86, 87
Tebault, Christopher H. **7**, **49**, 50, **62**, 94, **107**, 109, 139, 141, **142**, 146, **152**
Tebault, Christopher H., Jr. 39, 143, **152**
Tebault, Corrine Sallie (Harper) 143, **152**; *see also* Harper, Howard V

Tebault, Edwin 6
Tebault, Elizabeth 6
Tebault, Grantland L. 39, 86, 142, 143, *152*
Tebault, Major Edward J. 2, 5, 142
Tebault, Richard Mansfield 6
Tebault, Virginia Caroline 6
Tebault, William Gartley 87; see also "King of Royal Street"
telegraph system 119
10th South Carolina Infantry Regiment 1, 2, 14, 24–28, 41, 143
Tennessee 10, 67, 168
Tennessee River 17, 18, 25
Tennison, O.M. 86
Tenure of Office Act 75, 119
Texas 40, 44, 69, 73, 76, 167
Texas Cavalry 107
thermometer, medical 49
Thiébault, Paul Charles François Adrien Henri Dieudonné 6, 141
Thiele, Dr. M 63, 155
third grade teaching certificate 46
3rd South Carolina Volunteers 107
13th Infantry Regiment (Union) 21
30th Georgia Infantry 32, 142
Thompson, W.B. 144
Tichenor, Dr. G.H. *107*
Tilden, Samuel J. 89, 90
The Times Picayune 49, 79, 82, 86–89, 94–97, 136, 141–143
Tinsley, Samuel 39
Tinsley, Thomas 39
Tobin, John 144
Tompkinsville, KY 25
toothaches, treatment 169
Treatise on Practice 11
Trinity Church, New Orleans 144
tuberculosis 58
Tulane, Paul 50
Tulane Education Fund 50
Tulane University 6, 11, 35, 50, 138, 144, 146
Tullahoma, TN 28, 30
Tupelo, MS 23, 24, 143
Turner, Nat 79
turpentine 36, 37, 174–176
21st Louisiana Regiment 7, 17, 18, 24, 41
22nd Louisiana Regiment 107
typhoid fever 23, 34, 36, 62
typhus 46, 48, 59, 133

ulcers, treatment 169, 170
Uncle Tom's Cabin 15, 116
Underground Railroad 116
Union Leagues 78; see also Black Leagues
Union monuments 151
United Confederate Veterans 22, 37, 112, 120, 136–139, 141; reunions 2, 37, 41, 114, 123, 124, 134, 137–139, 144, 151, 155, 171
United Confederate Veterans memorial associations 138
United Daughters of the Confederacy 141, 142, 148
U.S. Board of Health 58
U.S. Census 44, 76
U.S. Congress 32, 39, 66, 72, 118, 142, 147; refusal to reseat southern legislators 67, 81; see also U.S. House of Representatives; U.S. Senate
U.S. Constitution 15, 17, 46, 80, 83, 85, 88, 104, 112, 115, 122, 124–126, 147; 2nd Amendment 84; 13th Amendment 44, 67, 104, 112; 14th Amendment 44, 67, 69, 104, 112; 15th Amendment 67, 112
U.S. House of Representatives 70, 71, 73, 76, 89, 112, 144; see also U.S. Congress
U.S. National Board of Health 55
U.S. Naval Home 104
U.S. Postal Service 97
U.S. Senate 71, 73, 75, 105, 119; see also U.S. Congress
U.S. Supreme Court 15, 66, 93, 104, 105, 114–117, 122, 125, 126, 147
University of Louisiana 22, 35, 46, 50; see also Medical College of Louisiana
University of Louisville 9
University of Nashville 13
University of Pennsylvania 7, 9
urbanization 60

vaccination 21, 22, 34, 37, 42, 58, 63, 64, 143, 155–159, 165
vaccination ulcers 156
valerian 169
Valparaiso (brig) 62
variola 22, 63, 64, 156–159; see also smallpox
Vautier, Charles 86
Vermont 10, 116
vesicatory 169
Vicksburg, MS 18, 24, 30, 69
Villepigue, Gen. John B. 17, *18*, 19, 20, 23, 24
Vinet, Gen. John Baptiste *107*
Virginia 10, 39, 116, 120, 124, 141, 167, 170
vomiting, as therapy 27, 51
votes, black 92, 101
voting requirements 100–103; see also disenfranchisement of Black voters

Wait, John 144
Walker, Elizabeth (Betsy) 6
Walker, Lady Mary 6
Wall, William Winas 144
war debt 66
war mortality 45, 113
Warmoth, Gov. Henry C. 68, *69*, 70, 81–84, 96, 98, 100; impeachment of 70, 71, 96
Washington, Booker T. 100
Washington, Frederick Stith 136
Washington, Pres. George 136
Washington, D.C. 12, 67, 84, 88, 125, 129
Washington Artillery 16, 107, 144
water, stagnant 50, 51, 60, 163
water supply 23, 26, 36–39, 55, 56, 132, 173, 175; New Orleans 54, 60, 163, 166
Watson, John W. *107*
Watson, Sir Thomas 58
W.B. Thompson & Company 144
Webber, Harriet 6
Weimar Republic 150, 151
Wells, Gov. James Madison 66–69, 72, 74
Weriein, Rev. S.H. 144
Wexler, Sol 144
Wheeling, (West) VA 11; prison 129
Whig 5, 32, 142
whiskey 40, 168
White League 2, 3, 71, 76, 77, *81*, 84–86, 88–90, 94, 146, 149
white supremacy 80, 83, 90, 91, 112, 149, 151, 153
Whitney-Central National Bank of New Orleans 144
Wight, Pearl 144
wild indigo 36
wild jalap 40, 169
Williams, Roger 120
Wilmington, NC 2, 40, 167
Wilson, Henry 119
Wilson, J. Moore *107*
Wilson, Brig. Gen. James H. 44; Wilson Raiders 44
Wilson, Pres. Woodrow 150
Winder, Brig. Gen. John 126, *127*, 130
Wirz, Henry 126, 129, 130, *131*, 148
Wisconsin 116
Wisconsin Territory 114
women, changing role of 65, 171
Wood, Dr. George Bacon 10, 11, 155; *Dispensatory of the United States* 11; *Treatise on Practice* 11, 155
Woodward, Capt. T.J. 144
World War I 149, 150; reparations for 150, 151

World War II 3, 149, 150
wound dressings, water 38, 173; *see also* bandaging
wounds 11, 13, 23, 33, 34, 37, 38, 43, 44, 90, 92, 107, 137, 146, 170–175; gunshot 11, 13, 38
W.R. Irby Tobacco Company 144

Yandell, Dr. David Wendell 13
yellow fever 7, 8, 36, 46–62, 103, 160–164; epidemics 47–49, 52, 54, 55, 103, 161; immunity from 52, 53, 55, 58; remedy 57; symptoms 50, 58; *see also* creolization; yellow jack

Yellow Fever Commission of 1879 36, **56**
yellow jack 50; *see also* yellow fever
yellow root 168
Young, Gen. Bennett H. 5

zinc sulphate 37

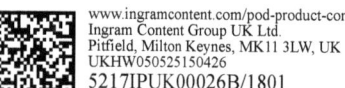
www.ingramcontent.com/pod-product-compliance
Ingram Content Group UK Ltd.
Pitfield, Milton Keynes, MK11 3LW, UK
UKHW050525150426
5217IPUK00026B/1801